EMPATHY AND HEALING

EMPATHY AND HEALING
Essays in Medical and Narrative Anthropology

Vieda Skultans

Berghahn Books
NEW YORK • OXFORD

First published in 2007 by
Berghahn Books
www.berghahnbooks.com

©2007, 2011 Vieda Skultans
First paperback edition published in 2011

Library of Congress Cataloging-in-Publication Data

Skultans, Vieda.
  Empathy and healing : essays in medical and narrative
anthropology / Vieda Skultans.
       p. cm.
  Includes bibliographical references and index.
  ISBN 978-1-84545-350-3 (hbk) -- ISBN 978-0-85745-138-5 (pbk)
  1. Medical anthropology--Cross-cultural studies. 2. Medical
anthropology--Latvia. 3. Traditional medicine--Cross-cultural
studies. 4. Traditional medicine--Latvia. 5. Mental illness--Social
aspects--Cross-cultural studies. 6. Mental illness--Social aspects--
Latvia. 7. Psychiatry, Transcultural. 8. Psychiatry, Transcultural--
Latvia. I. Title.

  GN296.S58 2008
  306.4'61--dc22

                                                2008008515

British Library Cataloguing in Publication Data
A catalogue record for this book is available from the British Library

Printed in the United States on acid-free paper

ISBN 978-1-84545-350-3 (hardback)
ISBN 978-0-85745-138-5 (paperback)
ISBN 978-0-85745-036-4 (ebook)

CONTENTS

LIST OF FIGURES

LIST OF TABLES

NOTE ON SITE OF ORIGINAL PUBLICATION

The following is a list of the original titles, places and dates of publication of the essays that appear in this volume. They are listed in order of appearance in the book and are reprinted here with the permission of the publishers:

- 'Empathy and Healing: Aspects of Spiritualist Ritual,' in J.B. Loudon (ed). *Social Anthropology and Medicine*, ASA Monograph 13. London, New York and San Francisco, Academic Press, 1976.
- 'Bodily Madness and the Spread of the Blush,' in J. Blacking (ed). *The Anthropology of the Body*, ASA Monograph 15. London, New York and San Francisco, Academic Press, 1977.
- 'The Symbolic Significance of Menstruation and the Menopause,' *Man* 5(4): 639–51, 1970.
- 'Women and Affliction in Maharashtra: A Hydraulic Model of Health and Illness,' *Culture, Medicine and Psychiatry* 15: 321–59, 1991.
- 'Overview: Anthropology and Psychiatry: The Uneasy Alliance,' *Transcultural Psychiatric Research Review* 28: 5–24, 1991.
- 'Remembering and Forgetting: Anthropology and Psychiatry: The Changing Relationship,' in V. Skultans and J. Cox (eds). *Anthropological Approaches to Psychological Medicine: Crossing Bridges*, London and Philadelphia, Jessica Kingsley Publishers, 2000.
- 'A Historical Disorder: Neurasthenia and the Testimony of Lives in Latvia,' *Anthropology and Medicine* 4(1): 7–24, 1997.
- 'Narratives of the Body and History: Illness in Judgement on the Soviet Past,' *Sociology of Health and Illness* 21(3): 310–28, 1999.
- 'From Damaged Nerves to Masked Depression: Inevitability and Hope in Latvian Psychiatric Narratives,' *Social Science and Medicine* 56: 2421–31, 2003.

- 'Looking for a Subject: Latvian Memory and Narrative,' *History of the Human Sciences* 9(4): 65–80, 1996.
- 'The Expropriated Harvest: Narratives of Deportation and Collectivization in North-East Latvia,' *History Workshop Journal* 44: 171–88, 1997.
- 'Narratives of Landscape in Latvian History and Memory,' *Landscape Review* 7(2): 25–39, 2001.
- 'Arguing with the KGB Archives: Archival and Narrative Memory in Post-Soviet Latvia,' *Ethnos* 66(3): 320–43, 2001.
- 'Varieties of Deception and Distrust: Moral Dilemmas in the Ethnography of Psychiatry,' *Health* 9(4): 491–512, 2005.

1

INTRODUCTION

When I first joined the Department of Anthropology in 1966 at University College London, social anthropology had a different face. That year two of my tutors published work that was to become highly influential. Mary Douglas's book *Purity and Danger* appeared in 1966 as did Ioan Lewis's article 'Spirit Possession and Deprivation Cults' in a journal that was then called *Man* (his thesis on deprivation cults was later to be developed in *Ecstatic Religion*, 1971). Thus two powerful advocates of structuralist and functionalist thought introduced me to anthropology. Both Mary and Ioan had, in their different ways, a facility for using the exotic to make sense of experience closer to home and always grounding highly abstract ideas in lived experience. Thus although fieldwork 'at home' had not as yet established a firm academic niche, when the possibility of doing some fieldwork in Swansea, on Welsh spiritualism, arose, it did not seem like a departure from the anthropological agenda to which I had been introduced. What was more of a problem was my interest in individuals.

Back in those days, individuals did not really exist in our theories. Geertz later described individuals in this earlier anthropology as mere 'outlines waiting to be filled' (1984: 132). In fact, the anthropological language of the time effectively eliminated the individual. In this language emotion, consciousness and experience only figured as social constructions. Moreover, to recognize the embodied uniqueness and particularity of individuals would have been seen as a lack of conceptual sophistication and a failure of theoretical nerve. I remember the uncomfortable grip this kind of position had on my own work among Welsh Spiritualists when I worried that the vividness of the people I met and the difficulty I had in damping down their individuality in my writing reflected a lack of theoretical grasp on my part. Informants were largely seen as instantiations of social rules and cultural beliefs and given little scope for initiative. There was even a fear then that to acknowledge individuality would blur the disciplinary distinctiveness of anthropology. Autobiographical knowledge had not been recognized as a resource. Self-reflexivity that reveals the situated nature of knowledge was not encouraged.

Indeed, I remember the perplexity I felt when John Blacking suggested that the connection between my refugee background and my choice of research among Spiritualists might not be altogether fortuitous. He was thinking, in particular, of my ethnographic focus on the creation of intimacy and how this might reflect a personal need and antidote to the experience of Soviet violence and displacement of the Baltic peoples. Since then I have periodically returned and reflected upon his comments. For four years my family and I were among the eight million displaced persons from the East who found themselves in a series of makeshift refugee camps in post-Second World War Germany. Until the age of nearly five, my idea of home derived, not from the changing floor space that we were allocated, but from the Latvian children's stories that spoke of and depicted an unchanging farmstead in a pastoral landscape. I can now see, as I have described in a chapter on displacement and identity, that the early importance that stories held for me, by creating a sense of belonging and permanence, came to influence my later approach and understandings of narrative (Skultans 2004).

My work among Spiritualist groups in Swansea set a serendipitous pattern that was to be repeated in subsequent academic work. I was initially employed as a researcher on a project financed by the then Ministry of Health to carry out a socio-anthropological study of doctor–patient relationships. I endured agonies of discomfort trying to figure out how I might insinuate myself into consulting rooms and get such a project off the ground. I had fully internalized the identification of fieldwork with participant observation and this made it difficult for me to see how I could fulfil my new professional duties without relinquishing my identity as an anthropologist. However, before my anxious ruminations reached monumental proportions I was alerted to a sign outside a Spiritualist church proclaiming 'Healing, All Welcome'. Of course, I knew that Spiritualist healing was not the same as a doctor–patient consultation, but there was enough of a family resemblance to encourage me to note down the time of the next healing session. Moreover, the conceptual remoteness of the beliefs and practices of these Welsh Spiritualists made me feel that I was, indeed, venturing into a territory no less strange than that of the spirit possession cults of Somali women or the pangolin worship of the Lele. I had no fear that shared, taken-for-granted assumptions would blunt my perceptions and critical awareness. The welcome I received on my first visit confirmed the course of my studies for the next three years. I attended Spiritualist meetings three or four times a week over a period of around thirty months.

I spent a lot of time 'hanging around' with Spiritualists and one particular Spiritualist became a close friend.

Those earlier classical paradigms of research had their limitations but they were also enabling in important ways. That distant paradigm held that we could, if given sufficient seriousness and time, understand all that we needed to know about the social. If the quest for a panoptic vision of social processes is an illusion, it can nevertheless promote the pursuit of thoroughness and the collection of data that may not seem immediately relevant. My earlier anthropological self, had it adopted an allegiance to narrative paradigms of research, might have been prevented, for example, from exploring processual issues such as the conflicts between Church and home circle and the competition for recognition and status. Those themes became central to my project.

The initial paper in this volume and its title essay was first presented at a conference held at the University of Kent in 1972. Mine was one of only two papers that were not based on research in remote societies. In my paper I tried to condense my ethnographic knowledge acquired over several years. The paper moves between three overlapping domains. It describes Spiritualist beliefs as a relatively homogenous body of shared knowledge. It describes the dynamics of Spiritualist communication and healing. And it offers an interpretative account of Spiritualist understandings of illness, pain and the sharing of pain essential to healing. In Spiritualist circles physical and emotional pain and painful stories are not private but are collectively owned and shaped. They are added to and amended by other members of the group and in the process they become more bearable to the sufferer. The technical term for this is 'taking on a condition', but it is just one example of a form of intimate communication that is found in many different illness settings. My account suggests that the beliefs and practices combine to alleviate the experience of isolation that accompanies physical and emotional pain. Spiritualist conceptions of the self break down the isolating boundaries of more conventional Western articulations of the self. They also enable others to reinterpret private troubles in a language of shared symbols thus aiding the process of externalization. It is worth remembering here that the semantic origins of the word empathy relate primarily to aesthetics and only by extension to a communion of souls. The philosopher Goldie (2000: 194) points out that the word empathy entered the English language at the beginning of the twentieth century and was a translation of the German *einfuehlung*, a term used to describe sympathy for a work of art. In other words, the genealogy of the word connects it firmly with issues of representation.

During my years of fieldwork among Spiritualists in South Wales participant observation was a taken for granted but relatively unexamined practice. The idea that observation might privilege the visual and confer a spurious objectivity was hardly discussed and I certainly was not aware of such arguments. I was, of course, a keen observer of ritual movements, enacted emotions and spatial configurations. However, many Spiritualist meetings take place in dimmed light or near darkness and Spiritualists are instructed to close their eyes. This blocking out of the visual world promotes a more concentrated and intense form of listening and I would date my interest in the narrative shape of experience from my time among Welsh Spiritualists.

My second piece of fieldwork from the South Wales period was carried out in a mining village and focused on women's use of menstrual and menopausal symbolism. Based on informal interviews with eighteen women who were aged around fifty at the time and a further eighteen aged between thirty and seventy, I tried to show how beliefs about menstrual loss were used to lay claim to a particular kind of feminine role. I put my informants into two categories: those suffering 'conjugal insufficiency' and 'irregularity of sexual and reproductive lives' and those enjoying seemingly conformist and traditional marriages. Women with an allegiance to a traditional role were more likely to attribute elaborate symbolic meanings to menstrual blood and see the loss of blood as vital to maintaining energy levels. Women with disturbed marriages had a more matter of fact approach to menstruation and its cessation. I have purposefully reproduced the language used to construct these categories despite the embarrassment it causes me. Back then, I used these 'experience far' categories because I thought of fieldwork, and data collection, as a scientific exercise. Only slowly did it dawn on me that I was trying to construct a narrative out of the narratives my subjects gave me, and that the real puzzle that fascinated me was the interplay of these oh-so-coherent narratives and the messy complexity of an individual's daily life. That puzzle only became apparent in my next project, in India.

In 1984 I went to Maharashtra. My fieldwork in Maharashtra focused on the gendered nature of beliefs about and the management of madness, affliction and trance and their practical implications for men's and women's lives. Part of the impetus for the research arose from my earlier studies of Welsh Spiritualism and my interest in the sharing of distress facilitated by possession. But my interest in this research was also fuelled by epidemiological findings of the time, which suggested that the preponderance of mental ill health among women in Western societies was not found in India. Indeed, it was thought that men were more likely to suffer from mental health problems. Subsequent research has shown this to be untrue and to result from the greater stigma attached to mentally ill women and the larger number of hospital beds occupied by men. More recent studies situate the greater stigmatization, poorer treatment and social extrusion of mentally ill women in the context of greater overall gender inequality. In many ways my findings from a Mahanubhav healing temple foreshadowed these later findings. In this chapter I wanted to document the lack of support and relative injustice that was the lot of mentally ill women whom I encountered. Whereas mentally ill men, however ill they might look to me, were perceived as getting better and their illnesses were not seen as an obstacle to the orderly progression of their lives, for women mental illness disqualified them from the usual expectations of family support and resulted in social exile. However, beyond the palpable gender injustices that my study of the Mahanubhav temple revealed, contested understandings of the nature of spirit possession and trance suggest caution in treating cultural beliefs as unified. Priests viewed women's propensity to possession as a gender-linked character defect, whereas women viewed possession as something they actively cultivated for the benefit of the families, particularly its male members.

In 1971 I had been appointed in Bristol's Department of Mental Health, later renamed Psychiatry. This has influenced the development of my ideas in different ways. On the one hand, daily conversations with my psychiatrist colleagues about their routine dilemmas and crises has protected me from some of the wilder assertions of social scientists about the nature of psychiatry and made me aware of commonalities of approach. On the other hand, it sharpened my awareness of inevitable differences.

The chapter 'Anthropology and Psychiatry: the Uneasy Alliance' reflects these divergent concerns and belongings. It documents the way in which socio-anthropological studies of the history of psychiatry have challenged what I describe as the 'intellectual purity of psychiatric ideas' and yet argues that many of the early anthropological ideas about 'primitive mentality' were just as intellectually impure. In other words, both psychiatric and anthropological concepts perform a social function and they cease to be used when their social task has been accomplished. Hacking introduces the apt metaphor of an ecological niche to describe the relationship between a psychiatric diagnosis and its social context (1998: 1). However, the anthropological enthusiasm for identifying ethnocentrism and intellectual imperialism within transcultural psychiatry largely excluded self-examination for signs of possible contamination. In this chapter I raise the issue of translation as a generic problem faced by both anthropology and psychiatry and see it as a challenge that must be addressed if we are to avoid the sterile and ultimately unworkable position of a thorough-going relativism. Substituting words like distress for more clinically flavoured terms like depression or anxiety does not solve the problem of interpreting one culture in terms of linguistic categories drawn from another. Immersion in another culture involves learning a new language. But as Gadamer points out learning a first language is radically different from learning a second one (1989: 453). If the first language is learnt largely through context, the second language necessarily harks back to the first and involves translation. Because fieldwork is not a first language, anthropologists can never approach the field as cultural innocents, but always through a filter of their own cultural lens. Much of this now sounds like a pseudo-problem, when self-reflexivity has been offered as a way out from the problems of relativism. But I would maintain that in the field of cross-cultural psychiatry, attempts to provide purely phenomenological accounts of mental illness may still serve to smuggle in ethnocentric categories in the guise of a clinically neutral language.

'Remembering and Forgetting' reflects upon the history of the relationship between anthropology and psychiatry. The large number of early anthropological studies carried out by medical men is generally acknowledged (see, for example, Loudon 1976). Less well known is what we might now describe as a kind of prescience in their acknowledgement of the individual on the one hand and a relaxed attitude to what Geertz famously described as a blurring of genres (1993: 19). An insecure concern over rigid disciplinary boundaries dominated anthropology for the best part of the twentieth century. These medical specialists were much more confident, and readily admitted anthropology's indebtedness to psychology.

Turner, in his introduction to Myerhoff's book *Number Our Days*, describes certain anthropologists as thrice born: born first into a natal culture, reborn into an exotic culture and thrice-born when they return to their own culture with new eyes (1979: xiii). This description comes close, but does not entirely fit my own position. I was born into a refugee and diasporic Latvian culture. My first visit in 1991 after the collapse of the Soviet Union and my fieldwork from 1992 onwards was in a society that had elements that were both intensely familiar and totally strange. Assumptions were made about my identity and to a certain extent I shared these. The terms coined by Kirmayer, but used differently by him, seem to best fit my experiences of identity in relation to fieldwork. He introduces the idea of the adamantine and the relational self in the context of refugee review tribunals (2003: 179). The *Oxford English Dictionary* defines adamant as 'an alleged rock or mineral of contradictory and fabulous properties. Now a poetical or rhetorical name for impregnable hardness'. This definition suggests endurance, secrecy and a certain mysteriousness in contrast to the fluid, adaptive and surface relational self.

When I went to Latvia in 1991, I discovered that my informants made use of both these notions of identity. When they wished to assert ethnic solidarity and sameness, an unchanging essentialist and adamantine self was evoked. But when they talked about particular events and social circumstances of the Soviet occupation they spoke of identity as changing and relational. By and large such uses of identity fitted my own implicit understandings of a Latvian identity laid down in early childhood through narrated family memories and children's stories of pastoral landscapes and lives (Skultans 1998a), and a British identity acquired through grammar school in north London, student life in 1960's London and an academic life in Bristol. But in my case, these two identities found a connection in that I made sense of narratives of the relational self by superimposing narratives of the adamantine self. Thus I perceived underlying fairytale fragments of place, character and plot in the narratives of expropriation, forced exile and imprisonment under Soviet rule. My readiness to approach culture through narrative and to identify literary paradigms in oral narratives is perhaps the result of my own Latvian identity being largely shaped through books. Reflecting upon my interpretative approach reminds me of Babcock's rejoinder to the criticism that self-reflexivity in anthropology is narcissistic. She argues by contrast that the problem with Narcissus was not that he was too taken up with his own image, but that he was not taken up enough, he did not look long and hard enough. In other words, he was not critical enough (Babcock 1980: 2).

In choosing to study neurasthenia in Latvia, I found like many anthropologists before me that my carefully thought out project was cast aside and reworked by my informants. Informants reworked my research questions so as to be able to tell me what they thought was important. Neurasthenia was the most widely used diagnosis in Latvia, but it was never adopted in lay discourse in the way that the Western diagnosis of depression has become part of popular discourse. Many of my informants who wrote to me started their letters by disconnecting themselves from the idea of neurasthenia and then going on to describe how the disorderly, unjust and violent events of their lives had made them ill. Among my informants were several doctors who saw, as did their patients, the oppressive events and circumstances of the Soviet occupation impinging directly and brutally upon the nervous system. Thus the accounts of doctors approximated more closely to those of their patients than to official textbook accounts. The chapter entitled 'A Historical Disorder' sets out to demonstrate how the shaping of experience by medical language may be contested. The history of neurasthenia in Latvia is an example of failed medical knowledge reflecting the endurance of resistance to fifty years of Soviet rule.

'Narratives of the Body and History' further develops this argument by suggesting that shared ideas about damaged nerves, damaged heads and damaged hearts are ways of representing the collective and patriotic body and using such representations to articulate a critique of the period of Soviet occupation of Latvia. In this chapter I have tried to convey the phenomenological richness of the body in a way that challenges its semantic thinness when used as one of a pair of dualistic opposites. For example, Luhrmann (2001: 8) characterizes the mind as belonging to the realm of morality and the body to lie outside this realm in morally neutral territory, at least in American culture and in American psychiatry. Interviews with psychiatrists and their patients showed this to be an overdrawn distinction for them. During the early 1990s there was an intense identification between personal narratives of the body and the grand narratives of history. Much as I admire and return to the work of C. Wright Mills he was surely wrong when he claimed that individuals are, 'Seldom aware of the intricate connection of the pattern of their own lives and the course of world history' (1970: 10). History may not be recognized as a force in all lives, but it dominates the lives of others and narratives seek to identify a historical and social genealogy for particular illnesses. I introduce Le Roy Ladurie's concept of an *événement créatrice* (1979: 130), a creative event, with some ironical reserve, to show how illness narratives are structured. For Ladurie these events are creative in the sense that they break down old social structures and introduce new ones. The history of Soviet Latvia has many such creative events and they form the building blocks both of a macro history and of an intimate medical history. It is interesting to note that my narrators who appropriated a share of a collective pathology for themselves, were not thereby incapacitated in the conduct of their lives. Rather like the French women described by Gaines and Farmer (1986) as 'visible saints', their condition attested to the nature of human life and suffering rather than to an individual inadequacy. Their accounts relate to what Das et al. describe as the importance of not 'essentializing, naturalizing or sentimentalizing suffering. There is no single way to suffer' (2001: 2). But the disjuncture between narrative and the conduct of lives also points to one of anthropology's most important tasks, namely mapping the complex relations between words and actions.

'From Damaged Nerves to Masked Depression' looks at the way in which changes in the Latvian economy and society have swept psychiatric theory and practice in their wake. Whereas in 1992 my informants complained about the disorder in society making them ill, in 2002 they spoke of a disorder within themselves and an inability to take control of themselves. This shift in the locus of control has been accompanied by guilt, shame and feelings of isolation for many. Equally, these changes have brought about a receptiveness to the new medical language of depression that the earlier language of neurasthenia did not enjoy. Hacking would describe these changes in terms of what he calls dynamic nominalism.

> The claim of dynamic nominalism is not that there was a kind of person who came increasingly to be recognized by bureaucrats or by students of human nature but rather that a kind of person came into being at the same time as the kind itself was being invented. In some cases, that is, our classifications and our classes conspire to emerge hand in hand each egging the other on (1986: 228).

The interesting question though is why some categories are readily accepted and not others. In other words, why do some kinds of medical knowledge succeed and others fail? Under what circumstances are people more ready to accept and make their own the reality proffered by the experts? (ibid.: 234). I suggest that the answer lies with Rose's account of the '*psy* technologies' (1998: 16) and the peculiarly penetrative power of their language. According to Rose this power derives from the importance that *psy* languages attach to the notion of personal freedom. This enables the *psy* experts to accomplish their project without its being felt as an imposition. 'The forms of freedom we inhabit today are intrinsically bound to a regime of subjectification in which subjects are not merely "free to choose" but ., to understand and enact their lives in terms of choice under conditions that systematically limit the capacities of so many to shape their own destiny' (ibid: 17). Hacking suggests that new psychiatric languages create new ways of being, 'Making up people changes the space of possibilities for personhood' (1986: 229). But I would suggest that not all languages create meaning and open up new possibilities; languages can also mystify. Mills reminds us of the complexities of freedom: 'Freedom is not merely the chance to do as one pleases; neither is it merely the opportunity to choose between set alternatives. Freedom is, first of all, the chance to formulate the available choices, to argue over them – and then, the opportunity to choose' (1970: 193). The economic superiority of the West, the idea of Europe as synonymous with civilization and knowledge and, not least, the new influx of psychopharmacalogical drugs all combine to make the new language of Western psychiatry difficult to challenge. The freedom it offers may be illusory. In this process individuals have been transformed from active commentators and critics of their life circumstances to passive recipients of diagnoses. Drawing upon a different social context Das et al. (2001: 10) describe how such pathologization helps to disguise the political and social sources of suffering, 'And in what way does the imagery of victimization as the pathology of an individual alter the experience – collective as well as individual – so that its lived meaning as moral and political memory, perhaps even resistance, is lost and replaced by "guilt", "paranoia".'

Participant observation seldom meets the needs of an ethnography of psychiatric illness because such an enterprise demands a more intense exploration of individual lives. We cannot simply wait for people to fall ill. Some illnesses involve spectacular behavioural changes, but many others take place quietly within the confines of a family or individual consciousness. New techniques must be developed or adapted from other disciplines. Marcus and Fisher's characterization of anthropology's object applies particularly to cultural psychiatry. They write:

> If anthropologists can no longer depend as certainly on their traditional media, such as public rituals, codified belief systems, and sanctioned familial or communal structures, for capturing the distinctiveness of a culture, then they must resort to cultural accounts of less superficial systems of meaning. The focus on personhood is an attempt to do just that (1986: 45).

Cultural accounts of the person and the vicissitudes of personhood can only be elicited through what I call a narrative ethnography because it focuses on the narratives of life history. Cavarrero pinpoints the way in which questions about identity so often collapse 'who' questions into 'what' questions (2000: 13). But she reminds us that these questions belong to different registers. 'What' questions concern external attributions, whereas 'who' questions are about subjective meanings. Who one is can only be answered by recounting one's life story.

However, the use of narrative seems to be a necessary consequence of seeing anthropology as doing ethnography and doing ethnography as 'thick description' (Geertz 1973: 5–6). Geertz gave Ryle's original concept a fame it might not otherwise have had and added meanings that are at odds with Ryle's dispositional account of the mind. Geertz uses the example of an eye twitching to argue that only a thick description invoking cultural rules, symbols and the actor's intentions can tell us whether the eye movement constitutes a twitch, a wink or a pseudo-wink. It seems to me that eliciting narrative accounts is one of the best ways of accessing thick descriptions of a culture and an actor's location within it. The man who taught me to do this was Joe Loudon, my PhD supervisor, who, before his conversion to anthropology, had specialized in orthopaedic surgery of the hand. He devoted the same kind of impeccable attention and interest to my ethnographic descriptions of Spiritualist groups as he must earlier have done to the anatomical workings of the human hand and he demanded of me the long, rich accounts now called life stories.

My goal has always been to come to understand other people's subjective meanings and above all the construction of identity. But identity is at one and the same time intensely personal and intensely social. Its achievement is, as Erikson reminded us some time ago, about making connections between the core of personal experience and the core of social experience (1975). In one way or another much of my work in Latvia has been about the difficult task of constructing personal identities when earlier social structures are violently destroyed.

Discussions of identity have been dismissed as 'little more than portentous incoherence' (Gleason 1983: 931). Memory has been described as 'the chocolate covered Madeleine on which we overdose' (LaCapra 1998: 14). Whatever the rights and wrongs of such accusations, we know that personal memory is unreliable and easily manipulated for political ends, collective memory is a reification, personal identity is but a comforting illusion of permanence or a culture-bound category conveying a false sense of agency to Western humankind, and national identity is an unjustified extension of individual identity. As Handler has argued, 'Collectivities in Western social theory are imagined as though they are human individuals writ large' (1994: 33).

So why venture into this deeply compromised theoretical terrain? My answer, as someone who aspires to practice a humanistic brand of anthropology, is that people's self-understanding of who they are and where they belong is of central importance in understanding human nature. Whatever the semantic histories of these concepts they are hugely important for individuals, indispensable conceptual tools for marking out the relationship between self and other. This is particularly true for people who have lived through a traumatic past since a core characteristic of trauma is that it 'disconnects the person involved from their relationship to the world' (Leydesdorff et al. 2002: 2). For this reason recovery from trauma is about reconnecting the personal to the social world and rebuilding social structures.

Memory and identity are privileged sites for exploring the relationship between self and other. Theorists fall into two categories: the primordial and the interactionist. 'For primordialists identity [and memory are] deep, internal and permanent; for interactionists/optionalists identity [and memory are] shallow, external and evanescent' (Gleason 1983: 920). Similarly a recent volume on memory entitled *Tense Past* (Antze and Lambek 1998) claims, 'Our book is less about memory than about "memory". That is to say about how "the very idea of memory" comes into play in society and culture and about the uses of memory in collective and individual practice. Put another way, it is less about the silent effects of memory than about the invocation of memory, including talk about the silent effects' (ibid.: xv).

The position I am advocating is less polarized and seeks to embrace at one and the same time both the deeply personal and the intensely communal aspects of memory and identity. The Italian oral historian Luisa Passerini, in her introduction to a volume on memory and totalitarianism, writes: 'We can remember only thanks to the fact that somebody has remembered before us, that other people in the past have challenged death and terror on the basis of their memory. Remembering has to be conceived as a highly inter-subjective relationship' (Passerini 1992: 2).

Latvian narrators frequently remembered dangerous situations by switching from a singular to plural first person pronoun, from 'I' to 'we', or by recalling folk or literary figures. Autobiographical and historical events are situated within cultural narratives. This kind of dialogic framing imbues the story-teller with moral courage. Thus in 'Looking for a Subject' Uldis intertwines his personal narrative of Siberian imprisonment with the story of *Sprīdītis*, the hero of a Latvian children's play, who becomes Uldis's invisible companion. The story of *Sprīdītis*, an orphan banished from home who wanders through the forest and rescues a princess from the devil but rather than marry her chooses to return to his farmstead, reassures Uldis and makes the possibility of his own return more real.

In 'Looking for a Subject' I examine the strategies used by one man to secure for himself an acceptable identity and place in his narrative of a terrible past. Uldis had spent much of his life exiled from society, namely, in prison labour camps in Siberia and Russia. I borrow Fernandez's terminology to present his story as moving from 'peripheral loneliness' to 'central sociality' (1995: 37). In order to describe a past that might have been experienced as eroding identity, Uldis introduces items of collective memory to buttress personal memory. Moreover, the story is no longer told in the first person singular but shifts to collective pronouns – hence the title of the chapter. Uldis's narrative provides a good illustration of the inseparability of form and content and the role of form in conveying meaning. As Riessman points out, 'Analysis in narrative studies opens up the forms of telling about experience, not simply the content to which language refers' (1993: 2).

'The Expropriated Harvest' pursues the theme of collective identity using as a starting point Bruner and Feldman's argument that the stability of collective identity depends upon the ability of a community or group to construct and commit to shared stories (1996: 294). The thesis starkly put poses problems for a nation such as Latvia whose history has created divided loyalties and deep schisms. The chapter looks at how the inhabitants of one parish in Vidzeme whose experience and role during the early period of the Soviet occupation were very different – some collaborated, some joined the resistance movement of forest partisans and still others were deported – all use the metaphor of the harvest both to describe actual events and to convey ideas of social disorder and injustice.

'Narratives of Landscape' looks at the way in which evocations of place contribute to the construction of a collective identity, particularly in the context of displacement. Narratives that freewheel across vast and empty Siberian landscapes return to the intimacies of an archetypal pastoral landscape that seduces the senses of both narrator and listener. I argue that figurative and literary representations of landscape, principally from the independence period, have shaped the way in which ordinary Latvians perceive the countryside and helped to create it as an ingredient of collective memory and identity.

'Arguing with the KGB' expands on Cohen's idea of an enlarged self (1994: 79), one that negotiates its identity and relationship to society on its own terms. In the context of my work with former victims of the KGB, this means above all the self as a creative source of values rather than one that mechanistically internalizes moral precepts. By taking my narrators to the KGB archive and together reading their old files I gave them the opportunity of challenging the past rhetoric of the KGB. In the context of a government that has introduced a system of rehabilitation without acknowledging wrong-doing or wrong-doers this opportunity is particularly important. It opens up the possibility of transforming personal misfortune into social distress.

The final chapter, 'Varieties of Deception and Distrust', explores some of the ethical dilemmas involved in researching psychiatric practice. Typically, ethical issues in the anthropology of psychiatry have focused on ideas to do with informed consent, autonomy and transparency of the research agenda.

My chapter argues that traditional ways of resolving these issues do not take into account the complexities of the psychiatrist-patient relationship and the anthropologist's allegiance to both. Furthermore, I argue that the ethical issues in carrying out an ethnographic study of psychiatric consultations transcend these issues. The more burning ethical issues are to do with the symbolic violence that a reified psychiatric language can wreak upon the experience of socially marginalized people.

Stories so readily break free from their telling and acquire lives of their own. Indeed, Bauman and Briggs argue that anthropologists have put so much emphasis on contextualizing story telling precisely because stories are so readily detachable from their context. They ask: 'What factors loosen the ties between performed discourse and its context?' (1990: 73). Allegiance to any one paradigm necessarily leaves in a shadow what would be highlighted by other paradigms. But much of anthropological research and writing is about making difficult choices about what to leave out. The question is rather how much context do we need in order not to distort or rob the narrative of its meaning?

Much of my writing raises issues to do with subjectivity. Despite the long established existence of both a subjectivist and an objectivist tradition in European thought and the accumulated critiques of objectivism, it remains true that these paired polarities are given different moral weightings. In lay language objectivity is still often elided with truth and subjectivity with unreliability. But our lives are not lived through the mediation of an external observer. As the philosopher Nagel points out, 'Life is lived from inside, and issues of significance are significant only if they can be raised from inside' (1991: 197). He argues that there is something irreducible about subjectivity and that it cannot be captured by causal or functional explanations. Nagel illustrates the non-reducibility of consciousness by using the example of the bat. 'Even without the benefit of philosophical reflection anyone who has spent some time in an enclosed space with an excited bat knows what it is to encounter a fundamentally alien form of life' (ibid.: 168). No amount of understanding of the brain mechanisms of the bat will tell us what it *feels like* to be a bat. There is an explanatory gap because physical accounts leave out subjectivity. Our own limited human experience precludes us from understanding the experience of the bat.

Experience is necessarily subjective and as Nagel points out the very idea of an objective experience is nonsensical. 'It is difficult to understand what could be meant by the objective character of an experience, apart from the particular point of view from which the subject apprehends it. After all, what would be left of what it was like to be a bat if one removed the viewpoint of the bat?' (ibid.: 173). Ignoring the viewpoint of the bat takes us further away rather than closer to understanding its reality. This discussion of the subjective experience of the bat points to the enormous advantage conferred by language in understanding human subjectivities.

Our experience may fall short of understanding the bat but it does not preclude us from understanding other human beings. We do this by observing what others do but above all by listening to what they say. This kind of understanding does not involve mysterious processes of identification but rather an ethnographic understandings of others and their projects as well as of ourselves: 'To interpret means to bring one's own preconceptions into play so that the text's meanings can really be made to speak for us' (Gadamer 1989: 397). This kind of anthropology transforms the autobiographical into an ethnographic self (Ryang 2000).

An awareness of the ethnographic self makes dissimulation more difficult. Were I doing fieldwork among Spiritualists now, I would be more cautious about systematically trading on different understandings of the focus of my research. I would, at the very least, weigh up the ethical implications of this position. All Spiritualists consider that they are doing research into the spirit world and thus introducing myself as a researcher eased my passage into the community of Spiritualists. I chose not to correct what I knew to be misconceptions about the nature of my research. I tape-recorded all services and used fragments of conversation formed by the triangulation of spirits, mediums and the afflicted to illustrate the way in which distress was dealt with. My indebtedness to one particular informant is not fully recorded nor the implications of my own role as a novitiate. If I had the chance to replay the past I would want to record the life stories of several of the Spiritualists and to give them more of an opportunity to speak for themselves. But at the time life stories were considered atheoretical and narrative theory was confined to literary studies.

My work also raises issues to do with emotion. Other writers have dealt with the question of how to find a balance between empathy and over-involvement and its threat to critical acumen. I would like to add my voice to the plea for vulnerability. Neurologists of a philosophical bent such as Damasio (1994) and Sacks (1998) have demonstrated the cognitive substitutability of different areas of the brain. If one area of the brain is damaged another area can take over its functions. But if the emotional centre of the brain is damaged then substitution cannot take place. All choices have equal value and the person becomes immobilized. Let me illustrate this position by recounting an incident from the film Iris. In the early stages of Alzheimer's, John Bailey, Iris Murdoch's husband, takes her to see a specialist neurologist. During the consultation the neurologist asks her who is the prime minister of England. Iris gives the question the kind of concentrated attention that she might devote to a complex philosophical problem, but finally has to admit defeat. She says, 'I'm sorry I don't know. But I'm sure somebody does.' Here she gives us the essence of what cognitive substitutability is about. As far as failures of factual knowledge are concerned, we can stand in for one another in a way that we cannot for failures of emotion. If my informant is demanding emotional understanding from me I cannot say 'I'm sorry I don't feel anything but I know someone who will.' Shotter (2004) calls this kind of understanding relational and distinguishes it from representational understanding.

Most fieldworkers, in recalling the emotional immediacy and power of the ethnographic encounter, will understand the distinction. Frank has identified this power in his distinction between 'thinking with stories' rather than 'thinking about stories' (1995, 2001). So what is the difference? As I understand this distinction 'thinking with' stories makes room for a greater degree of empathy with the storyteller which in turn makes demands upon our moral imagination. 'Thinking with' stories is an experiential and transformative process. When confronted with the pain and suffering of others, stories exert a moral obligation on the listener not to turn away but to acknowledge and share (Morris 2002: 197). Much of the literature on 'thinking with stories' derives from the work of Levinas and his concept of face.

And this kind of thinking is transformative. Shotter is very good on this transformative process: 'What the voices of others can do for us that we cannot do for ourselves, is that their otherness which enters into us makes us other. They can arouse a dialogically structured response in us, they can create possibilities of change within us that we cannot create within ourselves alone' (2004: 8). Our informants expect relational understanding rather than duplication in our responses. This kind of relational response is difficult to pin down but I suspect it determines the difference between research that yields thick and thin descriptions, or between rich and skeletal narratives. It also accounts for the way that we as ethnographers feel both enlarged and humbled by the experience of fieldwork, but in a manner that eludes description.

However, emotion is also an issue for our informants. Because medical and psychiatric ethnographies often involve stories of painful and disordered experience, the very process of telling elicits emotion in the teller. And the act of ethnographic mirroring of narrative experience by the fieldwork elicits further emotion. Thus, for example, Odysseus maintains composure in the face of his many misfortunes but breaks down in tears when he hears the story of his own life told by a blind minstrel. 'So the famous singer sang his tale, but Odysseus melted, and from under his eyes the tears ran down, drenching his cheeks. As a woman weeps.' (Homer 1965: lines 521–23). In other words, significance of past experience can only be fully apprehended when its telling has been heard and retold by another.

2

EMPATHY AND HEALING:
ASPECTS OF SPIRITUALIST RITUAL

This chapter deals with responses to pain and sickness among Spiritualists. It illustrates the close connections between the anthropology of medicine and of religion. Religious attention is frequently focussed on health and illness. Only by including ritual activity can a full understanding be gained of the meaning of sickness and pain for the patient. Spiritualism is one field where ritual matters and health matters are inextricably interwoven.

Before presenting the ethnographic material, the level at which sickness is being considered must be indicated. A theme in everyday thought as well as in theoretical discussion is one which recognizes a distinction between real pathology and socially defined sickness which may or may not have a basis in real pathology. From the point of view of the sufferer this is a meaningless distinction, since the experience of pain need not be affected by its basis, or otherwise, in real pathology. Spiritualist sufferers are concerned with their experience of pain irrespective of whether this has a basis in psychological disorder or psychological and social conflict. To ask whether spirit healing works in terms of removing the pathology is to alter the focus of attention. Spirit healing works in so far as Spiritualists claim no longer to have pain and insofar as they do not present themselves for treatment.

Given this approach to sickness, the term 'sociosomatic' illness is particularly useful with regard to my material. Illness which does not have a basis in real pathology has usually been labelled psychosomatic. I would argue that in very many cases this is an inappropriate label for which the term 'sociosomatic' could be substituted with greater descriptive accuracy. Reproductive disorders among women are typically among those most readily described as being of psychosomatic origin. I have argued elsewhere that statements about reproductive disorders and menstrual processes are symbolic statements about social roles and relationships (see Chapter 3, this volume). Menorrhagia, for example, can in many instances be looked upon as a 'housewife's sickness'. It is, therefore of 'sociosomatic' rather than psychosomatic origin.

Returning to Spiritualists, very many of their complaints are interwoven with difficult social or marital situations. This is born out by the way in which illness is presented within the Spiritualist group as one among a number of difficulties with which Spiritualists have to contend. This heterogeneity in the presentation of misfortune is echoed in eclecticism in explaining sickness. No one explanatory model predominates. Social, psychological and organic possibilities are considered as exerting a causal influence on sickness. Similarly, there is an eclectic approach to treatment. Spirit healing, herbal remedies, psychological insight, suggestions for social manipulation of difficult situations are each considered as methods worth trying.

This eclectic or 'sociosomatic' approach to sickness finds its focal point of expression in the Spiritualist concept of 'aura'. Everybody is thought to have an aura. It is half-physical, half-spiritual, rather like a rainbow that surrounds a person's body. Although not visible to the uninitiated it can be seen by 'sensitives' or those who are spiritually developed. A person's aura is like a barometer that measures social, psychological or physical balance and imbalance. This balance and harmony or their lack are reflected in colour. A good aura is white, blue or purple. A bad aura is a dark colour, especially red. The colour of the aura can be affected for the worse by an imbalance or state of conflict at any level, whether of social conflict, psychological stress or organic pathology. Blue is described as the 'healing colour' and is especially highly valued. The aura of a healthy and well-balanced individual who is at peace with him or herself and others is blue. Occasionally, when members of a Spiritualist group are in tune with one another and are temporarily freed from misfortune, a blue light is seen surrounding the circle.

In summary, this chapter concerns Spiritualism in South Wales and the response of Spiritualists to pain and sickness. Spiritualists lend themselves particularly well to this study since they consider themselves beset by a variety of disabilities and are preoccupied with the problem of the meaning of suffering and its communication.

General Ethnography

There are three Spiritualist churches in Swansea and numerous 'home' or 'developing' circles. It is difficult to give an accurate assessment of the total Swansea Spiritualist population, but I would put it at around four hundred. Of these most are working class; about three-quarters are women, middle-aged and older.

The 'home' or 'developing' circle is the most widespread and important form of Spiritualist meeting. Both terms are literally descriptive. The latter term refers to the group's functions; the former to its setting. Circles are run by mediums of long-standing and high reputation. The circle meets regularly, often in the home of the medium. Its aims are to develop the latent and nascent mediumistic powers of its members and thus produce fully-fledged mediums. In view of its intimate setting the circle can be seen as a private rehearsal for the grand debut which takes place at a Spiritualist service. This form of organization is a reflection of Spiritualist ideology which has as one of its basic tenets the belief that everyone possesses psychic power in a latent if not fully developed form. (This belief is, of course, consistent with the fact that most people never develop their mediumistic potential at all.) Entrance to such circles is difficult to obtain. Frequently this is achieved by making one's psychic gifts known publicly and especially to well-established mediums associated with the coveted circle. Continued and regular attendance is, it is thought, essential if good results are to be attained. Developing circles should never be large and the optimum number is thought to be about twelve. One of the underlying premises of developing circles is that progress in mediumistic performance achieved by one member affects every other member of the group in a positive way.

Although there is a written tradition of thought about Spiritualism and official doctrine is available at any one of the Spiritualist headquarters, its influence at the local level is insignificant. Practice and belief seem to be determined by local needs and inspiration rather than being documented by a central authority. This is explained in part by an explicit emphasis on individual inspiration and in part by an inherent weakness in organizational and co-ordinating abilities. This lack of influence of official doctrine is apparent in that few Spiritualists are aware of which national organization, if any, their church belongs to; let alone do they know the doctrinal differences consequent upon such membership.

Religious beliefs and practices are learnt from other more developed mediums, usually in the context of the developing circle. In fact, there is a stigma attached to learning about Spiritualism, especially mediumship and healing, from published material. The true path to Spiritual power, as, indeed, to much therapeutic art, is through regular contact with and encouragement from a small number of more advanced adepts. Spiritualist women in Swansea are frequently the daughters of Spiritualist mediums. Thus, first introduction to the movement takes place in childhood but a regular link is not established until later on in adulthood, usually after marriage.

Does Spiritualism Deal with a Peculiar Sector of Illness?

Much of Spiritualist activity is concerned with healing and giving advice about sickness. I shall describe this more fully later in the chapter. Before turning to the details of these activities, however, a summary of the types of complaints managed by Spiritualism and its relationship with orthodox medicine is necessary.

Unlike Christian Science, Spiritualism does not attempt to assert its supremacy over orthodox medicine. Spiritualists are seldom discouraged from seeing their doctor and are seldom given advice which contradicts that of the doctor. Indeed, Spiritualism does not see itself as an alternative to orthodox medicine but rather as its complement. It fills in the gaps and smoothes over the inadequacies of more orthodox treatment methods. Thus it does not deal with a peculiar sector of illness. It has a contribution to make towards the management of all sickness. Most frequently, however, spirit healing aims to increase a person's overall vitality, zest and resistance towards disease and the strains and stresses of life. In other words, one need not have a specific complaint to be able to benefit from spirit healing. However, healing is also given for specific complaints that have either been previously diagnosed by a doctor or are diagnosed within the Spiritualist setting by Spirit. In such instances spirit healing is always thought to help, in that it alleviates pain, and sometimes it is thought to cure. There are many first-hand accounts of such cures. Blindness, stomach ulcers, kidney stones have disappeared, it is claimed, by spirit healing. Thus within the context of Spiritualist ideology there is a tradition of curing and ready evidence for its success. Whether or not such cures would be recognized by 'scientific' medicine did not form part of my research interests, in that I was concerned with whether Spiritualists themselves considered themselves to be cured. Thus success was judged by their self-assessment of health.

The Spirit World

At this point perhaps an account of the structure of the spirit world should be introduced in order to bring out its relationship to earthly suffering. Two words are frequently used. 'Spirit' is a word commonly used to refer to the mystical, the non-empirical: it is used in such contexts as, for example, 'I am getting a message from Spirit, or, 'Spirit is very strong with you', or, 'Spirit is protecting you all the way'. Interchangeable with the word 'Spirit' in some contexts is the word 'Power'. Thus one can correctly say: 'The power is very strong with you'. However, it would not be correct Spiritualist usage to say either: 'I am getting a message from Power', or 'Power is protecting you all the way'. These examples show that 'Power' can be used as a synonym for 'Spirit' only in contexts when it is most closely related to and intermingled with human beings. Thus where Spirit is thought of as a discrete entity, distinct from human beings, it cannot also be referred to as 'Power'. However, in contexts where a person has already become an instrument of Spirit it is usual and correct to use the term 'Power'. In such contexts the word 'Power' is not only conventionally correct, it is also literally true. Messages that are agreed to come from Spirit are axiomatically true and, therefore, confer great power and prestige on the medium.

There is a similarity with Middleton's account of the Lugbara conceptualization of Spirit in terms of its remote and immanent aspects. The Lugbara words refer to Spirit in its remote aspects as being creative and infinite and to Spirit in its immanent aspects as being the cause of pestilence, droughts and famine (Middleton 1960). The parallel between the spiritual categories of Swansea Spiritualists and those of the Lugbara is not complete but it is there nevertheless. Although Power is not necessarily conceptualised as evil and hence is not the complete equivalent of the Lugbara term, nevertheless there is a distinct value for Spirit in its immanent aspect. However, it is only in its immanent aspects that Spirit can be bad or produce illness. In other words, the badness of bad spirits is only manifest on those occasions when they possess a person.

Spirits are hierarchically organized, there being a continuous upward movement from the time of death. Communication is usually with the spirits from the lower ranks of the hierarchy. Communication between human beings and the lower spirits constitutes a link of mutual interdependence. Immediately after death, spirits find themselves at a 'loose end' in the spirit world and still feel strongly attached to their 'earth conditions'. They are in a state of transition between the living and the dead. This state is ambiguous and, hence, dangerous. Spiritualists are able to help spirits who are trapped in the meshes of their previous existence by performing as mediums and acting out conditions of affliction. Through mediumship such spirits can be released from the previously painful conditions to which they were bound.

As instruments of Spirit, Spiritualists can provide the stage on which the circumstances of dying can be re-enacted: the medium becomes possessed or 'takes on the condition' of a dying person so that, in effect, a death scene is re-enacted in the midst of the Spiritualist circle. Thus the spirits in question are freed from the scene of their earthly pain and suffering and allowed to move upwards in the spirit world. Without the ready help of Spiritualist mediums, spirits would remain forever fettered to this life. This aspect of Spiritualist activity is known as 'rescuing' or 'rescue operations'. Most difficult 'rescue operations' are notoriously those which involve the spirits of deceased mediums.

However, the link between the spirit and physical world is one of mutual interdependence and help flows both ways. Human beings are dependent upon Spirit for help. This help takes the form of advice about health problems, emotional problems, protection in the face of difficulties and, most important, the power of healing. Such advice is not expected to come from the spirits of the immediately departed: it has been shown that they are themselves helpless. Neither is it thought to come from those spirits who have progressed far in the spirit world: they are no longer concerned with human beings and their material problems. Help is thought to come from those spirits occupying an intermediate position in the spiritual hierarchy. They are neither so involved in 'earth conditions' as to need help themselves, nor so distant as to be completely unconcerned. Perhaps the easiest way of indicating the scope of the spirit world is to list the categories of spirits that it contains:

1. There is a vast array of spirits who have ascended into the higher realms of the spirit world. No communication exists with these spirits and, hence, they are seen as an undifferentiated spiritual mass in which little interest is expressed.
2. The second category in order of spiritual prestige involves all those spirits who return to give advice. These range from the permanent and reliable spirit-guide to the casual spirit visitor with a single item of advice.
3. A third large-sized category of spirits covers those who, whilst not malevolent, are themselves in need of comfort and help as a result of some particularly distressing 'earth conditions' they have experienced and are unable to remove.
4. A fourth slightly smaller category includes all spirits who have died a violent or painful death. These are the spirits who call the 'rescue operations' mediums into action. Contact with these spirits requires a high degree of skill and control.
5. A final category, constituting a sub-category of category four, contains all those spirits, malevolently disposed, who actively inflict sickness.

Tambiah refers to this final category as those who have 'unnaturally escaped society'. He explains the evil nature of these spirits in the following terms: 'The belief in the violent spirit is thus a magnified and dramatized conceptualisation of a free-floating malignant force, which, however, does not find an expression as systematized cult behaviour. It represents the theoretical extreme of the concept of an unfulfilled life, the notion being transferred into the notion of an uncontrollable evil' (1970: 316). Thus it can be seen that the scope of spiritual categories is such as to provide an adequate mirror for the varieties of human distress. The range is between distressing conditions which can be managed with little active display of emotion, and those evoking strong emotional responses and acting-out behaviour. It is of interest that in the latter case the distress is located in the spirit world and the human agent is seen as taking on the role of a competent and generous helper.

Ritual Auctions: Illness as Currency[1]

When asked, most Spiritualists admit to physical disabilities. However, they do not regard this as unusual. Sickness, whether chronic, temporary or recurrent, is interwoven with Spiritualists' expectations of life. From this there stems a theme of sadness running through all Spiritualist activities. Spiritualists consider themselves different from others not in claiming more sickness for themselves, but in their management of it. Thus each occurrence in the medical and emotional history of a Spiritualist is a proper object of attention for the entire Spiritualist group.

An analogy using the idea of an auction will help to make clear the concerns of Spiritualist circles. The central importance of illness emerges from questions that such an analogy suggests. The questions to be asked include the following: What is the bidding for? Who are the auctioneers? In what currency is the bidding made? What rules govern bidding? At Spiritualist meetings bidding is for attention and status and all Spiritualists participate in the bidding. However, the participants are both auctioneers and bidders. Within the space of an evening Spiritualists both bestow concern and attention on others and demand it for themselves. The currency is in terms of physical or emotional complaint. However, there are well defined norms which specify what can and cannot be put up for auction and the manner in which this must be done. Conversation at meetings has as its focus the body and onslaughts on its well-being. Bidding for attention which becomes too frequent is critically received. However, a reserve is set below which bidding for attention is not tolerated. Physical impairment is thus almost a precondition of eligibility for group membership. Therefore, the degree and nature of participation by members in the activities of the group is controlled.

Illness and Pain

Much has been written by sociologists but little by anthropologists about the presentation of illness. Discussion has usually been under the heading of the theory of illness behaviour. Sociologists have aimed to identify social factors which are relevant to the way in which sickness is perceived and which determine the subsequent behaviour of the sick person. Medical sociologists have tried to show how behaviour in sickness is connected with a number of factors other than those relating to the severity or intensity of pain. For example, the values placed on endurance and self-control as opposed to the ready dramatization of pain have been cited (Zola 1966; Zborowski 1952). Behaviour in sickness has also been related to the social role of the sick person and the way in which the sickness can be accommodated to current obligations (Robinson 1971). Such considerations as these have directed attention away from the problem of pain and unease popularly regarded as being at the very heart of sickness. No doubt this is an attempt to focus attention away from the physical to the social and cultural. However, in the course of this shift of attention a very large area belonging to the cultural, namely the structure of pain experience, has, in fact, been relegated to the biological. Perhaps another reason why the connection between pain and sickness has been neglected is because it is too close and uncomfortable. It is the case, however, that little has been written about the influence that the structure of pain experience has on the presentation of sickness. The problem of examining the cultural and linguistic conventions that determine the perception and expression of pain has been left on one side. More importantly, there is no systematic study of how the perception of pain is reflected in subsequent definitions, management of sickness and healing procedures.

Privacy and Pain

The aim of this chapter is not merely to demonstrate a general concern which Spiritualism has with pain, suffering and its management, but to indicate the precise topography and content of Spiritualist pain experience and to relate this to their group activities. One approach is to consider certain key Spiritualist rituals and thereby infer the underlying attitudes to pain. A more direct approach considers overtly-expressed ideas about pain.

Spiritualist thought is diffused with anxieties about communication, that is, the inability to convey the precise quality of an experience to others and the sense of isolation when faced with pain and suffering. The activities of Spiritualist groups express these anxieties. Moreover, the development of mediumistic powers is one of the ways in which the quality of communication between people is improved. It is a way of penetrating the 'inner world' of others as well as the spirit world. One way of becoming aware of the Spiritualist experience of pain and the anxiety about its communication is by briefly considering a philosophical controversy about pain. The problems are definitional: should pain be defined as a sensation or an emotion? Jeremy Bentham (1970) treated both pains and pleasures as sensations. F.H. Bradley (1888), on the other hand, regarded pains as emotions. Pain, he thought, contributes the feeling-tone to an experience.

How pain is defined determines pain behaviour. Thus given our own linguistic conventions, pain defined as a sensation cannot be shared. One can *have* a pain, itch or throb, but one cannot be said to know it and neither can anyone else. Pain defined as emotion, however, relates to suffering. It can be communicated and hence shared. This philosophical digression in the middle of an anthropological text is justified if it reveals a variety of definitions of pain and, hence, ways of handling pain.

The teaching of Spiritualist mediums involves an implicit awareness of such definitional controversies. On the one hand they are taught to become possessed or 'to take on a condition'. On the other hand, they are taught to become 'impressed' or 'to listen to Spirit'. In possession or taking on a condition, the condition taken on is usually a painful one, such as, for example, backache, migraine, stomach ache. This is the condition suffered by one of the members of the Spiritualist group or by a spirit whilst it was on the 'earth plane'. However, according to Spiritualist theory, this condition may be experienced not only by the sick person but also by the healer and any other Spiritualists who are 'sensitives'. By 'taking on conditions' pains can be shared in much the same way as visual or auditory objects can be shared. The pain acquires some of the properties of a physical object, which several people can see, hear or feel at the same time, provided they are favourably situated. Pains taken on by 'sensitives' resemble the blurred contours of physical objects seen in a dim light.

'Listening to' or becoming 'impressed' by Spirit is a more complex activity. This procedure requires an active response on the part of the developing medium as opposed to a passive surrendering of one's conscious personality. It is a way of transmitting information and advice from Spirit to human beings. Such information and advice relates broadly to the fields of physical sickness and interpersonal relations.

These two types of activities can broadly be described as representing the overtly therapeutic and the didactic elements in Spiritualism. More advanced Spiritualists usually acquire a 'spirit-guide', that is, a spirit whose connections are confined to one particular Spiritualist. Such guides are frequently, though not necessarily, thought to be the spirits of deceased doctors and preachers. As such the healing powers that they are able to confer upon individual Spiritualists are especially strong. These spirit-guides resemble Tallensi ideas about 'good destiny'. Like good destiny a spirit-guide is not acquired before adolescence. Similarly, it makes its presence felt to the medium through a series of minor accidents (Fortes 1959: 41–55).

What I hope this description of ritual activities brings out is the basically solipsistic nature of the Spiritualist world-view. Spiritualists see each other as being rather like Ryle's 'ghost in the machine', each living 'the life of a ghostly Robinson Crusoe' (1949: 13). This epistemological outlook is one that at the emotional level, produces feelings of loneliness and isolation. It is also one that inclines towards seeking help from a mystical source in order to ease communication and overcome epistemological barriers. Most knowledge of others is gained by 'taking on a condition' or by 'listening to Spirit'. 'Taking on a condition' means complete identification with the other, in the sense of having their feelings and emotions. The implication is that any other form of acquiring knowledge of the states of mind of others by more empirical, everyday methods is bound to be incomplete, imperfect and, hence, disappointing.

The privacy felt to enclose one's inner world becomes especially hard to tolerate where illness or emotional hardship is involved. This may be because these are situations that most urgently require guidance or rules for understanding and acting, a feature that is conspicuously absent from a private world. However, these attitudes are not only implicitly revealed in certain ritual activities of Spiritualists; they are also openly acknowledged. Spiritualists admit to turning to Spiritualism 'out of pain and sorrow' and the need to share these.

This view of pain, which puts it in a domain of logically enforced privacy, is one which has implications for the classification of pain and sickness as types of misfortune. Gilbert Lewis argues elsewhere (1976) that sickness is a distinctive kind of misfortune in that it is contained within the body and threatens the continued existence of the self. I would argue that it is pain that has this distinctive quality, not sickness. Pain isolates and is difficult to communicate. Sickness, by contrast, breaks down this isolation in that diagnoses of sickness enable individuals to see themselves as one of a category of sick people.

This difficulty in tolerating the epistemological privacy of pain and the response of Spiritualism to pain is particularly interesting and unusual when considered in the light of psychiatric thought. Loss of psychological privacy, in the sense both of sharing thoughts, emotions and feelings and having them controlled by others, is taken as indicative of a loss of sanity. 'The loss of the experience of an area of unqualified privacy, by its transformation into a quasi-public realm, is often one of the decisive changes associated with the process of going mad' (Laing 1971: 36). This area of 'unqualified privacy' is, according to Laing, a reflection of the preoccupation with 'the inner/outer, real/unreal, me/not-me, public/private lines' (ibid.: 34). Traditional psychiatry refers to the loss of the privacy of experience and, hence, of ego boundaries and the identity of the self in terms such as 'ideas of passivity', 'ideas of reference' and 'ideas of influence'. Such terms are indicative of the psycho-pathological condition of the individual. By contrast, Spiritualism encourages such states of mind and they are achieved by mystical means.

The comparison is striking both in terms of the similarities and the dissimilarities that it shows. On the one hand, there is a similarity between the type of experiences sought by Spiritualists and thought patterns diagnosed as 'schizophrenic' by psychiatrists. On the other hand, opposed values are placed upon such experiences according to the context in which they appear. (Difficulties in the interpretation of experiences of loss of privacy become most acute when the same person is both a Spiritualist and a psychiatric patient.) Loss of psychological boundaries in the context of the Spiritualist circle seem particularly interesting when seen as a variation of the theme of loss of bodily boundaries. Values placed on bodily boundaries and their concomitants in social structure have received much attention (Douglas 1971). However, the boundaries of the 'self' and the experience of self have been neglected.

The Management of Illness

The way in which Spiritualists experience pain and illness can be shown in more detail by describing the way in which actual physical complaints are dealt with. The responses to illness can be roughly grouped under three activities, although each response has elements shared with the others. The activities may be distinguished as follows: 'Taking on conditions'; 'Healing'; 'Message giving'.

'Taking on conditions' has already been mentioned in relation to the training of Spiritualist mediums. It provides the backbone or element of continuity for all other Spiritualist activities. It is the mystical insight into the ordinarily hidden pains of others.

By the response of 'healing', Spiritualists refer to 'the power of healing', the greatest gift that Spirit can bestow on human beings. Most healers are men, although women can, in principle become healers too. Spirit healing involves the mystical discovery and identification of pain and sickness. It penetrates other bodies and unearths information otherwise available only to the patient.

It is believed that the healer is only an instrument or receptacle of the healing art of a spirit, frequently the spirit of a deceased doctor. Healer themselves usually knows that this possession has taken place by a peculiar tingling sensation in the fingertips. When this sensation is present the healer should place their hands on to that part of a person's anatomy to which they are guided by Spirit. Patients know that they are receiving this healing power by the intense heat which emanating from the healer's hands and penetrating the patient's body. This power, although it has physical attributes such as cause the sensation of heat to be felt, is itself non-empirical. The presence and the efficacy of the power are established *ex post facto*, when health has, in fact, been restored.

At the level of empirical description, spirit healing involves the laying on of hands by the healer on to that part of the body understood to be the cause of pain. Usually the healer's hands move in gentle stroking motions. Sometimes healers shake their hands after each stroke, thus symbolically discarding the sickness that has been drawn out of the patient's body. At sessions which are specifically and exclusively devoted to spirit healing several healers work at the same time. Healers wear white coats and stand or kneel by the patient who is seated on a chair. Each healer has a plastic bowl of water by his side in which they wash their hands after giving healing to each patient. In return, the patient, when he or she feels the healer's hands being placed upon him, says either 'Thank you' or 'Bless you'. Very frequently, women will murmur: 'Oh, that's wonderful', or, 'I can feel the power coming'.

The range of complaints treated by spirit healing is very wide; they vary both in their degree of severity and in duration. The efficacy of spirit healing is very highly valued. It is believed that the discomfort of chronic complaints such as rheumatoid arthritis can be alleviated through spirit healing; also that acute conditions such as ulcers, growths and kidney stones can be completely removed.

The activity described as 'message giving', insofar as messages from Spirit relate to pain and sickness, performs a labelling or diagnostic and explanatory service. The content of messages is obtained by 'listening to' or becoming 'impressed' by Spirit. This activity is a complex one since it demands an active and creative response on the part of the listener. Part of an aspiring medium's education involves training in the presentation of messages. It is thought that messages should be spiritual not 'material'. They should aim to sum up a person's situation or condition in a highly symbolic or eidetic form.

All Spiritualist meetings involve a continuous reinterpretation and reassessment of feelings, motives and relationships, especially insofar as these affect members' well-being or lack of it. This endless sifting of experience recalls Kafka's description of the Day of Judgement as a 'court in standing session' (1994).

Messages from Spirit define conditions involving pain and suffering in such a way that they can be managed and handled. The sense of privacy and isolation felt by Spiritualists to be a necessary corollary of pain gives rise to the demand that the sickness be seen as part of a more general pattern, that it be explained by being seen as one instance of a recurring series of events. In other words, that the painful event be defined and given a symbolic meaning. Detailed probing, both in the course of ordinary conversation and in the course of delivering messages, is made about physical ailments. Such probing is especially apparent during 'the unorganised phase' of the illness (Balint 1964: 2). Frequently it aims to locate the sources of tension in a person's social relationships insofar as these might be responsible for the lack of physical well-being. The establishment of a definitive reality is a mutual undertaking made by the healer and the sufferer and bears a close resemblance to the process, described by Balint, of bargaining for a diagnosis in terms of 'offers and responses' (ibid.: 21–36).

Perhaps an example of the management of pain and distress with reference to one particular woman, which brings into play the major Spiritualist activities can be described at this point. Ethel is a woman in her mid forties who has been a member of a developing circle for the past five years. She is married to an electrical engineer and has four adolescent children, the eldest of whom is married. The family lives in a large detached house in the suburbs of Swansea. Ethel's marital history is a tale of endurance in the face of conflict and despair. Her husband is, according to Ethel, irresponsible with respect to money, inconsiderate and inconsistent towards the children and sadistic towards herself. Throughout their married life he has been preoccupied with his involvements with other women. Ethel characterizes him as an aggressive and selfish man, utterly insensitive to the feelings of others. Apparently Jim is not altogether oblivious of her opinion of him, since he eventually agreed to consult a psychiatrist at a psychiatric hospital in Swansea. This man spoke to Ethel and told her that there was nothing at all wrong with her but that her husband was 'schizoid'. Since this consultation Ethel's life has been slightly easier, for she has realized that her husband is a 'sick man' and that he is suffering from an 'illness'. It is therefore her duty to stick by him and to help him even though her help may be rejected. Ethel's outlook is such that she now regards helping her husband regain his 'health' as her life's task and she approaches it with fervour. Despite her stoicism, however, her situation is not a happy one.

Ethel brings to the meetings her feelings of terrible loneliness, meaninglessness and despair. These feelings find frequent expression both during possession and during her non-mystical states of consciousness. Thus on one occasion, for example, Ethel had a very intense and uncontrolled fit of crying. It was not entirely clear whether or not she was in a state of possession. She turned to Mr Forde sitting on her left who had quite clearly 'gone' and was 'under control' by a spirit known as Sing Lee. What should she do? She had 'this heaviness, pain and depression'. Should she take pills? Sing Lee said she should not, that it was 'mental' and that pills would never remove the conflict. Upon hearing this Ethel was convulsed with heart-rending sobs. She screamed: 'Oh, my God help me!' and 'I don't want to be alone!' Mr Jones got up and laid his hands on her shoulders. Mr Forde, still 'under control', held her hands. The rest sang and prayed. All uncrossed their knees 'so as not to break the power'. In this instance, uncrossing symbolized the need to open up or the need for co-operation and help. This was done, with the exception of Mrs Russell, a competitive woman, who sat with her knees crossed. She was asked why she did not help in this obvious and simple way but replied: 'Ask a silly question, get a silly answer'. Subsequently she said that she herself had buried her brother and her brother-in-law that very week, but she did not bring the condition with her. In other words, her attitude implied that she begrudged the help that Ethel was getting and was, therefore, unwilling to take on the role of healer herself. However, other members of the circle showed a readiness to identify with Ethel. This was especially apparent in the healing that the two men gave Ethel.

Conclusion

The perception of pain and suffering as being, first, essentially private and hence divisive and, second, an integral part of life, especially a woman's life, influences not only the specific procedures developed for handling illness but also the setting in which these occur. In this context it is significant that most meetings, especially those that encourage the development of mediumistic powers, form an actual physical *circle* of sitters.

Like all good symbols the circle is significant at a number of different levels of meaning. First, at the level of social structure it reflects the ideal of equality between the 'sitters' expressed in the frequently repeated maxim: 'We all rise together'. This equality is with respect to access to spiritual power, since it is thought that everyone possesses mediumistic power in a latent, if not manifest, form. Spiritualists themselves way: 'The circle has no beginning and no end: it is perfect. That is why we sit in a circle'.

It is thus consciously thought of as a symbol of spiritual perfection. However, it is also an apt reminder of the permanence and continuity of suffering and pain. Thus in one sense the circle can be seen as a reconciliatory device. For, on the one hand, there is an explicit emphasis on continued spiritual progress summed up in the principle of 'eternal progress open to every human soul', whilst on the other hand there is a conspicuous lack of any real change in the lives of Spiritualist women. Spiritualism can, therefore, be seen as a ritual of reconciliation. The supportive and therapeutic nature of the groups is underlined by the fact that there is little, if any, interaction between members of a Spiritualist group outside that group.

To conclude, I want to suggest a cross-cultural approach, bearing in mind the associations suggested by my Spiritualist material. Is there a correlation between the degree of privacy or publicity felt to surround pain and a corresponding emphasis on mystical or secular methods of diagnosis and cure? The notions of privacy and of its essentially ruleless nature have not been singled out as significant concepts in understanding and explaining responses to illness and misfortune. Their consideration is needed.

Notes

1. I am grateful to Dr Basil Sansom for suggesting this analogy to me.

3

BODILY MADNESS AND THE SPREAD OF THE BLUSH

⁘⸎⸎⸎⸎⸎⁘

This chapter explores some themes and episodes in the emergence and development of the idea of insanity during the early nineteenth century. It considers the social and intellectual climate that was necessary for the idea of insanity to gain a public foothold. It also describes the peculiar bodily preoccupations which this new idea of insanity generated.

Several writers have sought to explain the growth of asylums and the elaboration of ideas about insanity which took place in the latter part of the eighteenth century. Foucault (1971), for example, sees the goals of the asylum as primarily intellectual and insanity as a residual category which is indispensable in an age glorifying reason. Rothman, in *The Discovery of the Asylum*, offers a more socially grounded view of the asylum: 'The well-ordered asylum was to fulfil a dual purpose for its innovators. It would rehabilitate inmates, and then by virtue of its success, set an example of right action for the larger society. ... The well-ordered asylum would exemplify the proper principles of social organization, and thus ensure the safety of the republic and promote its glory' (Rothman 1971: 4).

This view of the asylum as a model for society depends logically on an enlarged concept of insanity itself. Rothman does, in fact, describe such a process: 'Insanity was no longer the exclusive province of the raving lunatic or totally incompetent. Medical superintendents opened up the category and alerted the community to a whole new range of possibly deviant behaviour (ibid.: 123). Such deviance was thought of as the product of society's flaws and the deviant as its victim: 'Just as the first penologists located the origins of crime within the community, so psychiatrists linked mental illness to social organization. The epidemic of insanity, like the prevalence of crime, pointed to the most fundamental defects of the system, from mistaken economic, political and intellectual practices to grave errors in school and family training' (ibid.: 125). 'This approach to insanity gives little emphasis to heredity and predisposition and much to its exciting causes. For example, Samuel Woodward, an American alienist wrote: ' the strongest predisposition need not result in insanity' (1835).

Rothman very ably explores the relationship between this new, expanded concept of insanity and asylum organization in mid-nineteenth century America. I want to look more closely at the expansion of the concept and its consequences for symptomatology. Eighteenth century men and women suffered from an abundance of complaints such as hypochondriasis, melancholy, the spleen and the vapours. Whilst not recognized as varieties of insanity, they quite clearly had psychological as well as physical components. Implicit in such conceptions of disease is a view of man as an undifferentiated whole. Such distinctions as are made are between the contained and containing parts of the body, not between mind and matter. Complaints such as those listed above are used more or less inter-changeably. Hypochondriasis, for example, was a condition that involved both digestive disorders and discomforts, physical fatigue as well as a more generalized weariness and personality handicaps such as indecisiveness. The condition is movingly described by the anonymous author of *Confessions of a Hypochondriac or The Adventures of a Hypochondriac in Search of Health*. He writes: 'What is a hypochondriac, if not one who has no faith in himself, nor, indeed, in anyone else for two hours together? It is a state of being without a sense of security; a perpetual suspense, an expectation, a dread of an inevitable evil' (Anonymous 1849: 109). A rhetorical question expresses the case of the problem even more succinctly: 'Was I for ever to feel that sense of a vacuum, sometimes in the relenting heart and sometimes in the sensitive stomach?' (ibid.: 179). Although published in the nineteenth century, these confessions are written in what is essentially an eighteenth-century idiom.

These complaints gave the subject matter to many learned treatises. George Cheyne, Richard Blackmore and Robert Whytt were among the best known of English physicians who write on nervous distempers. The syndrome acquired the title of the English malady, and George Cheyne published a book by that name in 1734. This was the first, although not the last, time that a particular disease was claimed by the English as being peculiarly their own. Richard Blackmore begins *A Treatise of the Spleen and Vapours* with an affirmation of this:

> If the natives of this island either from the peculiar constitution of the air they breathe, or the immoderate quantity of flesh-meats they eat, or of the malt liquors they drink or any other secret causes, are more disposed to coughs, catarrhs, and consumptions, than the neighbouring nations; they are no less obnoxious to hypochondriacal and hysterical affections, vulgarly called the spleen and vapours, in a superior and distinguishing degree. And of all the

chronicle distempers that afflict the body, or disturb the mind, these two, consumptions and the spleen are the most rife and prevalent; and either directly or by their own power, or by introducing other diseases, make the greatest havoc and destruction among the people (Blackmore 1725: iii–iv).

George Cheyne, who counted himself among the afflicted, describes himself as suffering from 'head-ache, giddiness, watchings, lowness and melancholy' (Cheyne, 1734: 329). Unlike later writers, Cheyne sees these spiritual afflictions as inextricably bound up with physical distempers. 'I never saw any person labour under severe obstinate, and strong nervous complaints, but I always found at last, the stomach guts, liver, spleen, mesentery, or some of the great and necessary organs or glands of the belly were obstructed, knotted, schirrous, or spoiled, and perhaps all these together (ibid.: 184). This view of nervous distempers is in the earlier tradition of humoural pathology exemplified by, for example, Robert Burton. In his hands, melancholy becomes a catch-all of human ills and ailments and provides the archetype for later disease categories. Burton describes the condition in moving words:

> As it is with a man imprisoned for debt, if once in the gaol, every creditor will bring his action against him, and there likely hold him – if any discontent seize upon a patient, in an instant all other perturbations ... will seize upon him, and there likely hold him; and then like a lame dog or broken winged goose, he droops and pines away and is brought at last to that ill habit a malady of melancholy itself (Burton 1621: 18).

This contagious, all-embracing quality of melancholy is reaffirmed by the huge variety of causes and kinds of melancholy. Burton begins by considering the 'received' division of melancholy into three kinds: head melancholy, melancholy of the whole body, and hypochondriacal or windy melancholy, each of which proceeds from distemper in the named part of the body. Having located melancholy in the body, Burton then goes on to give an inventory of public and private miseries including poverty, ambition, avarice, love: in fact, a catalogue of human vices, failings and disappointments. Thus, although Burton pays lip-service to the distinctions between the infirmities of the spirit and those of the body, in practice he shows it an easy disregard.

In this approach Burton belongs to the medieval tradition expounded by Aquinas. It is perhaps best understood by contrasting it with the Cartesian view of the emotions. For Descartes, in *The Passions of the Soul* (1988), emotion is a purely private mental event that is only contingently connected with its bodily manifestations and its object. For the Medievals, by contrast, bodily manifestation of emotion is neither the cause nor the effect of emotion; it is its necessary condition or the *materia*. Clearly, Burton is medieval rather than Cartesian in temper, if not in time. Burton is equally at home in writing about the liver as 'the shop of humours' as he is in writing about the peculiar vulnerabilities of women, despite his charming avowals of modesty. He writes:

> For seldom shall you see a hired servant a poor handmaid, though antient, that is kept hand to her work, and bodily labour, a coarse countrey wench, troubled in this kinde, but noble virgins, nice gentlewomen, such as are solitary and idle, live at ease, lead a life out of action and employment, that fare well in great houses, and jovial companies, ill disposed peradventure of themselves, and not willing to make any resistance, discontented otherwise, of weak judgements, able bodies, and subject to passions, such for the most part are misaffected and prone to this disease (Burton 1621: 03).

But, then, suddenly recovering his sense of propriety Burton exclaims: 'But where am I? Into what subject have I rushed? What have I to do with nuns, maids, virgins, widows? I am a bachelor myself and lead a monastick life in a college. ... though my subject necessarily require it, I will say no more,' (ibid.: 304). Propriety forbids him to go on. But the next paragraph begins: 'And yet I must and will say something more, add a word or two ...' (ibid.: 304), and so on.

So much for *The Anatomy of Melancholy*. The writing of the eighteenth century remains within the same general theoretical framework. Cheyne, for example, introduces the all purpose term 'cachexia' to refer indiscriminately to either bad states of the body or the mind, or both. Again, as with Burton, the important distinction is between the contained and the containing parts of the body or, in Cheyne's terms, between solids and fluids: 'The human body is a machine of an infinite number and variety of different channels and pipes filled with different liquors and fluids, perpetually running, gliding, or creeping forward, or returning backward in a constant circle and sending out little branches and outlets, to moisten, nourish, and repair the experiences of living' (Cheyne 1734: 4). This anatomical picture suggests to Cheyne certain causes of insanity. These are (1) grossness of the fluids, (2) a corrosive quality of the fluids, (3) a too great laxity of the fibres. However, this location of nervous distempers does not put them beyond the individual's control. Cheyne is cautious about the common division of nervous disorders into original and acquired. He writes: ' a poor creature, born subject to nervous distempers, has no more reason to complain, than a child whose father has spent his worldly fortune and left him poor and destitute' (Cheyne 1734: 19). Thus health is within the reach of all provided a correct regimen and, in particular, diet are followed. Horse-riding and a daily pint of claret were commonly prescribed. On the other hand, the hypochondriac apologist 'was advised to take champagne moderately, a nutritious diet – exercise and amusement' (ibid.: 74).

Throughout this period the term 'complexion' refers alternatively to skin colour, disposition and character. The vocabulary of humoural pathology also follows this pattern. Words like sanguine and melancholic are used to describe complexion and appearance as well as styles of action and attitude. Such linguistic usage encourages an easy transition from emotional disposition to accompanying bodily characteristics. Throughout the seventeenth and eighteenth centuries, this is the background against which a continuing and familiar discussion of nervous distempers is set. For example, the essayists of the *Spectator* air common concerns and widespread fears. Boswell (1928) wrote about his hypochondria with an ease and readiness that have only recently reappeared in the women's pages of the national press. He prefaces his discussion with the phrase 'We hypochondriacks ...' David Hume, in a letter written to Dr Cheyne at the age of nineteen, admits to suffering from the vapours (1932). It was subsequently diagnosed as 'a disease of the learned'. Certainly, no stigma attaches to these disabilities. Cheyne, in his essay on long life writes: 'fine folks use their physicians as they do their laundresses, send their linen to them to be cleaned, in order only to be dirtied again' (Cheyne 1724: 182).

To summarize what I have said so far, terms like melancholy, hypochondria, spleen and vapours are used interchangeably in the medical literature of the seventeenth and eighteenth centuries. General literature also contains many references to these afflictions. They are diseases with spiritual and material components to them. This double aspect makes them both more distressing and more manageable. Cheyne has a memorable opening to his book: 'The Spirit of man can bear his infirmities, but a wounded spirit who can bear?' (1734: 1) This view of nervous distempers is, I suggest, in the tradition of medieval philosophy. It also makes it easier to acknowledge nervous disabilities. Hume, for example, in his letter to Dr Cheyne goes on to say: 'Tho I was sorry to find myself engag'd with so tedious a distemper yet the knowledge of it, set me very much at ease, by satisfying me that my former coldness proceeded not from any defect of temper or genius, but from a disease, to which any one may be subject' (Hume 1734: 14). However, the nervous distempers which were given so much attention in the eighteenth century were clearly distinguished from insanity. Hume was well aware of the difference: 'and there seems to be as great a difference between my distemper and common vapours as there is between vapours and madness' (ibid.: 70).

Clearly, this reading of the literature goes against the interpretation put forward by Michel Foucault in *Madness and Civilization*. In a simplified form, Foucault's interpretation goes as follows: until the seventeenth century madness was a recurrent ingredient of all experience. 'In the Renaissance, madness was present everywhere and mingled with every experience by its images and dangers' (Foucault 1971: 74). In the age of reason, however, the tone changes: 'All those forms of evil that border on unreason must be thrust into secrecy. Classicism felt a shame in the presence of the inhuman that the Renaissance had never experienced' (ibid.: 68). And this shame brings about what Foucault calls 'the great confinement'.

However, any review of the English literature of this period suggests, on the contrary, a personal and intimate treatment of that which is of universal concern.

In the early part of the nineteenth century the tone of writing changes. Moral management makes its first appearance and insanity is seen essentially as a disease of the will to which anyone can potentially succumb. Until this time, conditions such as the vapours and melancholy were attributed to an imbalance of bodily humours. This imbalance could be righted by following various prescribed regimens. With the changing conceptions of insanity and its change of locus from the humours to the will, possibilities for its rapid increase were created. The nineteenth-century view of man is dualistic and holds that the most important activities in a person's life are private and invisible. The workings of thought, emotion and the will take place in a private arena. Within this theoretical context it becomes more than ever important to identify the outward signs of inner states.

Once the relationship between a faulty will and insanity has been established, the numbers of those potentially susceptible to insanity are vastly increased. Many practical situations can be found which illustrate an inadequate or insufficient exercise of the will. In particular, civilization and an accompanying luxurious life-style present the will with temptations aptly described as 'the curse of polished life' (Burrows 1828: 21). Thus Maddock, writing about the spread of insanity, says' 'perhaps the rural and agricultural districts may claim some degree of exemption, over the more densely-crowded population of manufacturing cities' (Maddock 1854: 13). But then he goes on to write, in effect, that since England is the most educated and civilized of countries it suffers from the highest incidence of insanity: 'In no other country, compared with England, do we find such numerous and formidable examples of this extensive scourge. In some measure this may arise from habitual pride and hauteur of the English character; partly from the commercial greatness which it has long been her boast to enjoy; and partly from the unnatural style of living too generally adopted' (ibid.: 13). Whatever the incidence of insanity, it is clear that at the level of belief, early-nineteenth-century society is seen as presenting people with very special problems. These relate in particular to the demands made of individual endeavour or, in the idiom of nineteenth century physicians, to the trials of the will and its possible collapse. It is interesting to note that the recognition of insanity coincides with the discovery of childhood. For example, Coveney writes: 'Until the last decades of the eighteenth century the child did not exist as an important and continuous theme in English literature. Childhood as a major theme came with the generation of Blake and Wordsworth' (Coveney 1957: 29). The novelty of childhood as a separate category is echoed by Ariés: 'The idea of childhood is not to be confused with affection for children: it corresponds to an awareness of the particular nature of childhood, that particular nature which distinguishes the child from the adult, even the young adult' (Ariés 1960: 125). These two newly discovered categories of insanity and childhood emphasize individual malleability and growth and it is, therefore, not surprising that both categories emerged simultaneously.

Thus in the early 1800s the theme of moral management first appears. Moral managers urge the abandonment of physical restraint. Instead they advocate psychological techniques. Appeal to the conscience and will of the patient is suggested. In this way it is thought the power of self-control can be nurtured and the art of self-government furthered. In fact, the practice of moral management relies on a changed view of man and his emotions. The Cartesian disjunction between body and soul asserts itself. These theories emphasize the privacy and power of thought, feeling and emotion. At the same time they seek the external signs of these inner events. Within this context the study of facial expression assumes great importance. Many studies on physiognomy appear. Charles Bell (1806), Alexander Morison (1824), Thomas Burgess (1828) and Charles Darwin (1872) are all concerned with the physical expression of inner states. Even general texts on medicine contain sections on expression. Charles Bell writes, 'Expression is to passion what language is to thought' (1844: 52). The key to this grammar must therefore be sought. Paradoxically this interest in expression leads to the acceptance of a mechanistic view of facial expression and to stereotypes of physiognomy. Following the Cartesian approach, different blobs of emotion are thought to impress the face in different ways and thus result in different expressions. Johann Caspar Lavater's *Essays on Physiognomy* (1778) became a best-seller of the period. It was a standard possession of every self-respecting family who would not dream of hiring a cook or governess, let alone consider a prospective son-in-law, without consulting Lavater. This vogue for reading faces was beautifully satirized a few years later by George Lichtenberg (1783). The article, published in a German medical journal, supposedly sets out to be a study in physiognomic perception. It aims to increase students' awareness of physiognomy by an examination of pigtails. Firstly, it describes them, then it sets questions for further exercise.

Within this context it is not surprising that stereotypes of the physiognomy of insanity emerge. One of the most interesting aspects of the study of expression is the interest in blushing. In Thomas Burgess's *The Physiology or Mechanism of Blushing* (1828), the blush is seen as the distinguishing mark of the human and the supreme sign of man's spirituality. Burgess argues that unlike the other expressions of emotion, blushing cannot be caused by any physical means. The mind must be affected. In fact, Burgess believed that blushing was created by God 'in order that the soul might have sovereign power of displaying in the cheeks the various internal emotions of the moral feelings; so as to serve as a sign to others, that we were violating rules which ought to be held sacred' (Darwin 1872:

337–8). Others, like Charles Bell, saw the blush as the crowning touch to beauty. 'It adds perfection to the features of beauty' (Bell 1844: 95). Darwin saw the blush essentially as the product of self-awareness, and wrote: 'It is not the simple act of reflecting on our own appearance, but the thinking what others think of us which excites a blush' (Darwin 1872: 327). He cited Coleridge, who said that it is sufficient to stare hard at some persons to make them blush.

However, the theory that is most relevant to this paper is that of Burgess. He distinguishes between the true and the false blush. The false blush is due to a morbid sensibility or over sensitivity, whereas the true blush emanates from the conscience. He writes:

> After the impression is made on the sensorium which is to excite this phenomenon, we become immediately conscious of what is about to take place, we feel that the will is over powered – and, for the time being is rendered subordinate to the mental powers, and the emotions of sympathy. Now, from a feeling of our own helplessness, like a bad swimmer when out of his depth, we become flurried, and in our eager attempts to avert the threatened result, by endeavouring to expel from the mind or imagination that association of ideas which is about to bring it forth, we only fix it the more firmly, and ensure its full development, to the deep mortification and prostration of our will (Burgess 1828: 134).

This connexion between blushing, conscience and the prostration of will is particularly interesting in relation to contemporary theories of insanity which attached great importance to moral force and the power of the will to fight insanity. We would, therefore, expect the blush to figure also, and indeed the peculiarity of the idiot was said to be his inability to blush. The long-standing debate about whether negroes blush is to be seen against this background. The controversy is not so much a physiological one as one about moral development. The inability to blush was said to provide the outward feature of inner failing; but excessive blushing, on the other hand, provided evidence of inner moral derangement and very often betrayed the chronic masturbator.

This emphasized another, related area of physical activity that acquired importance during this period: masturbation. Again, this interest relates very much to the view of humanity current at the time.

Nineteenth-century medicine gained two diagnostic categories. They are spermatorrhoea and masturbational insanity. Both convey anxiety about loss of semen. The history of interest in this area is worth considering and requires some explanation. Why did masturbation come to be thought of as an activity of general importance, let alone of medical importance? And why did this happen in the mid-nineteenth century?

Literature contains few references to masturbation. John Aubrey (1950) is unusual in describing the young Duke of Buckingham's solitary pursuits. Otherwise one has to wait until the twentieth century before it becomes an acceptable literary theme. 'Scientific' interest in the subject can be given a precise date of origin. In 1710, an anonymous clergyman published a treatise on masturbation entitled *Onania, or the Heinous Sin of Self-Pollution*. Very many editions appeared in the course of the century. *Onania* is written with elegance and style. This terseness of style seems typical of eighteenth century writing and was lost by later nineteenth-century physicians. The flavour of the book may be caught by quoting the opening sentence: 'Self-pollution is that unnatural practice by which persons of either sex may defile their own bodies without the assistance of others, whilst yielding to filthy imaginations they endeavour to imitate and procure to themselves, that sensation which God has ordained to attend the carnal commerce of the two sexes, for the continuance of our species' (Anonymous 1710: 1). The first edition is just under one hundred pages long. Later editions are slightly longer and include a correspondence between the author and a critic of the book. The debate concerns the relative sinfulness of fornication and masturbation. The critic argues that self-pollution is the lesser of two evils since it avoids the debauchment of innocent women.

Onania was in many ways ahead of its time in that it appears neither to have reflected current concerns and anxieties nor to have influenced them. An easier, more relaxed attitude to sexual activity was the prevailing norm. In England, such ideas acquired their greatest popularity in the mid-nineteenth century. During the 1840s and 1850s there was a spate of books dealing with loss of semen. The works of Ellis (1838), Dawson (1840), Lallemand in English translation (1847), Milton (1854), Curling (1856) and Acton (1865), all dealt with this subject and appeared within a few years of each other.

Masturbation, or 'the primal addiction' as Freud was later to call it, is one focus of anxiety (1985: 287). Another more general and basic area of concern is seminal loss, which may, but need not, be caused by mastur-bation. A generally accepted, if not clear, definition of spermatorrhoea is given by Curling in his book *A Practical Treatise on the Diseases of the Testis*. He writes: 'The emissions may, however be more frequent than is consistent with health, and too readily excited, so much so, indeed, as to affect virility, and to give rise to constitutional symptoms of a serious character. These excessive spermatic discharges constitute the complaint termed spermatorrhoea' (Curling 1856: 386). This loss may be voluntary, as in intercourse and masturbation, or involuntary, as in 'nocturnal pollu-tions' or other emissions, for example, whilst at stool. Typically the picture presented is that of a dribbling penis. Throughout the 1840s and 1850s, physicians showed increasing concern that insufficient attention was paid to the dangers of seminal loss. For example, Milton writes:

> It has always appeared strange to me that this affection should remain abandoned by the profession to a few solitary specialists, and for the benefit of the vile harpies who prey on this class of victims. Surgery, which has wrested so

much from empiricism and ignorance, seems disposed to yield up this, as if it were, debateable land, to chance, philosophy, utter neglect or quackery (Milton 1854: 243).

Lallemand, the French specialist on spermatorrhoea, describes it as: 'A disease that degrades man, poisons the happiness of his best days, and ravages society' (Lallemand 1847: ii).

In part, these fears reflect uneasiness about sexuality as such, but a general coyness about sexuality does not explain the particular interest in seminal loss. Seminal loss in intercourse is set apart as being rather less harmful (cf. Spitzka 1887), but it is precisely the loss of semen involved in sexual intercourse, rather than the activity itself, which is considered pernicious. For this reason male masturbation is singled out for consideration. Spitzka writes: 'The effects of such indulgence are less serious in the female owing to the less exhausting nature of the discharges.'

In fact, beliefs about seminal loss constitute a distinct syndrome. Most writers on the subjects are agreed on the causes of spermatorrhoea. These include constipation, worms, piles, gonorrhoea, heat, heavy bedclothes, highly seasoned food, alcohol, intense application of the mind, and excessive indulgence in sexual intercourse, usually of a promiscuous kind. The effects of spermatorrhoea are similar to those of masturbation. In general these are debilitating. In particular, there is an intimate connection between seminal loss and the condition of the brain. There is an inability to sustain mental and bodily fatigue; a heaviness in the head; giddiness; sleeplessness. Interestingly, the appetite increases, often becoming voracious. Dawson writes: 'I have generally found unnatural seminal discharge accompanied with increased appetite, owing to the necessity which the system feels, of compensating the daily losses which it sustains' (Dawson 1840: 6). Long term effects, like those of masturbation, are more serious. Parched skin, loss of hair, stammering, deafness and blindness form part of the familiar list.

Masturbation forms a sub-category of the interest in loss of semen. The picture of the typical masturbator is one of extreme selfishness. Spitzka described a patient representing this category as follows:

> His demeanour was obtrusive, mean and selfish. He sat out all my other patients on the morning he called, withdrew to the waiting-room, under indignant protests, when I represented to him that I could not keep a physician accompanying patients, who had come a great distance, waiting any longer, he having already consumed two hours. He came in repeatedly, and finally, after I had finished, he took possession of the field, and as I hurried off to my much delayed lunch, he exclaimed, 'Hurry up, doctor, do not be long; I have a great deal to tell you yet. My case is of more importance than any other you ever had; I am the most important man in my family (Spitzka 1887: 239).

Maudsley describes the consequences of masturbation begun early in life as follows: 'we have degenerate beings produced who as regards moral character are very much what eunuchs are represented to be – cunning, deceitful, liars, selfish, in fact, morally insane; while their physical and intellectual vigour is further damaged by the exhausting vice' (Maudsley 1868: 156).

Another characteristic of the chronic masturbator is his shyness, timidity and, in particular, his inability to look others in the eye. David Skae, the Scottish physician who first identified a particular brand of insanity which he termed masturbatory, also singles out similar features of the masturbator:

> that vice produces a group of symptoms which are quite characteristic, and easily recognized, and give to the cases a special natural history. The peculiar imbecility and shy habits of the very youthful victim, the suspicion and fear, and dread, and suicidal impulses, the palpitations and scared look, and feeble body of the older offenders, passing gradually into dementia or fatuity, with other characteristic features familiar to all of you, which I do not stop to enlarge on, all combine to stamp this as a natural order or family (Skae 1863: 315).

The sad, psychological portrait of the masturbator is reinforced by the physical appearance of sallow complexion and dark ringed eyes. However, masturbation is not only one among the ingredients of a character type: it is also the cause of further disabilities. General weakness is a most common result, followed by headache, backache, acne, indigestion, blindness, deafness, epilepsy, and finally death. In fact, the syndrome produced is very similar to that of spermatorrhoea. Finally, an inability to participate in social life develops.

Although interest in masturbation persists into the latter part of the nineteenth century, there is a reinterpretation of its nature. Maudsley (1868) regards the activity with the abhorrence due to a form of moral degeneracy. It is worth quoting one of his cases at length.

> As an example of the high-pitched and absurd sentiments professed sometimes by these degraded beings, I may mention the case of a gentleman who had a plan for curing the social evil. He set forth with great feeling and energy the miserable and wicked thing which it was that many of the most beautiful women should be degraded to gratify the worst lusts of men; and professed himself to be grievously distressed by the sin and evil which were caused thereby. How were so much vice and misery to be done away with? His plan, which he practised himself and proposed that others should follow was to masturbate every morning into a tumbler of water and to drink it. He argued that the lust was thus satisfied without injury to any other person, while the man himself was strengthened by the nourishment afforded to his brain. Here, then, as in other cases, was a mind enervated by vicious practices, dwelling continually on sexual subjects, and concocting, not designedly, but with unconscious hypocrisy, an excuse for the vice which wrecked his life. It is a curious thing that to such a state of moral degradation have patients of this class come, that they will actually defend their vice on some pretence or other (Maudsley 1868: 160).

When Maudsley comes to reconsider the subject in *Pathology of Mind* (1879) he sees masturbation as a product of bad inheritance over which the individual has little control. In line with this reappraisal is the increasing insistence on preventive surgical measures in contrast to the earlier moral exhortations.

At first sight, the mid-nineteenth-century interest in spermatorrhoea and masturbation seems incompatible with the concurrent commitment to moral management. The 1840s and 1850s are also the period during which the major works of the moral managers appear. The moral managers urged the abandonment of physical restraint which had been central to eighteenth-century therapeutic practice. Instead they advocated psychological techniques. Appeal to the conscience and will of the patient was suggested. In this way, it was thought, the power of self-control could be nurtured and the art of self-government furthered. However, both areas of interest presuppose self-control and thus complement each other. Both must be seen as an expression of concern with continence in its widest sense. The disapproval of venery is but another aspect of the pursuit of moderation and discipline. Masturbation, one of the most solitary of activities, is regarded as the arch-vice precisely because of the hopes vested in the private endeavours of the individual. In typifying loss of control it is seen as the moral failure *par excellence*.

These ideas cannot be explained, as Szasz (1971) tries to do, as an attempt by the medical profession to control human sexuality (1971). Neither can 'the masturbatory hypothesis' be seen as a fallacy of reasoning, as Hare (1962) would like it, which is dispelled by the increasing clarity and coherence of medical thought (1962). Nor can it be explained as the product of the emotional immaturity and prurience of physicians as Alex Comfort claims (1968). One of the most illuminating works against which to set the masturbatory hypothesis is that of J.A. Banks, *Prosperity and Parenthood* (1954). As the title suggests, Banks examines the relationship between the postponement of marriage and expectations as to what constitutes an appropriate middle-class life style. According to Banks such ideas appear from the 1830s onwards. 'A "proper" time to marry! – more and more as the century wore on this became the theme of the middle classes, until the words "prudence" and "postponement" became the two most hackneyed in their vocabulary'(ibid.: 36). The situation is even more graphically described in an editorial taken from *The Times*:

> The laws which society imposes in the present day in respect of marriage upon young men belonging to the middle class are, in the highest degree, unnatural, and are the real cause of our social corruptions. The father of a family has, in many instances, risen from a comparatively humble origin to a position of easy competence. His wife has her carriage; he associates with men of wealth greater than his own. His sons reach the age when in the natural course of things they ought to marry and establish a home for themselves. It would seem no great

hardship that a young couple should begin on the same level as their parents began, and be content for the first few years with the bare necessaries of life, and there are thousands who, were it not for society, would gladly marry on such terms. But here the tyrant world interposes; the son must not marry until he can maintain on much the same footing as his father's (*The Times*, 7 May, 1857).

Late marriages may, in part, be responsible for the growth of anxiety about masturbation. However, beliefs about masturbation and the masturbator must also be set against the wider context of values and beliefs about the nature of man. Although, or perhaps because, beliefs about will-power deal with such an elusive and intangible area of human nature, they give rise to certain crude bodily stereotypes. The blush provides the outward evidence of a finely tuned moral sensibility. Similarly, the chronic masturbator embodies the antithesis of all the valued characteristics of the period. He is the polar opposite of nature's gentleman: the person who can get by on the strength of inner resourcefulness and outer accomplishments. He provides the prototype of uncontrolled and undisciplined behaviour. The full meaning of these ideas only emerges from a more general view of Victorian ideas about men and their place in society.

4

THE SYMBOLIC SIGNIFICANCE OF MENSTRUATION AND THE MENOPAUSE

This chapter is based on a medical anthropological study I conducted in 1970 in South Wales. I chose menstruation and the menopause as subjects of research for several reasons. Firstly, I noted that more than any other period of time in a woman's life, the menopause had gained popular attention as a topic of concern, apprehension and speculation. Furthermore, it has been selected by popular terminology as a period of transition *par excellence.* The corresponding processes of biological change at puberty, for example, have no such popular designation, nor do they command the same degree of attention. I, therefore, realized that there was a need to isolate and examine certain concepts relating to structural features of the female life cycle. An altogether different approach, and one not involving a consideration of the menopause within the female life-history, is one which would compare the differential emphasis put upon male and female sexual histories. Even though it may be admitted that the male reproductive system has no by-products as spectacular as those of menstruation, there is still, to the best of my knowledge, no comparable collection of beliefs and theories surrounding the male sexual life cycle. Yet perhaps a case exists for a comparative study of theories about changes in male and female sexual activities. More specifically, a comparative study of attitudes to 'losses' is called for which would relate such ideas to salient features of the male and female life cycle.

Such considerations as these led to the formulation of the main theme of this chapter. Namely, that at menstruation women are using a biological given, that is the loss of menstrual blood, in order not only to express their femininity, but also to reaffirm their acceptance of the female social role. The movement here is away from the biological to the social. This reaffirmation is expressed through attitudes towards and beliefs about menstruation. Furthermore, this analysis of a particular set of ideas about menstruation in terms of the reaffirmation of a particular kind of social role for women leads very easily to a consideration of the menopause or 'change' as a *rite de passage*, a passage from one kind of role to another. I shall return to a discussion of this topic later, after first considering the significance of menstrual loss *per se*.

This introduction should show that my analysis makes claims different from the one made by Mary Douglas (unpublished article). She writes:

> People's ideas about menstruation are part and parcel of their general ideas about how the relations between the sexes should be governed. If they take a very relaxed attitude to premarital sex and to family size they are not likely to think of menstruation as dangerous. The private instruction of European mothers might come somewhere near the scale one might draw of tribal reactions which vary from joyful congratulation, through solemn teaching to intense preoccupation with danger.

I would agree with the statement that ideas about menstruation reflect ideas about how relations between the sexes should be conducted, or the norms governing inter-sexual behaviour, but would go on to qualify this statement differently. I have not found much evidence which would tend to support a relationship between the degree of danger attributed to menstruation and attitudes towards family size or towards premarital intercourse. The connection which I shall try to establish, however, will be one between the dangers of menstruation on the one hand and, on the other, the reaffirmation of one's social roles as sexual partner, mother and housewife.

This connection between the polluting qualities of menstrual blood, the subsequent need for purging and the fulfilment of the duties regarded as traditional for married women, was suggested not only by the results of research directed specifically towards the topic of menstruation and the menopause, but also by previous research on spiritualism which I had been carrying out in Swansea. In the first place it was noted that membership of Spiritualist meetings was largely female. Secondly, that most of the women were at least middle-aged. Furthermore, a high proportion of the messages received from Spirit could be most obviously interpreted as referring to menopausal troubles, especially to the feelings of uncertainty and lack of direction which are described as frequent accompaniments of the physical symptoms of the 'change'. Moreover, it was painstakingly explained to me by Spiritualists that what they termed the menopause, or at least menopausal symptoms, could occur at any time in a woman's life from the age of twenty-three onwards; and that it is not necessarily associated with an impaired capacity for childbearing, nor with the disappearance of this capacity nor with the cessation of menstrual bleeding. Such assertions made me realize that my own conception of the menopause had hitherto been a far too literal one, at least by the standards of Spiritualist women, if by no others. It became apparent that the concept of the 'menopause' was a cultural rather than a biological one and that the concept was being used to express a cultural or social rather than a biological truth. This judgement was confirmed by subsequent research. However, in keeping with the general orientations of the research, which viewed Spiritualism as an expression of dissatisfaction with the female sexual role and a substitute for it, the presentation of menstrual symptoms such as backache, flooding and tiredness were treated as revealing 'a deep-seated rejection of woman's basic roles' (Deutsch, 1944: 304). In fact, it was found that subsequent evidence did not support this theory. It was found that many Spiritualist women had problematical relationships with men and it was, therefore, originally thought that Spiritualism was a further retreat from men. Now, however, I would regard Spiritualism, for those women I studied at least, as an attempt to understand and accommodate oneself to an at times uncomfortable role.

Another topic which figured very largely in my thinking about menstruation and the menopause was that of hysterectomies. I was told by a general practitioner in south Wales that there exists a large body of medical literature which claims that in a substantial percentage of cases the hysterectomy was not justified on strictly medical grounds but was performed at the woman's insistence, whose reasons were psycho-social rather than medical. This suggestion gains plausibility if it is borne in mind that, in the case of hysterectomies, assessment of the need for operation relies more heavily upon the verbal presentation of symptoms which could counterweigh medical examination. Estimates of the percentage of unnecessary hysterectomies, that is cases recording no pathological condition, have varied from 30.8 per cent (Miller 1946) to 12.5 per cent (Doyle 1952). Since 1844, when the first hysterectomy was performed, enthusiasm for the operation has increased continuously. Miller says: 'Indeed, extirpation purely as a measure of preventive medicine is by no means unheard of'. Doctors are frequently confronted with such bald statements as: 'I want to have it all out', or 'I want to get rid of the lot' (personal communication from the general practitioner). Such choice of expressions would indicate the wish to put a definitive end to one's sexual life and even one's female identity, rather than the simple rejection of one particular organ. The extreme attitudes of the unnecessarily hysterectomized will, therefore, provide a theoretical model around which the residual category of women who attach no special value to menstruation can be grouped.

The Fieldwork Setting

Research was carried out in a mining village in south Wales with the very generous co-operation of a local general practitioner. The village in question established its character as a mining community in the 1870s at the same time as the mining communities of the Rhondda were set up. Its population of 1,700 is contained in uniformly-neat terraced houses. At the centre of the village, occupying the same patch of fenced-in land as does the athletic club, lies the health centre.

Fieldwork began in January 1970. Working from an already-compiled age/sex register, the names of all the women born between 1919 and 1921 were extracted. These were judged to be the three years producing the highest proportion of women presenting menopausal symptoms. A total of thirty-one fifty-year-old women were approached. Of these, only eighteen agreed to be interviewed. There was, in other words, a refusal rate of 42 per cent, showing a reluctance to discuss menstruation, which is itself in need of explanation.

Interviews were structured, in the sense that they aimed to establish the salient features of the life history of each woman, how long she had been married, how many children she had had and so on. They also aimed to establish a brief medical history of the woman, with special emphasis on present and past menstrual and menopausal complaints. The medical cards of each of the women were later examined in order to see how the patient's self-image differed from that of her own doctor.[2] However, the most important part of the interview, that which sought to determine the woman's attitudes to her husband and to 'men' generally, to menstruation and the cessation of menstruation, was conducted less formally. Women were asked, for example, whether they thought men treated women fairly or whether they thought men understood women. The quantity and quality of answers to such questions obviously varied enormously. Interviews lasted between thirty minutes and two hours, depending very much upon individual volubility.

After a few weeks of research it became apparent that one of the most crucial items of information related to attitudes concerning the loss of blood in menstruation and the permanent or temporary cessation of bleeding. It was found that women could be divided into one of two clear-cut categories. The first category contains women wishing to lose as much blood as possible and to menstruate for as long as possible, believing this to contribute to the good of their overall health. The second category contains women fearful of 'losing their life's blood' and wishing to cease menstruating as early as possible, believing menstruation to be damaging to their general health. This latter category expressed itself in quasi-scientific terms, saying that they did not, for example, make a fuss about menstruation, 'I just carry on as usual'. By contrast, the former category regard menstruation as a time at which a woman is particularly vulnerable and exposed to dangers, especially through the possibility of an obstruction of the menstrual flow.

It is, of course, known that menstrual blood is not the only kind of fluid around which such ideas have collected. Spitting, for example, is a custom illustrating a similar belief which stresses cleanliness and the importance of ridding oneself of saliva. However, it is of significance that the fluid be menstrual blood, which is clearly distinguished from inter-menstrual discharges and bleeding from piles. It was found that the mere discharge of a fluid, irrespective of its source, did not produce a feeling of being cleansed and restored to a former state of efficiency and vigour. Having separated out these two distinct categories of women, an attempt was made to discover what other features were unique to each category. The only correlation which could be found was one between the need for purging through menstruation and a relatively undisturbed conjugal relationship. Conversely, the absence of this need and the viewing of periods as a nuisance seemed to be associated with an irregular or disturbed conjugal relationship.

Tolstoy has said that all happy families resemble one another but each unhappy family is unhappy in its own way (1980). It was decided, however, that the criteria for assessing 'happiness' in marriage were so many as to yield a final category which was unmanageable. Instead an attempt was made to isolate obvious cases of conjugal deficiency under the heading 'irregularity of sexual and reproductive lives'. Under this term are included such conditions as permanent or temporary separations from the husband including widowhood, as are such conditions as childlessness, spinsterhood, as well as extremes of marital conflict. This kind of definition enables us to distinguish a norm for satisfactory marriages which entails the absence of certain negative features. In fact, this division between women having a regular and those having an irregular conjugal relationship is very fruitful, for it emphasizes the importance which women not having an irregular sexual or reproductive life attach to the uterus and menstruation. It also highlights the considerable number of gynaecological complaints to which such preoccupations give rise.

These findings, therefore, lead to a conclusion apparently opposed to much of that currently expressed in the medical literature on the subject. Recent literature has pursued a strand of thought which refers pelvic and menstrual complaints to personality difficulties. Estimates of the percentage of emotionally-based pelvic complaints range from 31 per cent (Miller 1946) to as high as 65 per cent (Johnson 1939). Incidentally, these figures are almost identical to the estimates for neurosis in general practice (J.B. Loudon, personal communication). Johnson (1939: 374) has claimed that: 'Bodily processes are the common ways in which unconscious attitudes find expression'. Sixty-five per cent of all pelvic complaints are, he claims, of functional origin, revealing upon examination a healthy uterus and being instead the expression of social or sexual maladaptation.

This examination of the kind of role to which menstrual and gynaecological complaints are assigned in medical literature requires a restatement of the main theme of this article, namely, that gynaecological symptoms, rather than being the expression of social or sexual maladaptation are, on the contrary, the expression of social conformity and sexual adaptation. However, we must, of course, allow for the fact that some, if not many, gynaecological symptoms are related to physical conditions such as, for example, fibroids.

The significance attached to menstruation finds expression in a system of related beliefs concerning menstrual bleeding, including the notion of menstrual blood itself, considered as a separate category. The most easily recognizable theme in these beliefs is that focusing on 'bad blood' and the process of menstruation whereby the system is purged of 'badness' and 'excess'. This 'badness' and 'excess' is subjectively experienced as acting as a kind of cog in the wheel, slowing down one's activity, making women feel huge, bloated and poisoned. Surrounding these ideas of female 'badness' and the consequent need for purging are a number of prohibitions to ensure that the body does, in fact, succeed in ridding itself of the 'badness'. Women stated that they would not have a bath for fear the period might 'go away', although they hastened to add that they would, of course, wash. Many would not wash their hair for fear they might go 'funny'. One woman was more explicit, saying that she had once tried to wash her hair whilst menstruating, but had afterwards 'fancied I was not losing as much'. The emphasis here is on losing as much menstrual blood as possible because this is thought to be 'natural' and is a means whereby 'the system rights itself'. The symbolic content of these beliefs appears to be so high as to warrant their description as 'magical'.

In replies to questions about the significance of menstruation, certain key words emerged. These are 'to lose', 'to see' and 'natural'. The analysis of these words which follows is, I am aware, a bit of a linguistic struggle but I attempt it nevertheless. First, the term 'to lose'. When women refer to the process of menstruating, they most frequently do so by the intransitive use of the verb 'to lose". Thus, for example, 'I think it is good to lose'. Alternatively, women say 'I think it is good to see them'. Finally, one of the ways in which all such statements are sanctioned is by reference to their being 'natural'. I do not think it is stretching meanings beyond their natural sphere of reference to say that these words, by their very lack of precision and by their ambiguity, are particularly well-suited to convey certain features of the female social situation. The verb 'to lose', for example, can be used transitively, as in 'to lose blood', and, intransitively, in the sense of losing a game. I would maintain that it is this double sense which contributes to the recurrent appearance of the word. Thus in referring directly to the importance of losing large quantities of menstrual blood, they are referring indirectly to the importance of coming to terms with their role as 'losers' in a much wider sense. This sense of loss is expressed most acutely when talking about 'men' generally as a distinct category from women. 'Men' are thought to lack understanding about and consideration for women, especially as regards the constraints which childbearing and housekeeping impose upon a woman. As a category they are thought to be selfish and lacking in responsibility and sensitivity towards their female partners. A similar type of analysis can be given for the word 'see'. For one cannot only be said to 'see' one's periods, but one can also be said to 'see', in the sense of understanding a situation. Finally, the necessity of 'losing' or 'seeing' one's periods is justified on the grounds that 'it's natural' or, alternatively, 'it's got to be'. The felt element of constraint inherent in an external, non-subjective reality would lead me to substitute the word 'social' for 'natural', thus completing the chain of inter-dependent meanings.

My interpretation of these recurrent words, in terms of which menstruation is talked about, gains added plausibility from the explanatory clauses which qualify the initial statement about the necessity of losing menstrual blood. For example, women say they feel huge, bloated, slow and sluggish if they do not have a period or if they do not lose much. One woman said she felt, 'really great' after a heavy period, whilst most insist on the value and importance of having a 'good clearance'. In more practical terms the side effects of not having a 'good clearance' express themselves in inactivity, especially in the inability to get on with the housework. One woman in particular, who had already arrived at the menopause, said that she used to find it much easier to do the cleaning whilst she was still menstruating regularly than she did now in her post-menopausal state.

What has just been said requires an amendment of the previous quotation which claimed that bodily processes were the expression of unconscious emotional attitudes. They may indeed be the expression of such attitudes but, in the case of menstruation, these attitudes will be determined, not by individual conflicts, but by a shared common role which women themselves see as generating a particular type of conflict in women.

Perhaps what has been said about attitudes to the loss of menstrual blood and cessation of such a loss can best be illustrated by giving the case histories of two women. Their names are, of course, fictitious.

Mrs Olwen Jones has lived in the village all her life and was born two doors from the house where she now lives. Her father, now dead, was employed as an undermanager in a pit and her husband, Fred, is a coal merchant. Mrs Jones has just turned fifty, having been married for twenty-five years. She has two children, a son aged twenty-one and a daughter of eighteen. Mrs Jones leaves the impression of being quick-witted and an energetic woman. She takes an obvious delight in saying the unexpected or, to her mind, shocking and then slowly savouring the effect this produces on me, her audience. She considers herself a happily married woman who is devoted to her husband, Fred. Her worries have been of the common variety, centring on money and anxieties over the children's education. Nevertheless, her speech is permeated with an aura of dissatisfaction which is never quite fully identified. She says she is always depressed, more especially since the children have grown up and her husband has taken to going out in the evenings and leaving her at home by herself. She feels 'sorry for herself'. Her experience of life, and hence her view of the world, is such that she sees it bisected by an insurmountable communication barrier. Men can 'never in this world of God' understand women. Men she thinks are like animals, although she would exclude Fred from this characterization. Amplifying on this verdict she said: 'I'm not very fond of my sex life'. She considered it ridiculous at her age. Asked why, she said it was just ridiculous. However, this did not prevent her from acceding to her husband's demands in bed, ridiculous and frustrating though she finds these episodes. Contrasting with this background of ill-defined dissatisfaction about her feminine role, Mrs Jones has very emphatic and definite views about the importance and value of menstruation in her life. She says she would feel very old and 'frustrated' without her periods. Frustrated because she would not be able to get rid of blood, because she would feel unclean. Frustrated also because she would not feel like doing anything about the house and the washing and cleaning would be left undone, almost as though the energy for housework was generated as a by-product of the process of losing menstrual blood. For the same reasons, Mrs Jones would dread any gynae-cological operations in case they disturbed the menstrual flow.

A very different and contrasting life history and attitudes to female physiological processes are presented by Mrs Leah Thomas.

Mrs Thomas was born in the village in the same year and as Mrs. Jones brought up there. In contrast to Mrs Jones, who had only one sister, she comes from a large family of seven children. Her father's occupation was that of blacksmith, whilst her husband has had a succession of occupations, more recently being employed as an ambulance driver and then a bus driver. Mrs Thomas has had a total of five children, four of whom are still living. The youngest girl is still at home, the others all being married. In comparison with Mrs Jones's married life, Mrs Thomas's conjugal relationship has been highly unstable. Although she is still legally married and has been for over thirty years, her conjugal relationship has been punctuated by the intermittent and regular disappearance of her husband. She has now been separated from her husband for four years. At present he is living with another woman on the outskirts of a northern city. This woman he met some twenty years ago whilst he was working as an ambulance driver. Their liaison started then and has been pursued ever since. Mrs Thomas, however, claims she was totally ignorant of the fact that Frank had 'another woman'. She claims that she considered herself a happily married woman during the years of her marriage, despite the fact that her husband was very little at home. She describes him, somewhat euphemistically, as being 'not a very domestic sort of man'. From her reminiscences and descriptions of her husband it emerges that she regards herself as still very much in love with him. His sexual prowess and his powerful and melodious voice are still very much sources of admiration and wonder to her. After he had left her to 'live tally' with his friend, Mrs Thomas had made it clear to him that she was willing to forgive him and have him back. Frank, however, had said that he did not deserve such gentle treatment. He had, he said, 'made his bed and must lie in it'.

However, not only is there a difference in the patterns of married life between Mrs Jones and Mrs Thomas, there is also a striking difference in attitudes about menstruation. Mrs Thomas possesses no theories whatsoever about the value of menstruation or the need to lose menstrual blood. She says she cannot wait to stop menstruating because she is losing such a lot. She said, 'I'm sure I'm no better in health by seeing them'. Menstruation to Mrs Thomas is an unmitigated source of annoyance and discomfort. Prior to and during menstruation, Mrs Thomas feels extremely weak, suffers from sick headaches, dizziness and vaginal irritation. A hysterectomy would not worry her in the least, in fact, she thinks it would provide a welcome relief.

Contrasting with this lack of emphasis on menstruation, merely wishing for its absence, Mrs Thomas expresses marked concern about and attaches great significance to other bodily ailments. Her complaints are numerous and of such a nature that they lend themselves to lengthy, detailed descriptions. According to her own account, and her doctor, she suffers from high blood pressure, headaches, dizzy spells, palpitations, backache, indigestion, nervous rashes, sleeplessness and, lastly, depression. In comparison the list of Olwen Jones's ailments is very meagre. Her ailments centre on headaches which she attributes to high blood pressure and depression.

These two case histories, although obviously each unique, illustrate one of the main themes of this article. Namely, that it is the women with relatively undisturbed, though by no means necessarily problem-free, married lives who emphasize the loss of large quantities of menstrual blood, who are more sensitive to bodily changes or menstruation and who regard such processes as essential to producing and maintaining a healthy equilibrium. Relationships with other features of a woman's social situation, for example, family size, religion and education, were found to be incidental. In other words, no constant relationship could be established within a larger number of women.

Before concluding this preliminary discussion of menstruation, it may be useful to contrast my approach with that of the psychoanalysts. Freud, not surprisingly in view of his male-centred approach, has very little to say on the subject. In his essay on female sexuality (1931), the subject is significant by its complete absence. In *Civilization and its Discontents* (1930), Freud refers to menstruation in a footnote. In the context of a discussion about the foundations of the monogamous family which results from the transformation of the need for genital satisfaction from the status of 'an intermittent and sudden guest' to that of a 'permanent lodger', Freud draws attention to the changed importance of menstruation. He says: 'the taboo on menstruation is derived from an "organic repression", as a defence against a phase of development that has been surmounted' (ibid.: 36). By the term 'organic repression' Freud is referring to 'the diminution of the olfactory stimuli' as a significant element in sexual attraction. In other words, Freud is saying that woman is at her most attractive during menstruation and that for some unknown reason the natural process of this attraction has been stemmed, with the result that rigid barriers have been erected against the possibility of experiencing consciously this original attraction. Hence, there is a prevalence of taboos surrounding menstruating women. Freud's final comment on the significance of menstruation is perhaps most telling. At the menopause, the absence of menstruation is re-experienced by woman as the psychological loss she once felt in early childhood, when she compared her body to a boy's for the first time and concluded that she had been castrated.

Other psychoanalytic writers, among them Horney (1967) in her chapter on premenstrual tension, links menstrual disorders with ambivalent or contradictory attitudes towards motherhood. (For example, where the fear of childbirth or the fear of coitus is coupled with a simultaneous, strong desire for children.)

However, the interpretation which is sociologically of the greatest value is that offered by Deutsch (1965). Deutsch singles out menstruation as being the most interesting gynaecological occurrence, 'and this *par excellence* "biological event" is to a high degree influenced by psychological factors' (ibid.: 311). One of the chief aspects of menstruation Deutsch concerns herself with is dysmenorrhea, this being the term used to refer to cases of excessively painful menstruation. Of this she states: 'Women suffering from dysmenorrhea assume a priori the attitude toward menstruation that all occurrences in the female genital region are an orgy of painful suffering. The physical discomfort of menstruation mobilizes and substantiates this feeling. Often a feeling of death accompanies the pain' (ibid.: 311). A concomitant of dysmenorrhea is the belief in the 'poison theory of menstruation'. According to Deutsch this is generally held to consist in the belief that: 'The sexual processes produce poison which is eliminated from the woman's body through menstruation' (ibid.: 312). The psychoanalytic interpretation of these ideas and symptoms is one which links the poison theory with antecedent guilt feelings surrounding sexuality and a resultant personal need for purification of the body and thus the expiation of sins. In other words, the claimed pain of menstruation serves as a punishment and an outlet for guilty feelings. She concludes: 'Here can be seen the apparent paradox: that women who suffer from dysmenorrhea are hypersensitive to pain, but at the same time, have strongly masochistic tendencies' (ibid.: 312). Briefly, Deutsch considers all such struggles for purification as an expression of guilt feelings and as attempts to escape the feminine destiny, that is, as an incomplete adaptation to the female identity.

Whilst allowing that, of the psychoanalytic interpretations of menstruation so far considered, Deutsch's comes nearest to grasping its symbolic weight, I should nevertheless like to suggest a rearrangement of the elements in her explanation. It may be true that there exists a category of women who regard all occurrences in the female genital region as a 'painful orgy', but my sample did not in any way corroborate the connection of this attitude with guilt feelings. Neither did the occurrence of painful menstrual symptoms entail the experience of more directly and obviously sexual experience as painful. Indeed it seems more likely that emphasis on pain at menstruation is among other things a way of safe-guarding the smooth functioning of sexual activity at other times. One is reminded of Harris's (1959) article on possession hysteria among the Taita. It is as though the symbolic destruction of one's inferior status (the insistence on 'a good clearance') left one better prepared to accept the vicissitudes and constraints of being a married woman.

Menopausal Beliefs

Having considered the part menstruation plays in the symbolic or emotional world of women, it becomes necessary to ask what happens to this when menstruation ceases.

Bearing in mind the importance which menstruation had as a means of conveying a feminine social role, this second part of this chapter will go on to consider whether the climacteric, in terms of the standardized modes of experiencing it and in terms of the conglomeration of beliefs associated with it, can be better understood when viewed as a *rite de passage*. However, this approach will be exercised with caution. The climacteric may not conform completely to the pattern of a *rite de passage* in the sense of, for example, puberty rituals among what were earlier described as 'primitive peoples', but it may nevertheless share sufficient of the features of transition rituals to make an examination of their basic elements worthwhile.

First, however, a description of the surface features of the 'change' which immediately bring to mind a *rite de passage*. For a start there is the expectation of unknown dangers to be endured, with the emphasis on the uncertainty as to what these dangers actually consist of. Furthermore, these dangers are given a value in themselves. Many women expressed the belief that it was good to experience 'hot flushes' as frequently as possible, otherwise there was a chance of dangerous complications developing. Hence, the saying current at the time of my research: 'A flush is worth a guinea a box'. I was told that to anyone who was literate before the Second World War, the association with an advertisement for Beechams laxative pills would be immediate. Flushes were thought to 'carry you through the change more quickly and safely'. Again the reference here is to a 'passage' through which one is carried. Some women who were 'on the change' even voiced a regret that they did not flush enough. Asked whether they suffered from hot flushes, they admitted their failure by saying': 'No I'm not very good'. Hot flushes were thought to be the result of menstrual blood rushing to the head so that an absence of flushes implies a deficiency of menstrual blood. Prohibitions surrounding the climacteric incorporate a mixture of medical and magical information. Women were advised not to touch red meat for fear it should 'go off'. They should not attempt to make bread because the dough would not rise. They should not touch salt. Finally, women envisaged 'the change' as a period of time when certain ill-defined anatomical or structural changes are taking place within their bodies. This was the reason most often cited to me in answer to the question as to why 'the change' was called the 'change'. One seventy-year-old lady told me that at the menopause women turned into men inside. She herself had, she said, been aware of this process taking place, and had experienced it as a 'turning and tightening' of the thigh muscles.

The description of menopause attitudes and beliefs will, I hope, justify the analysis of the structure and function of transition rituals which follows. However, it was realized that women who have attached little importance to menstruation, having already had disturbed sexual lives, are unlikely to feel that they are moving from one role to another. They have already mentally forsaken their sexual role. Thus of the eighteen fifty-year-old women interviewed, it was the eight women whose sexual lives were described as irregular who adopted a quasi-scientific attitude both to menstruation and to the menopause. These women experienced fewer menopausal symptoms, as well as feeling that the cessation of menstrual bleeding would not be disturbing to their mental or physical equilibrium.

Van Gennep (1909) in his study of rites of passage elaborates one basic theme: namely, that all rites exhibit the same underlying pattern and that this pattern serves a primary function wherever it is found. The bare bones of his argument can be summarized as follows: change exercises a disturbing influence both upon the individual and upon the society; the solution provided by society to deal with these disruptive effects is to ritualize the processes of change, thus minimizing the danger inherent in all transitions. 'An individual is placed in various sections of society synchronically and in succession; in order to pass from one category to another and to join individuals in other sections, he must submit from the day of his birth to that of his death, to ceremonies whose forms often vary but whose function is similar' (van Gennep 1909: 189).

The pattern which van Gennep claims to perceive underlying all ritual activity is divided into three major phases: rites of separation from the original environment, rites of transition, and rites of incorporation into the new environment. This does not, however, mean that each phase is equally accentuated in all rites, as van Gennep himself stresses. (In fact, it is one of the factors which lends stress to the menopausal situation that rites of incorporation or ritualized ideas expressing incorporation into a new group are remarkably lacking from a time when attitudes and beliefs are otherwise highly ritualized.)

Gluckman criticizes van Gennep for lacking 'a clearly formulated theory of society' (1962: 14) and himself wishes to make rites of passage a class of the more general category of rituals effecting role specialization. However, it is difficult to see how, for example, rites of pregnancy and childbirth could in the first instance be said to differentiate roles, which are not already secularly defined. The analysis might apply to the case of a man changing his activities, but it hardly seems necessary to use mystical means to identify a pregnant woman, or for that matter a pre-menopausal or a post-menopausal woman.

Gluckman's criticism is centred around the notion of a 'role'. Had van Gennep realized the importance of this concept for his analysis, he would have been in a far better position to work out the implications of his theory. However, this does not mean that the analysis of ritual has to take an entirely new direction and concern itself with ritual as role differentiation. The notion of a role can be introduced in such a way that van Gennep's thesis is merely expanded and not rendered otiose.

Parsons defines role in the following way so that it becomes the Archimedean point for the whole theory of society: 'it is a distinctive feature of the structure of social action, however, that in most relationships the actor does not participate as a total entity but only by virtue of a given differentiated "sector" of his total personality. Such a sector which is the unit of a system of social relationships has come predominantly to be called a "role"'. A page later he says: 'Role is the concept which links the sub-system of the actor as a "psychological" behaving entity to the distinctively social structure' (ibid.: 35). The notion of a role, therefore, being distinct from the individual, is defined by reference to a norm which is built into the very concept and by means of which it is identified. The rites of passage can thus be seen as not merely marking the transition from one status to another in the passage through society, but as expressing the demands of the new role and the expectations of society on the incumbent of the new role.

Van Gennep's analysis of ritual, therefore, as movement from one status in society to another, or as movement from one group of individuals to another, can be left intact. However, we can supply a fuller answer as to why such rites decrease the danger of change. Change is dangerous precisely because one can recognize that the individual, *qua* individual, and not merely as a member of society, is not exhaustively defined by the sum total of their roles in society, even though in practice it may be difficult to refer to them other than via one of their roles. The point being that the aspect of individual identity which has been neglected by or has eluded role definition increases ambiguity.

If we use van Gennep's analysis of rites of passage together with my amendment we find that it is a peculiarly well-suited theoretical tool with which to approach the climacteric. The very term 'change' is an unambiguous reference to the nature of the climacteric.

The transition in this particular instance is from woman in her reproductive role to woman in her non-reproductive role. In view of the central position which female fertility occupies in the public image of the adult female, the disappearance of this reproductive capacity is bound, at the very least, to present the women with problems. A little girl is taught to expect that she will fall in love, get married and have children, preferably in that order. However, the story tails off rather inconclusively and unsatisfactorily by saying that she will live happily ever after. Again no provision is made for alternatives to this pattern. This theme, of the intrinsic connection between fertility and 'female adulthood' in our society is extensively dealt with by Kirk (1964) in his study of childless marriages and adoption.

It is also very fruitfully explored by Becker (1963). Becker's article deals with menopausal depression. The question he asks is: 'Why does a woman who to all appearances, has led a satisfying life, suddenly break down at the menopause and decide that her life is not worth living?' (1963: 355). The answer he gives is as follows:

> Women become depressed at the menopause because ... they do not have enough reasons for satisfying action, and when they lose the one apparent reason upon which they predicated their lives – their femininity – their whole active world caves in. Let us be brutally direct: Menopausal depression is the consequence of confining woman to a too narrow range of life choices or opportunities. It is a social and cultural phenomenon, for which the "designers" of social roles are to blame (ibid.: 358).

In that quotation, Becker is referring to psychiatrists and psychoanalysts when he uses the term '"designers" of social roles'. 'We create menopausal depression by not seeing to it that women in their forties are armed with more than one justification for their lives' (ibid.: 359). Becker illustrates his analysis of menopausal depression by a re-examination of Freud's case study of a 51-year-old female patient. This woman came to see Freud because she had found that her life was suddenly 'flooded' by an insane jealousy of a young career girl with whom she imagined her husband to be having an affair. Freud's interpretation of the situation was that, through the use of this jealousy language, the woman was trying to conceal her own libidinal urges felt towards her handsome young son-in-law. Becker's view of the situation is very different. From his point of view the significant elements in the situation are, firstly, that 'this woman senses the decline of her only value to men – her physical charm', and, secondly, the difference as between the patient's status as compared with the young girl whom she imagined involved in the affair with her husband. The jealous wife had played the social game according to all the conventional rules, but something had gone wrong. She now found herself alone, without usable skills, no longer with children, without her accustomed beauty. However, the situation is rendered doubly poignant by the fact that the woman is 'without words in which to frame her protest'. The protest against 'helplessness and potential meaninglessness takes the form of jealousy accusations'. This jealousy language is an indirect reference to the woman's exclusion from the man's world. Indirect, of necessity, because the exclusion is so complete as to deprive the woman of the language in which a direct protest could be voiced.

Acknowledgements

I wish to express my gratitude to Dr J.B. Loudon for his help during the research and to the general practitioner who wishes to remain anonymous.

Notes

1. Permission to look at medical cards was obtained both from the doctor and in writing from each woman concerned.

5

WOMEN AND AFFLICTION IN MAHARASTRA: A HYDRAULIC MODEL OF HEALTH AND ILLNESS

Beliefs about the nature of spiritual affliction, its epidemiology and aetiology vary according to gender, family structure and position within the family. One manifestation of affliction is thought to be madness. However, the experience of mental affliction is very varied; for example, the number of family members accompanying an afflicted person, the amount of money made available for treatment, the length of treatment, as well as the less tangible but equally important aspects of treatment such as the degree of empathy and concern felt, all vary according to the afflicted person's gender and status within the family. The inferiority of women's position in society and their precarious belonging in their husband's family comes to the fore in cases of mental illness. The greater shame attaching to women's mental illness means that more women seek temple treatment alone and that the level of family support and involvement is less for women. Recently married women and older childless women fare particularly badly in the division of concern and responsibility for the afflicted. In Maharashtra the recognition and experience of mental affliction varies according to the stage of family development and, most importantly, according to the gender of the patient.

Introduction: Theme, Sources and Methodology

This chapter explores the relationship between mental affliction and family structures in rural Maharashtra.[1] The relationship is reciprocal and many stranded. It is both simple and complex. At a simple level gender, status within the family and family composition influence the experience of mental affliction and determine such things as the quality and amount of care and financial provision made available to the afflicted person. Conversely, mental affliction has implications for family structure, and these implications differ according to the gender of the afflicted person. At a more fundamental level, gender and position within the Maharashtrian family influence the development of a theory of mental affliction which emphasizes female vulnerability to affliction, produce an almost exclusive preponderance of women in certain categories of affliction such as trancing, and result in much inferior forms of care for mentally afflicted women, while at the same time emphasising women's 'natural' qualities as care givers.

Fieldwork was carried out in a Mahanubhav healing temple in western Maharashtra during two separate periods: for six months in 1984 and 1985 and for three months during the summer of 1988. The temple provides shelter and accommodation for those who are spiritually afflicted as well as their families if they choose to accompany them. Families come from the whole of Maharashtra, though the majority are from within a radius of one hundred miles. The accommodation provided is of the most basic kind. The inner portion of the temple is surrounded by a courtyard and this courtyard is flanked by thirty-nine cubicles. The cubicles are roofed and each is individually separated from the next by a pole. Two sides have a beaten earth floor while one length has a stone floor. The temple provides two water taps. Thus the temple literally offers supplicants a roof over their heads. Families come with their belongings consisting chiefly of bed-rolls and cooking utensils. Each dormitory space also contains a clay cooking space so that each family unit can cater for itself.

The temple population consists of all castes apart from Brahmins. However, poverty and illiteracy are typical characteristics of supplicants. The majority do not arrive with an intended length of stay in mind. They come prepared to stay until the affliction has been lifted. In practice the average length of stay can be reckoned in months rather than days or weeks. A handful of supplicants who had been at the temple in 1985 were still living there in the summer of 1988. Thus embarking on a cure is a long-term enterprise. The temple also caters to the needs of large numbers of extra mural visitors: at major festivals thousands of supplicants return in order to safeguard and promote family health. Earlier temple dwellers return for occasional brief visits very much with a prophylactic intent. Thus the temple has a central core of resident supplicants and a peripheral following of part-time attenders.

The existence of two categories of supplicants facilitated my own role as a non-resident participant observer. There was, therefore, a precedent for my pattern of visiting and level of commitment. During both fieldwork trips I lived in a bungalow a mile away from the temple and visited daily. My investigations were greatly furthered by the help of a very able research assistant whose house abutted the temple complex and whose family had had long connections with the Mahanubhavs. My acceptance by the supplicants was, therefore, made easier. My continued presence did, however, create anxieties amongst the priests. My first visit coincided with an interest by the national press in the Mahanubhavs and my enquiries were sometimes perceived as a kind of investigative journalism. Nevertheless, my visits and questioning were in no way curtailed. The slow speed of enquiries related to the low priority which was put upon answering my questions compared to the importance attached to cooking, eating, resting and carrying out various devotional activities. Despite occasional impatience with my importunity and slowness to grasp what was obvious to them, supplicants were by and large remarkably helpful and ready to talk about painful family issues.

All the supplicants in the temple were there because they, or a member of their family, were suffering in some way or other. The purpose of the temple stay was to arrive at a diagnosis of the nature and causes of the suffering as well as to effect a cure. The exact historical antecedents of this healing tradition are difficult to establish. However, the history of the Mahanubhav sect has been recorded by a number of writers (Feldhaus 1983; Raeside 1976; Sontheimer 1989). It was founded in the thirteenth century by Cakradhara in opposition to the ritual authority of the Brahmins. The Mahanubhavs emphasize the possibility of direct communication with God and have traditionally welcomed deprived sectors of society such as untouchables and women. Raeside (1976: 587) mentions that many of the founder's most devoted disciples were women. Sontheimer writes that Cakradhara was 'aware of the religious aspirations of women and sudras.' He emphasizes the fact that Cakradhara was sensitive to the material problems of dependent women. Moreover, Sontheimer mentions that 'a number of destitute women ultimately found their security as followers of Cakradhara' (ibid.: 349). No doubt this association between the Mahanubhav sect and the disadvantaged contributed to its 'peripheral status in Marathi society' (Raeside 1976: 585). Thus there is a long established tradition of accommodating marginal individuals and, whilst the exact history of the association between the Mahanubhavs and the mentally afflicted cannot be established, the compatibility of the two has clearly existed from the beginning.

In contemporary Maharashtrian society the Mahanubhav temples have a reputation for diagnosing, sheltering and ultimately curing the mentally afflicted. While this reputation extends to all Mahanubhav temples, Phaltan is thought to be a particularly appropriate destination for the mentally ill since it is the birthplace of the founder of the sect, Cakradhara. While this fact of religious geography accounts for the spiritual potency of the place, its precise association with mental affliction is unclear. No information could be gleaned regarding the origins of this association beyond the general assertion that the mentally afflicted had been coming to Phaltan for a very long time. Only a tiny minority of the temple dwellers would describe themselves as Mahanubhavs. In most cases personal need and the reputation of the temples for effecting cures combined to attract supplicants to the temples.

During the period of the study the temple provided shelter for a total of 31 afflicted persons and their carers. Thirteen of these were women who were unaccompanied, 8 were women with an accompanying family member and 10 were accompanied men. If we combine the figures with those of an earlier field trip the following picture emerges. In all there were more than 32 families accompanying an afflicted man, 20 families accompanying an afflicted woman, and 21 afflicted women who had no carers. Put another way, we could say that afflicted men had no risk of being unaccompanied whereas women had a fifty-fifty chance of being on their own. Tables 5.1, 5.2 and 5.3 give details of the individual's affliction and family circumstances and show that the social response to illness and affliction varies dramatically for men and women. The total temple population during this time was somewhere in the region of sixty persons. Daily visits to the temple throughout this period allowed the circumstances of the afflicted and of their families as well as their ideas about affliction to be recorded in detail. While the outward circumstances of the individuals varied considerably, the underlying cause was thought to be *karani* ('witchcraft') and/or *bhut bhada* ('spirit possession'), and such explanations lent a unifying theme to the temple's activities.

The explanation of mental illness as supernatural affliction does not appear to lessen either the attribution or the experience of stigma. All the temple dwellers see themselves as the victims of *pida* or 'affliction'. Unlike *karma*, which is one's properly apportioned good and bad fortune or destiny inherited from earlier incarnations, *pida* is perceived as entirely unmerited, unwanted and far in excess of the ordinary troubles of life. It is perceived as a form of unsolicited attention from and victimization by malevolent spiritual forces. *Pida* is recognised more by its cause than its manifestations. *Pida* is the result of *karani* or *bhut bhada* or quite frequently a combination of the two. *Bhut bhada* is thought to be more readily cured, and five weeks is often cited as the required period for a cure. It does not result from human malevolence but comes out of the blue by an unlucky constellation of circumstances. Through an unfortunate coincidence of time and place a person may become possessed by *bhut bhada*. By contrast, *karani* is invariably the result of human malevolence, most frequently coming from other family members. In nearly all cases, the *karani* is done by the husband's brother or brother's wife or the husband's father's brother or his wife. Such quarrels between brothers are recognized to be frequent and inevitable and are thought for the most part to be triggered by the wives, who are not bound by ties of childhood affection and loyalty and are, in any case, thought to be more quarrelsome by virtue of being women. Sometimes the joint family splits up as a result of these quarrels; in other cases the family has already divided into separate households, often adjacent, but disputes over the inheritance of land and property persist. Many temple families felt that they had been wrongly deprived of their share of family wealth and as a result the very survival of the family unit was under threat. Where the family is threatened by mental illness, *karani* explanations link the crisis of mental affliction to the earlier economic crises occasioned by inheritance disputes.

Attendance at the temple plays a central role in unravelling the causal sequence and nature of affliction. Part of that attendance involves submission to trance. The Mahanubhav temples, especially those in Phaltan, have a reputation for inducing trance, and (for a combination of reasons discussed later) trancing occurs more frequently in women than in men. By virtue of the powers they acquire through trance women play an essential part in the understanding and management of family affliction. Temple trancing is instrumental in arriving at true knowledge concerning the family's suffering. The occurrence of trance is in itself an indication of the spiritual nature of the affliction, of *pida*. However, it is also the means whereby further information is gleaned about the sources, desired management and prognosis of the affliction. Thus because of their predisposition to trancing women are able to achieve a position of some power as diagnosticians of the family's trouble.

The power attributed to *karani* points to the importance of family ties and the destruction which ensues when such ties go wrong or break down. In some cases the discovery of *karani* serves to consolidate the family structure as it closes ranks around the mentally afflicted individual. In other cases, the *karani* provides an opportunity for the family to regroup, extruding the afflicted individual, usually a woman. *Karani* is generally recognized as being difficult to cure. It seems that these ideas about the intractability of *karani* reflect the difficulty of finding ways of remedying the breakdown of family relationships. Mental illness is almost invariably attributed to *pida*. By contrast, physical illness is not for the most part thought to be related to family conflict or *karani*. It is simply one's *karma*, the result of one's actions in previous lives. However, the universality of belief in *pida* or *karani* does not appear to lessen the stigma of mental illness. Rather, stigma appears to be related to gender and family structure.

Mental Affliction and the Family: The Differential Impact of Gender on Attitudes and Structural Dynamics of the Family

Because of the different expectations and evaluations of men's and women's behaviour, mental affliction in women is likely to incur a greater amount of shame, discredit and dishonour for the woman herself and her family.

Secondly, the woman's pivotal role in the family is cited as a reason for greater shame. Because the woman is in charge of household affairs, particularly cooking, her affliction is likely to affect the whole family. Thus the three cornerstones of the Maharashtrian stereotype of madness – namely, tearing of one's clothes, violence towards other family members, and lack of attention and irreverence towards the preparation and consumption of food – are all behaviours which are more severely condemned in women than in men. Women are supposed to be modest and gentle and their most important household task is the provision of meals for the family. Mentally afflicted women are not able to fulfil these expectations.

However, it is noteworthy that although this stereotype of mental affliction recurred regularly in all the accounts given of sick family members, the actual behaviour of the mentally afflicted within the temple precincts did not always conform to the stereotype. This may have been due to a discrepancy between my perception of the manifestation of the affliction and the families', or because an improvement in behaviour had occurred after arrival at the temple, or most probably a combination of both reasons. Whatever the cause, the actual behaviour of the afflicted appeared to be at odds with the stereotype. Rather than being violent, afflicted men and women were apathetic and listless in the extreme. The only suggestion of violence came from the presence of iron chains which bound the ankles and sometimes the wrists of the afflicted, but this hardly constituted evidence of violence. Furthermore there was little sign of dishevelled or torn clothing. Only two cases (out of a total of 41 studies in 1984/85 and 31 in 1988) could be found which conformed to this stereotype. Finally regarding attitudes to the preparation and eating of food, these fell into two categories. Most afflicted women did seem to have lost interest in food preparation and cooking. However, afflicted men, rather than disregarding and devaluing mealtimes, demanded to be fed with predictable and discomfiting regularity. Mothers, in particular, complained that while their sons earned no money, they yet expected their meals to be routinely presented. One mother who cleaned the temple in return for a small monthly sum talked particularly bitterly of her son's expectation of three large meals a day. These women's attitudes appear to make use of an implicit equation of the male duty to provide cash for food with the female duty to prepare food.[2]

Thus although behaviour may have occurred in the past to support the stereotype of mental affliction, there was not much of it in evidence at the time of the study. The focus on these particular behavioural markers of madness conforms with the suggestion that in many non-European societies altered behaviour rather than altered subjective experience is characteristic of madness (Lipsedge and Littlewood 1982: 191). The nature of the stereotype points to the importance of family ties in Maharashtra. Like the seventeenth-century men and women described by Macdonald, who 'to

show that a person was insane [they] examined his relations with his family
with an intensity that mirrored the importance of those ties in their own life
(1981: 165), so Maharashtrians cite the destruction wrought by the
mentally afflicted within the family and within the home. Attempts to sever
emotional ties, particularly through the beating of mothers and wives by
afflicted men, are described. Also cited are examples of individuals
absconding and the physical destruction of the home by, for example, the
tearing out of electric wires. However, within this pattern there is room for
individualism. One wife, when questioned about her husband's behaviour
before and after mental illness, confessed that, while he used to beat her
when he was well, he did not beat her in his madness. Thus, here as
elsewhere, there are exceptions to the rule.

The recurrence of disrespect for food or inappropriate eating habits as
evidence of mental illness indicates the central importance which the
preparation and sharing of food occupies in family life. The mentally ill are
described as rejecting food prepared at home, begging food prepared from
other houses and indiscriminately eating dirty things. Often they are
described as having voracious appetites and consuming inordinate quantities of *bhakris* (a round unleavened bread made of millet flour and the
staple food of Maharashtra). In the temple the mentally ill are sometimes
accused of stealing food from others. Thus the afflicted are seen as either
undervaluing family resources or overtaxing them. Their behaviour
threatens the nurturing function of the family and their own role as
recipients of that nurture.

Finally, appropriate clothing is one of the ways in which the family's
standing in the community is judged. By their dishevelled dress the afflicted
endanger this standing. Here too there appears to be a similarity with
Macdonald's description of seventeenth-century England. He writes:
'Nothing signalizes the rank of a person more plainly than dress and Tudor
and Stuart observers paid inordinate attention to the clothes – or lack of
them – of madmen. Nakedness was included among the symptoms of mania
in ancient and medieval times' (ibid.: 129). Contemporary Maharashtrian
and seventeenth-century English mad people are alike in their wanton
destruction of the institutions which succour them. In particular, the
mentally afflicted temple dwellers are seen as trying to undermine, through
their behaviour, the family and its standing in the community.

Different aspects of this stereotype of affliction apply more to one sex
than the other. Mental affliction in women manifests itself as a withdrawal
of support and services to the family and a threat to the honour and privacy
of the family by the woman's shameless behaviour. Mentally afflicted men,
on the other hand, are thought to indulge in behaviour which is more
actively destructive of the family. Maharashtrian family structure has been
described as patrilineal and patrilocal (Orenstein 1965: 37; Karvé 1965:
183). Descent is traced in the male line, and on marriage a girl moves from

her *maher* (parental home) to her *sasar* (in-law's home). Orenstein emphasizes the low status of the incoming bride: 'The position of a recently acquired wife in a joint family was the lowest in the group' (1965: 45). This assignment of low status is already apparent at the outset of marriage negotiations: 'the delicately wrought balance of priorities involved in the search for a spouse distinctly reveals the superiority of the groom's side to the bride's' (ibid.: 48). The girl's character and appearance are rigorously scrutinized, whereas for the boy such scrutiny was usually omitted and information was sought solely on his financial and educational standing. The superior position of the groom is extended to his family and is expressed in 'the good treatment and deference' (ibid.: 97) which they receive. This is endorsed by Dandekar who writes: 'The institution of arranged marriages makes a woman a burden to her family, but not a man to his' (1986: 105). However, Orenstein also suggests that the converse of the new bride's lowly position is the responsibility which the senior members of the in-law's household should feel for her. Indeed, dominance and responsibility are the two axes along which family relationships are distinguished. Thus, 'the oldest male of the highest generation was supposed to receive the most respect and obedience. The female at the opposite pole [should receive] the most protection and care' (Orenstein 1965: 47–48). Orenstein concedes that whilst these ideas about ideal relationships are clear cut, the reality may not always attain the ideal: 'The ideal 'daughter' status did not usually last long' (ibid.: 60). The lowly status of the new wife is manifest both in the heavy burden of housework which she bears and also in the absence of responsibility for her welfare.

This inferiority of the woman's position is painfully evident in cases of mental illness, and it is only somewhat alleviated by recourse to the matrilineal principle. Karvé (1965) emphasizes that Maharashtra is a transitory zone in which features from the social institutions of northern and southern India combine, and that Maharashtrian family structure can best be understood as a fusion of northern and southern principles. Thus although 'The family in Maharashtra is patrilineal and patrilocal it has many customs unknown in northern India, but which are found universally in the south' (ibid.: 183). Unlike in northern India, a girl visits her parents' house frequently after marriage, and traditionally the husband and his family have much difficulty in persuading her to rejoin them. While the girl may maintain frequent contact with her *maher*, Karvé does not mention that among the high caste Marathas it is not considered proper for the parents to visit her in her *sasar* until after the birth of a son. The girl's brother is the only person who is traditionally permitted to visit her. However, welcome and support from the parental home are conditional upon the girl's maintenance of her honour. In cases of mental illness the girl's and the family's honour are severely threatened, and sources of help and care are therefore drastically reduced.

In Maharashtra an individual's well-being and in many cases his or her survival are dependent upon the existence of an intact family. For women the problem seems to centre not so much on the intactness of the family as on her acceptance by the husband's family. As many writers have pointed out, perpetuating the lineage and leading a life of selfless devotion to her husband and his family are important factors contributing to acceptance. Hence the seemingly endless interest and questioning about one's family circumstances. For despite the threat to the family's honour, socially approved expectations of care in mental illness persist. Expectations of familial love and care are high and appear to invoke an ideal family structure. Conversely, the existence of this powerful shared ideal opens up the possibility of disappointment, and this disappointment is frequently expressed in terms of _karani_.

Within the temple there was a general consensus that while 'shame' (the term used most often was _laaj_) and 'honour' (_abru_ and _hizaat_) are associated with all mental illness, it was more shameful for a woman to become mentally ill than a man. In Phaltan a woman's honour is thought to be more 'fragile' (_nasuk_), and even slight misconduct on her part will bring shame upon the 'household honour' _gharachi abru_. One informant quoted the Marathi saying that 'a woman's honour once broken, is broken forever' (_Baikanchi abru manje kacheche bhande ekda putle, ki kayamche putle_). Another young woman living alone in the temple suggested that a woman's mental illness entailed a public enquiry, or _panchanama_, on the whole family. If a woman has younger unmarried sisters at home, her parents may find it difficult to arrange their marriages. One young widow who was accompanying her afflicted sister said that the sister's affliction had provoked a hundred questions from neighbours who also came to observe her in the temple. Their visits were prompted not by solicitousness for her welfare but by malevolent curiosity, she thought. The recurrence of this theme of shame recalls descriptions of the _purdah_ complex, where male honour depends upon female veiling (see, for example, Mandelbaum 1988). At the heart of the veiling complex lie notions of privacy and modesty which are destroyed when women become mentally ill. Many informants cited the talk of neighbours and the public gaze as the most difficult aspects of the family's affliction.

While most parents and wives admitted that they felt shame when their sons became mentally afflicted, this was thought to be less severe than that incurred by women's mental affliction. A man's affliction was described as a cause for sorrow rather than shame. Whereas mentally afflicted women endangered the marriage prospects of their young sisters, this was unlikely to be the case for mentally afflicted men, particularly where their younger brothers enjoyed a good financial position.

A few informants insisted that mental illness involved no shame, but was simply a 'misfortune' (_durdaiva_) for both sexes. The mentally ill person was simply a victim of *karani* and had done nothing to incur such misfortune. However, the majority of informants while recognizing the operation of *karani* saw shame and the loss of family honour as yet another of the evil consequences of *karani*. The reasons given for the differences in the amount of shame accruing to the family are of two kinds. First, the behaviour of mentally afflicted women is perceived as inviting sexual exploitation. Tearing one's clothes and going about naked or scantily clad are among the commonly cited symptoms of mental affliction and in women such behaviour is seen as diverging further from required feminine behaviour than from masculine behaviour. Lack of proper attention to appearance and care of the body are seen as shameful. Furthermore, wild and violent behaviour is also more at odds with the ideal of femininity than of masculinity. Because of these implications it is thought that a young woman suffering from mental affliction incurs a far greater amount of shame than an older woman similarly afflicted. She is more likely to be sexually exploited. It is thought that if an older woman becomes mentally afflicted, few questions will be asked. She can simply be kept in a room and fed, whereas a younger woman's affliction is likely to provoke a multitude of questions. An older woman will already have fulfilled many of her duties, whereas a younger woman still has to bear children, to look after them and to cook for the family. She is described as the pivotal point of the family (*kutumbacha madhyabindu*). Shame and dishonour are incurred equally by unmarried and married woman. It is thought that for the unmarried woman there will be great difficulty in getting her married, whereas for the married woman there is the problem of who will look after her and support her. All were agreed that the in-laws were extremely unlikely to look after the young woman. One old informant said that if a woman becomes mentally ill after marriage then only one out of ten in-laws will look after her. Her own parents will feel shame on her behalf and anxiety lest the dishonour is passed on to any of the unmarried sisters. Thus young women appear to be in a particularly vulnerable position with regard to mental illness. Not only does their affliction pose a greater threat to family honour, but also the stigma is more likely to be passed on to other younger female members of the household.

Women, it seems, absorb stigma more readily than do men. In this particular context the transmission of stigma is considered to be wholly negative and therapeutically unhelpful. Differences for men and women in the experience of stigma have implications for the family response to affliction. Thus, for families with afflicted men, stigma, if it occurs at all, is muted. The more typical response is that of sorrow rather than shame. Sorrow is more readily shared and leads to a display of family solidarity. Carers drawn from both affinal and blood kin are rallied to the support of the afflicted man. The sorrow of male affliction leads to an expansion of the family in the form of a loosening of internal boundaries and codes of conduct between affinal and blood kin. Parents-in-law and brothers-in-law as well as parents and siblings take an interest in the plight of an afflicted man. All the resources of the extended family are brought into play and the tensions between husband's and wife's family are submerged in the overwhelming concern with the man's welfare. Women cultivate trancing in order, it is thought, to shift the affliction from their men folk onto themselves. The nature of this transference is discussed later.

Women's affliction, however, evokes a different set of social responses. The stigmatised nature of women's mental affliction and its association with shame and dishonour result in an unwillingness to share it. Under these circumstances the family closes in upon itself to contain the stigma and family sympathies contract. In the case of married women the fragile alliance between the husband and wife and their respective families is severed and the woman is left to look for support from her parental home. Thus the woman is forced to fall back upon the uncertain resources of the narrower matrilineal kin group. The ideology of affliction posits that trance in other family members may shift or lessen the original affliction. In the case of women, this mechanism is rarely brought into play. The different impact of affliction and madness on men and women is summarized in Figure 5.1.

The Family and the Afflicted: Ideology and Reality of Familial Carers

An attempt was made to discover the nature of the ideal Maharashtrian family. Temple dwellers were asked to describe the size and composition of a happy family. Twenty temple inhabitants answered questions. Informal conversations took place at quiet times of day when people were generally sitting about chatting and passing the time of day. Informants were asked to imagine a typical Maharashtrian family and say how many children, brothers and sisters a wife should have in order to be happiest and conversely, how many children, brothers and sisters her husband should have to be optimally happy. For some informants the required hypothetical leap away from their own family circumstances proved too difficult an exercise of the imagination. However, most informants enjoyed the imaginative exercise and produced an ideal family structure which looked somewhat like that indicated by Figure 5.2A or 5.2B.

These ideals are common to both men and women. (The only slight discrepancy which occurred was in the number of sisters the husband should have, wives preferring their husbands to have fewer sisters.) The size of the family varied, but a required excess of males remains constant in both figures A and B. To be happy it is thought a married couple should have double the number of male than female children. The wife should have

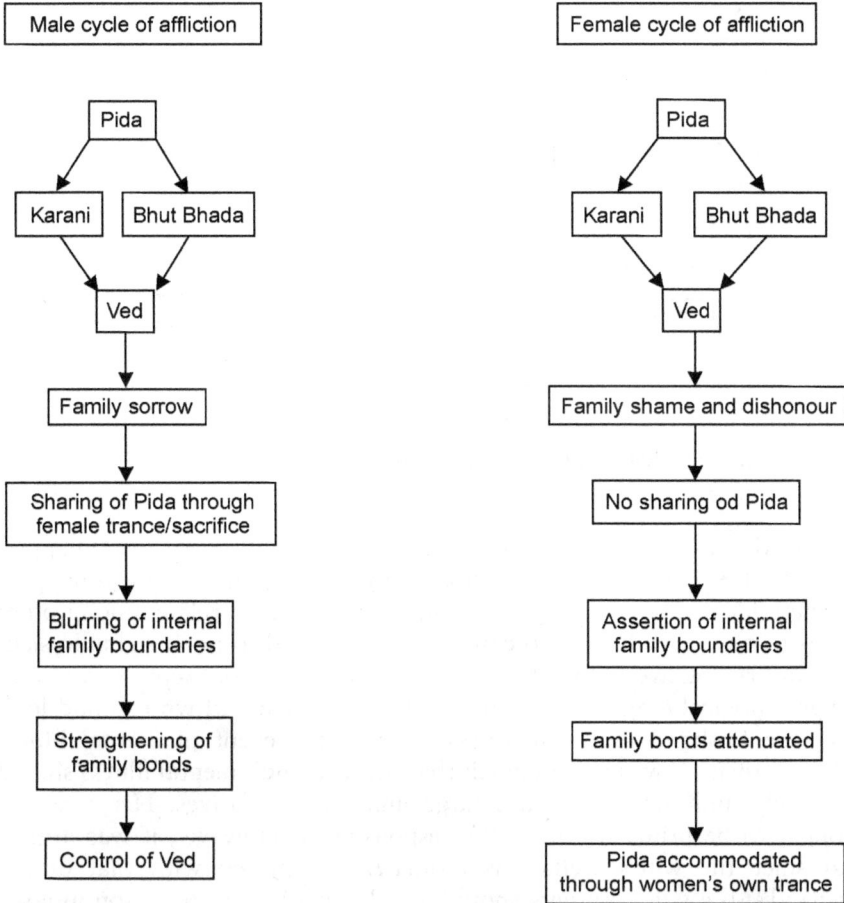

Figure 5.1: Gender Differences in Cycles of Affliction

many brothers – at least twice as many brothers as sisters. This wish appears to relate to Sacks' (1979) argument that women's status – in this case, health status – is improved if women can exercise their rights as sisters. However, the husband's happiness is not thought to depend upon the existence of brothers. Indeed, many informants stated quite explicitly that one brother was quite enough and that many brothers led to many quarrels between the brothers, but especially between the brothers' wives. There was a tendency for informants who themselves came from smaller families to idealize larger families whereas informants from large families preferred smaller families. There was no consensus about whether joint or separate households were happier, although there was a tendency for those

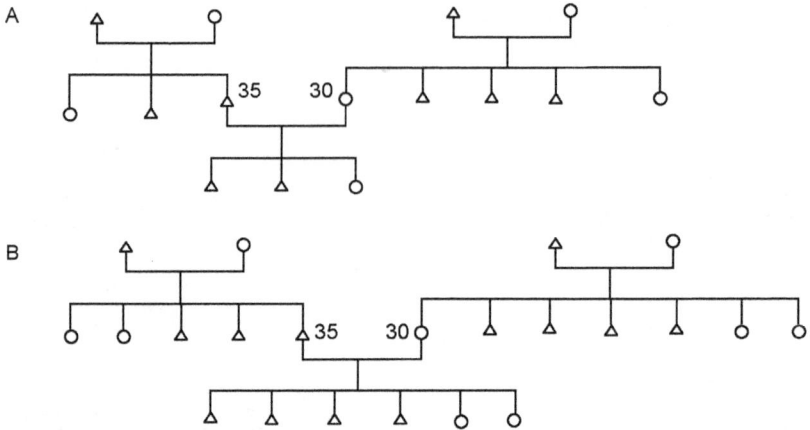

Figure 5.2: The Ideal Maharashtrian Family

who lived in joint households to say that separate households were happier and those living in separate household to think that joint living was happier.

These ideals about family composition appeared to relate among other things to one's entitlement to care and nurture and to one's rights in sickness. Informants were, therefore, presented with pictorial representation of the genealogical diagram in Figure 5.2B and were asked who should look after the husband and wife respectively in the event of mental illness befalling them. It was generally felt that the husband's mental illness should elicit help and concern from a large number of relatives. His care was thought to be primarily the wife's responsibility. However, it was argued that since the wife's welfare is intimately bound up with that of her husband's, the wife's parents should also be involved in their son-in-law's treatment. The care and concern which his own parents should give him appeared to be taken for granted. Thus relatives both from his side of the family and his wife's were seen as appropriate carers.

Mental illness in the wife elicited a different response and was tempered by a sharp sense of realism. In such an event there was a consensus that the wife should be looked after by her parents and brothers. While it was felt that the husband *should* look after his wife, it was thought to be highly unlikely and only to happen if he were exceptionally kind-hearted.

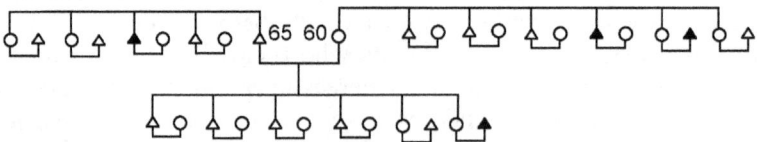

Figure 5.3: An Idealized Maharashtrian Family, Late in the Life Cycle.

The same couple were shown in a later stage of their life cycle, now both in their sixties. (A pictorial representation of Figure 5.3 was drawn.) At this later stage the health of both the husband and the wife was thought to be primarily the sons' responsibility, and it was agreed that sons should look after either or both the parents in case of mental illness. Thus the ideal family structure where parents have more sons than daughters and where the wife has many brothers is one which is theoretically able to fulfil the expectations of care and concern in case of mental illness. These shared expectations of help and succour conform with the formal kinship system as described by Karvé (1965) and Orenstein (1965). The importance assigned to sons as providers of support is in line with the emphasis given to patrilineality by Orenstein. The hope that a woman will have many brothers conforms with Karvé's emphasis on the bilineality of the Maharashtrian kinship system.

In practice, expectations of family care and concern are not always met; where they are met, help does not necessarily come from the expected sources. First, nature does not provide the desired abundance of male benefactors. Actual genealogies of temple dwellers show an enormous variety which takes no account of the overwhelming preference for male births. Second, even where existing family structures do conform more or less to the ideal, mental illness does not always evoke the desired patterns of help. Few of the afflicted families conform to the ideal patterns of care and many diverge completely from them. A considerable number of the women have no husband (owing to death or remarriage) and no children. However, even where the family includes husband, wife, sons and brothers, care in illness is rarely forthcoming from the expected sources. The divergence between normative expectations and actual practice, between what should happen and what does happen, is greatest for women. However, for mentally afflicted men too there is a divergence between publicly avowed expectations and the practices of care.

Tables 5.1, 5.2 and 5.3 show details of family circumstances and affliction. The figures show the different circumstances of affliction for men and women. Table 5.1 shows the circumstances of unaccompanied women, Table 5.2 of accompanied women and Table 5.3 of accompanied men. Case material of typical temple dwellers may help to focus on some of the more salient findings and distinguishing features of each category.

Mangal (Table 5.1, A2)

Mangal was living alone in the temple during the period of my fieldwork. She looked very depressed and apathetic and, indeed, her entry in the temple register described her as suffering from *dukkha*, or 'sorrow'. The psychiatrist whom I persuaded to visit her described her as suffering from schizophrenia in remission. Of all the women in the temple she seemed least

Table 5.1: The Circumstances of Unaccompanied Women Sufferers in the Temple

Name	A1	A2	A3	A4	A5	A6	A7	A8	A9	A10	A11	A12	A13
Sex	F	F	F	F	F	F	F	F	F	F	F	F	F
Trance	12 yrs	No	Yes recently	3yrs	2yrs	15yrs	Yes in temple	No	None last 2yrs	5 yrs	6 yrs	*drishtant*	20 yrs
Age	50	28	20	35	50	50	55	36	45	55	60	60	55
Marital status	Married	Married/ 2nd wife	Married/ 2nd wife	2nd wife	Married husband 80	Widow	Married	Married	2nd wife	Married	Widowed	Widowed	Widow
Children	2m/1f	None	None	None	None	2m/2f	3m 1 died	None	6m/3f	3m/3f	3m/3f	6m 2f died	1m/1f 2m/4f died
Care givers	None	None but mother visits	None	None	None	None	None	None	None	None	None	None	None
Temple diagnosis	Pida	Dukkha Pida	Pida	Veda	Pida	Pida	Pida	Pida	Pida	Pida	Pida	Pida	Pida
Previous medical/ psychiatric diagnosis	Asthma	Schizophrenia in remission	None given	None	None	None	None	None	None	None given	None	None	None
Chained	No	No	No	No	No	No	No	No	No	No	No	No	No
Other treatment sought	No improve- ment from inject.	None	None	None	None	None	None Worse	Many drs. - no help	None	Hospital treatment for son	None	None temples	Holy ahs & water from other

Duration of affliction	12 yrs	10 yrs	5 yrs	12 yrs	11 yrs	16 yrs	15 yrs	15 yrs	12 yrs	23 yrs	11 yrs	14 yrs	10 yrs
Length of stay	13 months	1 month	3 yrs	2 months	2 yrs	5 weeks	1 month	8 days/18 months earlier	4 yrs	10 months	1 year	9 yrs	Many years stay. This time few days visit
Source of financial support	Husband and sons	Mother brings food/money	Works in temple	Works in temple	Eldest daughter's husband	Brothers	Husband	Husband gives money	Works as cleaner outside the temple	Husband brings money	Son brings food	Sons	Worked in temple
Cause of trouble	Karani from husband's brother's wife	Not known	Karani from guardian	Karani from fusband's brother's wife	Karani from duaghter's husband's borther's wife	Bhunt bhada	Karani from husband's brother	Karani from f-in-law's brother's wife	Karani from father's brother	Karani	Un-identified karani	Karani from f-in-law's brother	Karani from f-in-law's mistress
Reason for coming	Breathing trouble	Not eating or talking	Tears and yawning	Kind of madness crying/dizziness	Quarrel-cursing	Crying, dizziness trembling	Dizziness/crying	Headache tiredness anxious	Dizziness/weakness	Oldest son mad & elder brother	2nd son was mad	Son mad	Son has fits

Table 5.2: The Circumstances of Accompanied Women Sufferers in the Temple

Name	B1	B2	B3	B4	B5	B6	B7	B8
Sex	F	F	F	F	F	F	F	F
Trance	No	Yes 1 month after arriving	Yes since arrival	Yes 12 months	No	No trance last 12 yrs	No	No
Age	65	25	80	35	65	16	55	15
Marital status	Married	Married	Married	Married	Married	Single	Married	Single
Children	1m/2f	4f	3m/3f	2m/3f	1m/2f, 1m died	None	1m/2f, 1m/2f died	None
Care givers	Daughter	Husband and 4 daughters (2–6)	2nd son	Mother	Widowed daughter	Widowed mother (nun)	Daughter	Maternal grandmother trances
Temple diagnosis	Pida	Pida	Natural illness	Pida	Natural illness	Pida	Pida	Pida
Previous medical/ psychiatric diagnosis	None	Psychiatric illness	None	None	Cancer	None	None	None
Chained	No	No	No	Yes	No	No	No	No

Other treatment sought	Medical treatment no help	Yes, medical & psychiatric	Doctor's injection made condition worse	Kidney and hysterectomy operations	Operation	Doctors/ dispens. made condition worse	Doctor no help lost weight	Dispensary no help
Duration of affliction	10 years	4 years	4 months	1 year	5 months	4 years	3 months	12 years
Length of stay	1 week	3 years	1 month	6 months	5 days	4 years	1 week	2 months
Source of financial support	Husband	Husband	Son	2 brothers	Son	Brother	Husband	Parents
Cause of trouble	Karani from m-in-law (deceased)	Karani from father's brother's wife	Karani from husband's brother	Karani from neighbour	Karani	Bhut Bhada	Karani or Bhut Bhada	Karani
Reason for coming	Breathing trouble	Dizziness trembling weakness	Swollen hands and wrists	Hungry but can't eat. Restless, beats herself	Worse after operation	Won't eat – very thin	Stomach swelling shaking trembling	White skin patches

Table 5.3: The Circumstances of Accompanied Male Sufferers in the Temple

Name	C1	C2	C3	C4	C5	C6	C7	C8	C9	C10
Sex	M	M	M	M	M	M	M	M	M	M
Trance	No	No	No	No	No	No	No	No	No	No
Age	20	20	22	35	29	35	35	30	35	35
Marital status	Single	Single	Single	Single	Single	Married	Single	Married	Single	Married
Children	None	None	None	None	None	1 female	None	2 female	None	2f/1m, 1m died
Care givers	Sister stays & trances, parents visit	Parents visit (not trance yet)	Parents visit monthly	Mother (trance)/father/sister	Mother (trance) father	Wife	Mother (separated) trances 18 months	Wife (trances)	Mother (widow) no trance	Wife
Temple diagnosis	Pida	Pida (Veda)	Pida	Pida (Veda)	Veda	Pida	Vedepan	Pida	Veda	Veda
Previous medical/ psychiatric diagnosis	Schizophrenia	None	None	Schizophrenia	Paranoid reaction	None	None	None	None	None
Chained	Yes	Yes	No (chained earlier)	Yes	Yes	No	Yes	No	Yes	Yes
Other treatment sought	Hospital treatment	Hospital/ clinic ECT	Doctors didn't help	Hospital treatment	None	Doctor has given ECT	Taken to disp. ECT & devrishi	None	Devrishi	Devrishi

Duration of affliction	4 yrs	2 yrs	7 yrs	9 yrs	(Last 9 yrs particularly bad) 20 yrs	5 yrs	17 yrs	8 yrs	15 yrs	6 yrs
Length of stay	3 yrs	6 weeks	4 yrs	3 yrs	18 months	18 months	2 yrs	6 weeks	10 yrs	1 week
Source of financial support	Father	Sold land to look after son	Parents	Father	Father mortgaged land	Wife, father, brother give money/little from own parents	Mother works in temple to get help from brother	Wife's ygr brother gives some money. Husband makes bricks	Works in temple	Wife's mother and brother have given money
Cause of trouble	Karani from father's brother	Karani source unknown	Karani from father's brother	Karani from father's brother	Karani from father's brother wife	Karani from brother's wife	Karani from brother's wife	Karani from sister's m-in-law	Karani from mother's sister's daughter	Karani from paternal grandparents
Reason for coming	Hitting/abusing family, running away	Hitting mother, destroying house, running away	Dizzy, restless, headache, fighting		Hit parents, undressed, ran away	Tears clothes, runs naked	Tearing clothes, eating night soil, roaming about	Husband roams about, doesn't eat, beats wife	Son runs away, curses/abuses her	Beating people and wife, wouldn't live in house
Siblings	1 brother (ygr) 1 sister	1 brother (ygr) 2 sisters	2 brothers 3 sisters	3 sisters	1 brother 1 sister	2 brothers 2 sisters	None	1 brother	2 brothers (died)	4 brothers 1 sister

able to care for herself and most disassociated from her surroundings. Mangal was 28 at the time I knew her and had been married 12 years ago. She had a son who died in infancy. After the death of her son she started having 'trouble', *tras*, and refused to eat or talk. As the trouble persisted Mangal was taken back to her parental home by her husband's brother, who stated that the husband and his family did not want any further responsibility for her. The husband subsequently remarried and had two sons by his second wife. Mangal did not receive any hospital treatment since the trouble was not physical and her family did not see such treatment as appropriate in her case. Meanwhile Mangal had to rediscover a niche for herself in her parents' home. She was lucky to be the youngest daughter and to have two elder sisters already married, otherwise she may not have been accepted back. However, Mangal had four brothers, three of them living at home and her position, particularly vis-à-vis the brothers' wives, was not likely to be easy. It is significant that although she was one of the two most severely incapacitated women in the temple, she was nonetheless left to fend for herself. She was brought to the temple by her elder brother, and although she expected him to visit, this did not take place during the period of my fieldwork. The mother did visit and the transformation in Mangal's appearance and demeanour at this time was remarkable. She became more active and talkative in behaviour and neat in appearance.

Although Mangal did not receive the level of care which is theoretically deemed necessary for cure, she was lucky that her parental family could afford not to disassociate themselves completely from her. Her relative youth was an advantage, as also was the fact that both her parents were still alive. However, unlike many of the young men she has had neither hospital treatment nor the full ingredients of traditional treatment. No family member was staying with her and there was no question of shared affliction through trance. Mangal herself appeared to be too disassociated to be able to benefit from trance herself.

Parubai (Table 5.1, A9)

Parubai provides an illustration of the way circumstances change for women as they get older. She was about 45 at the time of my research. She was not sure exactly when her trouble started but she knew it had gradually become worse over the twelve years since her husband took a second wife. For five years she had lived in the temple and when I spoke to her, her trouble consisted solely in involuntary cyclical motions of the head and yawning. She also said she feels swollen and has no strength in herself. However, earlier she had suffered from dizziness, restlessness and crying. She said that when she became 'nearly mad' her parents could not visit her because it was not their tradition and her brother was sent to fetch her home. After a short stay living with her mother and brothers she was brought to the temple. This was now her third stay in the temple. During the earlier stays her mother and brothers visited her, but later she had no visitors. She said quite matter-of-factly that her family were village people and, therefore, a bit harsh and not concerned about her welfare. Although she received no visitors, she did sometimes go home. She received no money from home but earned about 200 rupees a month by going to clean for people outside the temple. Although she started having *hajeri* (trance experiences) after first coming here, she later had no *hajeri* and felt harshly deprived in this respect. She questioned whether her devotional activities and expenditure are insufficient and might, therefore, account for the lack of *hajeri*.

Bapu (Figure 5.3, C5)

Bapu was 29 during the first period of fieldwork and the eldest of two brothers. His elder sister was married and living elsewhere. When I first spoke to the family they had been living in the temple for one week. Bapu was brought to the temple by his mother and father, both of whom were staying with him. His trouble was described as being twenty years old. His father described the original trouble as trivial – disobedience to small orders. The family were farmers but clearly had high aspirations for Bapu. Bapu was sent to a prestigious private school in Pune and then admitted to a homoeopathic medical college there. But after the age of twenty, Bapu's behaviour became very troublesome. When he came home he would sleep a lot, he would not work, he showed no interest in day to day affairs and he threw away his clothes. The father tried to take him to hospital but the son insisted there was nothing wrong with him. When he was taken to a doctor he behaved perfectly normally. Eventually he was enticed into going to the temple by the ruse that they were going sightseeing. The family attributed the son's trouble to *karani* from the father's brother's wife, who attributed her husband's death to Bapu's father. Thus the parents saw Bapu's affliction as part of a wider family quarrel. Even the farm animals were affected. When Bapu's problems intensified the mother started trancing, initially at a local temple and later in the Mahanubhav temple. The family made considerable financial sacrifices to fund the temple stay. Much of their agricultural land is lay idle and they took out a loan of 25,000 rupees. The younger son was sending the family 150 rupees a month. However, the parents were confident that their devotion would bring about a cure, and that the son's recovery and eventual rehabilitation as a doctor would save the family from its difficulties.

Narain (Figure 5.3, C4)

Narain was the only son among four children. He was thirty-five when I knew him and had been troubled for nine years. He had been living in the temple for six years with his mother, and his father and younger sister as frequent visitors. He was described as having become suddenly afflicted. One day he came home laughing in a state of madness. Thereafter he beat his parents, ran away and refused to work. His mother claimed that she neglected her home and other children in order to look after Narain, but felt that he was her prime responsibility. After arrival at the temple the mother suffered frequent trancing but this gradually decreased and the family attributed the general deterioration in Narain's condition to his mother's infrequent trancing. Narain had had hospital treatment also, including ECT treatment and two days in psychiatric hospital. During his stay in the temple he had regular consultations and treatment from the local psychiatrist. Narain's condition was seen as being part of a general family misfortune whose source is *karani* performed by the father's brother. However, despite temporary setbacks in Narain's progress the family were confident of his ultimate recovery. When this happens Narain will be married and the family would be able to recoup its losses.

Suman (Figure 5.2, B2)

Accompanied women tended to stay for shorter periods in the temple than either accompanied men or unaccompanied women. In this respect Suman was not typical of the accompanied who staid on average for a few months: she had been living in the temple for three years. She was, however, typical in that her affliction nevertheless left her very able to cope with daily life. Suman was twenty-five years old and married with four daughters. Her husband and four, children aged between two and six, lived with her. The elder two girls went to school from the temple. Although Suman had earlier received a general diagnosis of her condition as mental illness, in my eyes she betrayed no signs of such illness. She was one of the most articulate and outgoing of the inhabitants. The visiting psychiatrist, after a five-minute interview, diagnosed her as having an immature personality, but I suspect his diagnosis was based largely, if not solely, on the fact that she suffered from trance. Her self-professed symptoms of dizziness, trembling and weakness were not in evidence. On closer acquaintance it emerged that Suman had two secret anxieties. The first related to the fact that she had only daughters. This has placed her in an enormous quandary in that she would like another child but fears it may be a girl yet again. She and her husband feel they cannot afford another female child. Her second anxiety related to an ulcerous tumour in her armpit. Although I was eventually able to arrange medical treatment for this, it had clearly been a major source of worry for some considerable time. Suman derived considerable benefit from trancing. Trancing was her reason for being in the temple and she looked upon it as a kind of work, a duty to be carried out. After trancing she felt refreshed and charged with energy. She also found that the anxiety of her personal problems diminished in intensity.

These case studies illustrate some of the differences typically found between men, accompanied women and unaccompanied women. Although these cases are united by common residence in the temple and a shared terminology of affliction, they in fact represent quite different problems, different levels of severity and different methods of dealing with these problems. The majority of women are unaccompanied and, while they complain of mental affliction and describe themselves as suffering from a variety of symptoms, they are not for the most part incapacitated by their symptoms. Women with more incapacitating afflictions seldom appear in the temple. Thus, rather than forming the majority of the afflicted population as has sometimes been claimed (Kakar 1981; Obeyesekere 1981), there is a surprising absence of severely mentally afflicted women. While the presence of mildly afflicted women and the absence of mildly afflicted men suggests that the temple is differently weighted as a source of help for men and women, the absence of severely afflicted women cannot be explained solely in these terms. My study was not able to supply any definite answers as to their whereabouts. Afflicted women were not to be seen roaming the countryside or streets, and my experience in this is similar to Bhattacharyya's Bengali study which found that 'Those who do live on the streets are men' (1986: 171). Many of the women referred to their problems as a 'secret trouble', or *gupta tras*, by which they seemed to mean not so much that they were unwilling to disclose the nature of their trouble but that it was peculiar to themselves; that it was their personal problem. These personal problems are alleviated through trance. Those women who are unable to trance see this as a kind of curse or punishment, the result of bad *karma*. One woman speculated that perhaps her inability to trance was due to the fact that she was not spending enough money on devotional activities. Many of the unaccompanied women have lost the right to a position within the family. The financial situation of most unaccompanied women is precarious. Four of the women in this category are working either in the temple or outside at menial cleaning jobs.

A further four women were previously living in the temple with their sons. Whilst their sons' health improved and they returned to their native villages, the mothers have chosen to remain in the temple as a means of safeguarding the future health of their sons. Their continued presence in the temple was, they felt, a guarantee of their sons' continued well-being. They have offered themselves as spiritual hostages to God. They are thus conforming to the gist of the folk saying: 'One can pay back the father's debt by making the holy pilgrimage to Benares, but one can never hope to repay the debt of gratitude to the mother' (quoted by Karvé 1965: 206). Women who stayed behind in order to safeguard their family's health and to protect their sons from madness are looked after by their families in return.

Referring to the data in Tables 5.1, 5.2 and 5.3, A11, for example, is visited daily by her sons and is brought food. However, A13, who is a widow and has only one son, has to fend for herself. The contrast between men and women is most striking in the case of younger women such as A2 and A3. Of all the women in the temple, A2 appeared least able to look after herself and yet she was left to fend for herself despite the generally accepted principle that family care is crucial to a successful outcome. She did not cook for many days and, therefore, went without food. She sat listlessly with her back to everyone and her physical condition seemed to deteriorate as a result of her mental state. A3 was also left to fend for herself. However, whereas A2 was brought food and money by her mother, A3 had to fetch water and sweep the temple in return for 200 rupees a month. Perhaps her lowly role in temple life may have been because she was of untouchable *Mahar* caste converted to Ambedkar's Buddhism.

By contrast, the men all had at least one carer and sometimes several. Of the three married men (C6, C8, C10), all were accompanied by their wives. Two had brought young children with them as well. One, Dattu (C6), was originally accompanied by his wife, father-in-law, father-in-law's brother's son, wife's sister's husband as well as by his own brother's son, thus supporting the claim that the wife's welfare is so bound up with that of her husband's that his health should be as much the concern of her family as of his own. Of the seven unmarried men, two were accompanied by both parents, their pattern of care thus conforming to shared expectations. However, of the remaining five, one was cared for by his younger sister and one by his mother and younger sister. These two examples reverse the official ideology that brothers should look after sisters. The following folk song alludes to the difficulties of the sister/brother relationship. 'The rain comes in torrents and vanishes as suddenly. My brother too has forgotten me since the birth of his daughter' (quoted by Karvé 1965: 208). The other three men were looked after by their mother alone. It is significant that all the young men cared for by their mother or mother and father are either only children or eldest sons. C2 is the one exception, being the second born son, and it is significant that his parents do not stay with him continuously. Moreover, he does not appear to be as severely incapacitated as the others and this, taken together with the fact that he trances, puts him into an altogether different category. All the families appear to have made con-siderable financial rearrangements to accommodate the men's mental affliction, even to the extent of mortgaging or selling land. In the case of the two widows, both worked in order to support their sons. An interesting psychiatric hospital study in Bangalore (Bhatti et al. 1980) looked at patients' preferred accompanying relative and duration of stay. They found that staying with the preferred relative shortened the hospital stay. How-ever, irrespective of preference, the father's presence shortened the hospital stay and the mother's presence lengthened it. The authors suggest this may be because of the tendency of mothers to reinforce the sick role by over protection. My own study found that the two mothers accompanying their afflicted sons had been staying at the temple a very long time (two years and ten years respectively). However, this seemed to be an expression of their commitment to the caring role and identification with their sons, rather than of over protection.

Of the older women only one, B3, who was suffering from swelling of the limbs, was accompanied by her unmarried son. Of the younger women only one, B2, was accompanied by her husband and four daughters. Of the other six accompanied women the three older ones were accompanied by their daughters, and two of the younger ones were accompanied by their mothers and one by a grandmother. So for most women the socially sanctioned sources of help are not forthcoming. For younger married women their acceptance by the in-laws' family appears to be contingent upon fulfilling their required duties and upon good conduct. The woman's right to belong to the in-laws' family depends upon producing male offspring. Dandekar writes:

> The security of a woman's position in her marital home depends upon her loyalty to the family. In this the bearing of a son to perpetuate the family is critical. If she does not bear a son, the husband may remarry with the full force of societal sanction behind him. In this case the first wife becomes almost an outcast and is forced to return to her father's house (1986: 107).

However, this return to her parental home is at best 'an uneasy compromise' (ibid.: 108) for she brings with her dishonour for the parents and must occupy a lowly and dependent status. Mentally ill women are not able to fulfil the requirements upon which their acceptance depends. The position of women who have not yet borne a son or any children is particularly difficult. The problematic nature of the woman's relationship with her in-laws is acknowledged in the Marathi term *saserwas*. The literal meaning of the term is in-laws' dwelling, but the term is commonly used to describe 'in-law trouble'. One woman recalled her husband bringing her to the temple and leaving her with the words: 'For me she is dead.' The more common pattern is for some member of the in-law's household, often the husband's brother, to return the women to her parental home. The embarrassment which such women then pose for their own parents is reflected by the absence of parents looking after their daughters at the temple and by the fact that the women who are there are less severely afflicted than the men. It is also significant that four of the eight women who fall into the accompanied category are there because of physical rather than mental conditions. Yet another proverb refers to the difficulties of the parents *vis-à-vis* their married daughter: the father says, 'My daughter I have given you to others but I cannot stand guarantee for your future' (Karvé 1965: 205). This description also applies to the old women who appear to be suffering from anxiety and depression resulting from their loss of family and position. Indeed, Ullrich (1987) writes of Havik Brahmin women living in constant fear of widowhood. Older women, even when they have sons, seldom receive assistance and even less frequently care from their sons. Vatuk notes the 'dominant tone of pessimism' (1980: 300) despite the general expectation that sons should look after elderly parents. Insofar as women receive care, it tends to be from mothers or daughters, although this is not officially acknowledged.

When confronted with the contradiction between the ideology of male caregivers and afflicted women and the practice of female carers and afflicted men, temple dwellers gave two explanations for this state of affairs. One related to the social roles men and women are expected to play and the second to the "natural" qualities of men and women. Women, it is thought, have a greater capacity to bear suffering. Men tire more easily of caring for the mentally afflicted and find the practical chores more shameful, whereas women can care for the physical needs of the mentally afflicted no matter what the age of the child without feeling embarrassment. One man said that men have more of a role to fulfil in society and therefore cannot devote themselves to the care of the mentally afflicted child to the same extent. To do so they would have to neglect their job and then who would provide for the family?

Gender Differentials in Perception and Diagnosis of Affliction and its Severity

Although the Mahanubhav temple is renowned for curing *pida* through hajeri, and the *diksha* (or monks) maintain that all the problems brought to the temple are fundamentally the same, acquaintance with the temple population revealed a multiplicity of problems. When questioned about differences between the afflicted, the monks confessed that they had not observed their behaviour so minutely. Individual differences in the family background, behaviour and attitudes of the afflicted are not of interest to the temple officials. Such differences are glossed over in temple theories of *pida* which emphasize women's proneness to affliction and trance. The official unifying doctrine promotes a stereotype of feminine susceptibility to mental affliction and trance which distorts the perception and, indeed, the recording of cases of affliction, as discussed later. Such stereotyping also glosses over the variety of personal needs and circumstances to which the temple caters.

Among the afflictions brought to the temple there is also physical disease. However, where medical advice is rarely sought and treatment is at best sporadic, it is not always easy to distinguish severe life-threatening physical illness from mental affliction. Severe asthma (*damma*), particularly where its occurrence induces anxiety in the sufferer, is difficult to distinguish from certain types of mental affliction or psycho-neurotic behaviour. High fever, trembling and shaking in the old may be a symptom of terminal illness rather than a sign of mental affliction. There certainly were cases of physical disease which the sufferer or his family thought were due to *pida*, whereas the monks maintained that such conditions were 'natural' (*naisargic*). Included in this category was a woman suffering from severe and chronic asthma, a case of a woman who appeared to be suffering from terminal cancer, and another of a woman who appeared to be dying of an unidentified illness. While it is difficult in the absence of a medical examination to establish exactly how many cases of physical disease were categorized as mental affliction, it is likely that a few such cases regularly found refuge in the temple. Since it is the family who decides on the nature of the affliction, those cases are included in the temple population even though the religious experts might query their categorization.

The temple keeps a register with entries for each new case admitted to the temple. The entry consists of the name of the afflicted person, village, date of arrival and nature of trouble. In the vast majority of cases the nature of the trouble is recorded as *pida*. In a few cases the terms used are either *ved*, 'madness', or *mental* written in Devanagari script. There does not appear to be any underlying logic or consistency in the choice of these terms, in that some obviously mad persons are described as suffering from *pida* and not *ved* or *mental*. Indeed, all madness and mental illness are seen as being the outward expression of *pida*. *Karani*, it is thought, is more likely to damage the mind than the body, although physical disorders are occasionally seen as a sign of affliction. Thus all persons registered in the book are seen as suffering from *pida*. However, in many instances a female carer's name appears in place of the person on whose behalf the family has come. This lends support to the monks' view that the majority of the mentally afflicted are women. Kynch and Sen claim that the 'Non-perception of disadvantages of a deprived group helps to perpetuate those disadvantages' (1983: 365). Similarly, it should be added, their systematic misperception blocks change. Writing about India, the authors discuss the so-called unsplittable compound notion of family well-being and ask whether it may not include 'systematic biases in favour of fulfilling the needs of some members of the family e.g. the males' (ibid.: 364). With regard to the women in the Mahanubhav temples, they are systematically misperceived as constituting a majority and their disadvantaged treatment is not recognized.

During the period of my second study there were twenty-one cases of afflicted women and ten cases of afflicted men. Although it was not possible to carry out a systematic evaluation of the mental health status of temple dwellers, my own impressions, the rapid assessments made by the local psychiatrist on his visit to the temple, and the assessment of the temple priest and of the accompanying carers all converged on the opinion that the men suffered more serious forms of affliction and were more seriously incapacitated. The temple diagnoses entered in the register book on arrival describe only one woman as being 'mad' (*ved*); all the others are described as suffering from 'affliction' (*pida*). Six of the ten men are described as suffering madness and from *pida*. In other words 60 per cent of men but only 5 per cent of women receive a temple diagnosis of madness. Of the ten afflicted men, eight had been chained at some time. Of the twenty-one women only one was chained and that was at the woman's own instigation. (For the mathematically minded, eighty per cent of the men were chained compared to five per cent of the women.) The evaluations of the relatives concurred with that of the temple priests. There was no instance where a diagnosis of madness was entered in the register book which was disputed by the family.

The behaviour of the afflicted was no doubt affected by the strength and unanimity of the judgement against them, and indeed my own perceptions may have been influenced by these views. However, the men did seem to be considerably more impaired. My own judgements were based on two sets of criteria. First, on willingness to talk: the severely afflicted were largely mute. And, second, on their level of participation in everyday and religious activities: the severely afflicted participated hardly at all and either slept or sat staring vacantly. None of the women were mute although A2 had some days when she was reluctant to talk. Similarly, all the women were fairly active though some had their off days. B4 felt that being possessed by a spirit made her hyperactive and, therefore, asked to be chained so as to feel more comfortable. All but three of the ten men were mute and inactive.

Several attempts were made to obtain a psychiatric diagnosis for the temple population. There is one psychiatrist practising in Phaltan and several of the temple residents are already patients of his. However, it was extremely difficult to effect a meeting at the temple for reasons which never became quite explicit, but were probably related to the stigma of the place and the implications which such visits might have had for his status. Five meetings were arranged but only one materialized. The general direction of his diagnoses confirmed my impression that the men were more severely afflicted than the women. The woman with a temple diagnosis of madness was described as suffering from schizophrenia in remission, while several of the women who tranced were diagnosed as having immature personalities.

This overall picture is consistent with earlier findings (Skultans 1987). Previous fieldwork had found that although the majority of the temple population was female, there were more cases of male than of female affliction. Although the overwhelming female appearance of the temple engenders initial anxiety about the validity of earlier interpretations, closer investigation and questioning still shows the majority of severely afflicted to be men, thus dispelling the nagging doubt that one's interpretation may be based on a purely fortuitous constellation of circumstances rather than part of a more enduring pattern. Chaining is perhaps the most important means of registering the community's assessment of the severity of affliction. Certainly, according to this local evaluation men are more seriously afflicted. Thus, although monks and priests talk of women's weakness and proneness to affliction, the composition of the afflicted temple population belies such descriptions. Indeed, the differences between afflicted men and women raise issues about the relative rating given to temple care for men and women. It appears probable that the rating may be different for men and women: residence in the temple may be lower down the 'hierarchy of resort' for men than for women. This is borne out by the information about earlier treatment sought. Of the men, six out of ten had had previous psychiatric treatment. Of the twenty-one women only one had done so. A further nine women had had medical as opposed to psychiatric treatment. This leaves a further nine women who had received no other treatment. In other words, the temple is likely to be a first resort for women, particularly if they are unaccompanied, and a last resort for men.

Hajeri – Its Meaning and Significance

Stereotypes of women's weakness are also cited to explain the distribution of *hajeri* or trancing among carers. Women's nature, the fact that they are thought to have less self-control and will power than men, is thought to account for the greater incidence of trancing among women. In other words, shortcomings of character are held to account for women's trancing. According to this view trancing is a form of illness for which temple residence is a cure. This theory is cited to explain the preponderance of women in the temple. However, this official theory is by no means universally accepted. An earlier paper (Skultans 1987) described the different interpretation which women themselves give of trancing. In this account trancing has a somewhat flexible if not ambiguous meaning which varies between priests and temple dwellers and from woman to woman. While some women emphasize the suffering which they willingly inflict upon themselves, others emphasize the benefit which they derive from trancing. Thus the one term possesses a variety of overlapping meanings which might be described as constituting a set of family resemblances, to use Wittgenstein's term (2001: 66). Trance has one meaning for the temple priests and for men with afflicted womenfolk in their families, another for men who are themselves afflicted and for their female carers, and a third meaning for women who see their own affliction as the primary problem. Temple priests and to a lesser extent men whose assumptions have not been challenged by the problem of male affliction within the family opt for the comforting view that there is a natural affinity between women and trancing. Second, trancing among the carers of the afflicted is seen as being self-inflicted, in that wives and mothers pray that they themselves may become the targets of affliction, thus diminishing the malevolent intensity of the affliction besetting their men folk. The onset of trancing is seen as part of a process of redistribution of affliction. No cases of men undergoing self-imposed trance were recorded. Third, women who come to the temple alone and whose problems appear to stem from lack of family support welcome trancing as a means of containing and standardizing their private sorrows. Thus a single term covers a variety of circumstances and behaviours and enables the differences between them to be masked.

Although there are a few cases of men trancing, these cases are not associated with the affliction of another family member, but with their own diverse symptoms of a psychological nature, of which trancing is one. When questioned as to why men do not suffer from trance when others in the family are mentally afflicted, the reasons given again relate to their social role. If men were to go into trance they would have to neglect their job and their standing in society would be impaired. Whilst men acknowledge the value of trancing among their female kin, when questioned in general terms they say they are not inclined to believe in such things. One informant summed up attitudes succinctly by saying that for a father to trance would be a disadvantage, whilst for a mother to trance is the fulfilment of her duty, her *kartyava* (literally 'the thing to be done'). Further questioning elicited the responses that God simply grants trance to women and not to men. Spiritual affliction (*pida*), or more generally trouble (*tras*), has a greater affinity for women than for men. It is thought that this is simply how things are.

The different configurations of the meaning of trance are linked by the element of constraint which appears in each setting. Thus trancing is not simply natural for women; there is also an emphasis on trancing as a woman's duty. Women who came to the temple because of their own affliction are required to trance regularly as part of their cure. Women carers also experience a feeling of constraint about trancing. In this case trancing is thought to be of direct help to the afflicted family member. This help takes two forms: firstly, it lessens the severity and amount of affliction, and secondly, through trance a diagnosis and information about the causation of the affliction are obtained. In all instances the expectations of required performance engender feelings of anxiety. One mother, Venutabai, who had remained in the temple after her son was cured and had returned home, expressed anxieties because she had not been trancing for the past fortnight and feared she might be asked to leave by the trustees. Another man, Tukaram, who had been asked to leave the temple ten months earlier, suspected that this might have been due to the fact that neither he nor his son suffered from trance. Several women expressed a regret that although they tried to trance they could not. Such individualists seem to me to support rather than refute the hypothesis that trancing among carers is a means of sharing the burden and shame of the affliction. For example, Venutabai, mentioned above, said that although she was unable to trance she did have a 'vision' or *drishtant,* at *arati* or 'ceremonial worship' during which she was able both to experience what her son had gone through in his illness and to understand the causes of the illness.

This sense of constraint and required performance is evident in the terminology used. The more learned Marathi word for trance is *sancara.* My first assistant also started trancing and the term her mother used to describe the condition was *sancara.* However, this word is never used in the setting of the Mahanubhav temples. The word employed here is *hajeri,* and it is given an altogether local meaning with which outsiders, that is townspeople, are not immediately familiar. For the Mahanubhav devotees *hajeri* means the presence of spirits or trance. However, for outsiders the term has a range of meanings and connotations which make its use in the temple context particularly interesting. *Hajeri* can mean a roll call, register, daily wages, attendance record or a required reporting of one's presence. For example, certain nomadic castes such as the Ramashi and Pashepardi, who had a reputation for thieving and bad conduct generally, were, until recently, required to report to the police twice daily. This act of registering their continued presence in the town was known as *hajeri.*

The feeling of required performance also comes across on the actual occasions of trancing, that is at *arati*, which appear to be carefully orche-strated events. During *arati* monks play the role of master of ceremonies carefully setting the scene for the trancers. It is they who perform all the ceremonial aspects of worship, such as beating the cymbals and drums, waving incense and beating the feathered fans. Thus the monks provide the required setting for trancing, and indeed trancing seldom takes place outside that setting. However, the explanation for the readiness with which women comply with the expectation that they should trance should be sought in the precariousness of their position within the family structure and, in particular, in the tenuousness of their link with the husband's family. For many women it is not so much the family which is under threat as their right to belong to it.[3] Through trance women carers are sharing the family affliction and thereby affirming the legitimacy of their connection with that family. Orenstein (1965: 54) is surely wrong when he claims on behalf of his villagers that the wife has the religious advantage since she cannot assume the sins of the husband while his merit can be shared by her. Women appear to be particularly ready to share the affliction of their husband and sons, thereby emphasizing their loyalty and their right to belong to the husband's family.

Women who see themselves as sharing the affliction of their men folk both actively assume trance and see it as a threat to their health. This approach to their own trancing is to be explained in terms of the import-ance of their sons' health for their own acceptance and rights within their husband's family. What we have in operation is a hydraulic model of family as opposed to individual health with women playing a pivotal role within that model. The term hydraulic is an apt one because it suggests both the fluidity of affliction and its convertibility. It also suggests that there is a determined amount of affliction which remains more or less the same (unless there is a leak in the system), although its site can change. Women's trancing constitutes such a leak, in that regular and vigorous trancing is thought to bring about a gradual diminution of the total amount of affliction. Symptoms and family members can replace one another. Women physically take on the symptoms of their male kin through trance. Their role as scapegoats is both a reflection of their lowly status within the family and a procedure for enhancing this status. The hydraulic model is necessarily modified where women are themselves the targets of affliction. Where the afflicted women are unaccompanied this is because they are powerless to enlist the support of others. Such women are socially isolated and the affliction cannot be passed on to others. Instead, there is a transformation of the actual nature of the affliction.

Such women experience considerable satisfaction through trancing. Their various earlier symptoms decrease or lessen in intensity. Here trancing could be described as a public way of dealing with private sorrows. Informants' accounts frequently contrast the burden and pain of symptoms experienced prior to arrival in the temple and the sense of release which trancing and spiritual diagnosis can afford. Many of these women describe trance as something which keeps them going and enables them to deal with life.

Within this model trance provides the element which enables it to become a fully functioning ideology. Trance is the mechanism whereby affliction is shifted from one member to another and whereby the stereotypes of male fortitude and health and female weakness and ill-health are reinforced. The precise nature of these transformations emerges more clearly by considering the information from Tables 5.1, 5.2 and 5.3. Of the eight afflicted men, only one trances. However, five of their carers have started to trance. In a sixth case a mother felt she was about to start trancing. In other words, 75 per cent of female carers of an afflicted man went into trance. Of the eight accompanied afflicted women (Table 5.2) three had started trancing themselves and one carer had started trancing. Thus 12 per cent of female carers of an afflicted woman went into trance. Of the thirteen unaccompanied women (Table 5.1) only two had no experience of trance. All the others were trancing regularly. One spoke of her failure to trance for the last two years. Yet another saw her *drishtant* or 'vision' as having the same function as trance. Thus 85 per cent of the unaccompanied women tranced. This distribution suggests that trancing relates to the vulnerability of the afflicted within the family. The most vulnerable group, namely unaccompanied women, are most likely to trance.

Accompanied women form an intermediate group. Afflicted men being the most protected by their female kin are least likely to trance. This category of unaccompanied women share the characteristics of the women studied by Claus in Kanara District. He writes: 'Men, that is a woman's father, brother and husband, are responsible for her well-being, the control and regulation of her sexuality and fertility and the protection of her reproductive potential from outside malice. Lacking protective male control and support, a woman feels defenceless against spiritual attack' (1979: 36). However, in the Mahanubhav temples women who lack male support see this lack of support as itself part of their affliction.

Pfleiderer writing about afflicted women consulting a Muslim healing shrine has emphasized that 'women in a polluting state are vulnerable to spirit attacks' (1988: 419). In the Mahanubhav temple official ideology regarding trance and affliction also implicates women's sexuality and reproductive functions. However, this vulnerability is more particularly grounded in Maharashtrian family structure and the specific circumstances of a woman's family life. What we find, therefore, is that women's position within the social structure gives rise to distinct yet inter-related aetiological theories regarding women's affliction, to different patterns of trancing and of care.

Conclusions

This chapter illustrates the different impact which men's and women's mental affliction has on family structure. Mental affliction in men provides an opportunity for the strengths, endurance and cohesiveness of the Maharashtrian family to be demonstrated, whereas mental affliction in women reveals the weaknesses of the family, in particular the tenuousness of women's rights to family membership. Alongside these differences in family structure are differences in the amount of shame accruing to mentally ill men and women, and differences in rights to family care and financial support. Most importantly, there are differences in stereotypes of male and female susceptibility to affliction which serve to disguise the real differences in men's and women's experiences of mental affliction.

While these stereotypes of affliction are common to all the temple users they are held with varying degrees of conviction. Since women share a social world which accords them low social and ritual status it is not surprising that they concur with the dominant view regarding their proneness to pollution and susceptibility to affliction. However, women and their families also ascribe to an alternative model in which they play a more respected role and in which trance and affliction are given a more positive interpretation. Ardener wrote about the existence of 'muted categories' (1975: 1–17). Women in the Mahanubhav temples seem to be a semi-muted category, in that their account of affliction is not universally acknowledged and is often ascribed to ignorance. I have described the female version of affliction as a hydraulic model. This model persists despite its disparagement. Thus I am arguing that there are systematic differences in the explanatory models which relate to individuals' location within the social structure. My position is, therefore, more far reaching than that of the study carried out by Weiss and his colleagues in Bombay and other cities (1988: 471–77). They found that family members adopted different explanatory models according to their individual experience and involvement in the illness.

Trance is often attributed religious importance, spirit possession well nigh universally so, and both are closely connected to illness. Illness may be the outward manifestation of hitherto undetected spirit possession, or it may be a consequence of spirit possession or trance which are thought to have debilitating effects on mind and body. Trance and spirit possession offer alternative, highly personal forms of religious experience and healing technique. In both the religious and medical context their status and function have been the subject of disparaging interpretations which cast doubt on the mental health of those experiencing trance and spirit possession. However, those directly involved may have a quite different interpretation, and thus several interpretations of the same religious/healing activities may coexist.

These characteristics of the settings of trance and spirit possession prompt a reassessment of the nature of pluralism both in the religious and medical contexts. The differing interpretations of the experience, cause and purpose of trance suggest that the term pluralistic applies not only to the coexistence of several religious belief systems within a society, but also serves as an apt description for the coexistence of several distinct orientations within a religious group. This kind of pluralism has been largely ignored by social anthropologists who have tended to concentrate on intercultural difference. As a result intra-cultural differences have been neglected and this has also been encouraged by the fact that anthropologists glean their information from a 'single' expert source. The culling of expert opinion coupled with a disregard for alternative views may be promoted by an ideological resonance which favours the selection of a particular account of a religious or medical institution. The commonplace distinction between traditional and scientific medicine provides one ideologically based example of the neglect of intra-cultural differences. The interpretation of trance and spirit possession as a response to women's psychological ill health provides another example where one native view is promoted at the expense of others because it forms an ideological link with an entrenched view about the nature of women held by the social anthropologist or researcher. Thus the truly pluralistic approach would resist an analysis of religious and healing systems as harmonious and mutually compatible sets of beliefs and activities. Indeed, the term system is inappropriate since it does not take account of the different and sometimes conflicting beliefs and experiences which go to make up a single religious group or healing practice.

The perceived distribution of affliction between men and women and its association with shame and stigma for women appears to be a reflection of women's subordination within the gender hierarchy. This subordination occurs at both an ideological level and a behavioural one. Rogers has suggested that 'sex differentiation may exist in a variety of forms' (1978: 154) and that certain combinations of this differentiation are less likely to lead to inequality between the sexes. She suggests that 'where both ideological and behavioural differentiation exist a balance of power is most likely to occur' (ibid.: 155). On the other hand, 'where behavioural differentiation exists without ideological differentiation, a hierarchical relationship between the sexes – with a clear imbalance of power – becomes more probable' (ibid.: 156). In the Mahanubhav temples, men and women are perceived as having different personal attributes which befit them for different roles and which determine their susceptibility to affliction and illness and the form which such affliction takes. This ideology promotes trancing among women which in turn reinforces the association between mental affliction and women. Thus ideology and behaviour are inextricably linked and feed on each other, both contributing to the subordination of women. In the course of this process the alternative perspective of women and the families is lost to sight. The indigenous epidemiological understanding also hides from view the differences between men's and women's preferred treatments. It appears that whereas the temple is the preferred treatment for women who also bring less incapacitating afflictions, it comes much lower in the hierarchy of choice for men. These findings are related, though not identical to those of a study carried out by Singh and others in the Punjab. Their study of eleven Punjabi villages examined 615 deaths and the medical care sought prior to death. The study found 'that fewer females had medical care in fatal illnesses than did males, and generally by attendants of a lower level of competence' (Singh, Gordon and Wyon 1962: 874). Men received more care than did women from all categories of practitioners. However, whereas among high caste patients women and men sought help from indigenous practitioners and spiritual healers in equal numbers, among low caste patients more men than women sought help from these sources. This pattern of seeking help suggests that women will be the lesser users of the preferred or dominant mode of treatment and that what is considered to be the dominant mode in any setting will vary. My study found that the dominant mode of treatment varied for men and women from the same social background.

While the particular ritual and medical expression of female inferiority are related to Maharashtrian family structure, the images of femininity and mental infirmity deployed are related to women's subordination within the caste system. A number of writers have suggested that the universal devaluation of women is to be explained by their closer association with nature (Moore 1988: 120–21). The association of women with madness can perhaps be seen as a manifestation or elaboration of this more general theme. Women's alleged instability is explained in terms of their pollution proneness and both characterisations appear to emphasize women's affinity with nature. However, the recognition of these negative stereotypes should not divert attention from the very real mental health problems of Maharashtrian women. Kynch and Sen found that the general health of women in Calcutta was worse than that of men (1983: 376) and that throughout India there is a 'sex differential in sustenance and survival' (ibid.: 377). While one might, therefore, expect women to have poorer mental health also, evidence from Maharashtra should caution against substituting stereotypes derived from and buttressing the social structure for more careful empirical evidence. Kynch and Sen (ibid.) are surely right in claiming that Indian women experience considerable discrimination and neglect in health matters. While fieldwork in the Mahanubhav temple did find evidence of discrimination and neglect against women it could not provide a basis for conclusions about the epidemiology of mental illness. Fieldwork did, however, unearth local epidemiological theories which were buttressed by shared images of male and female nature and which were held despite being completely at odds with the events of daily life in the temple. The priestly image of weak and valetudinarian women is contradicted by the role they play in health care, whether their own or that of others. Moreover, the distribution of illness within the temple showed men to be more severely afflicted than women. Thus in certain respects there is a discrepancy between official beliefs about illness and affliction and how things are. Indeed, the official line actively represses alternative, competing theories of affliction and reinterprets behaviour in a way to suit itself. However, it also has a more far-reaching effect in actively promoting trance in women. Thus the priestly view of affliction is a true ideology: it moulds behaviour to its requirements and decries the reality of behaviour which is incompatible with its views. In this process the true complexity of temple activities, the varieties of affliction and responses to male and female affliction are hidden. The complexity of the temple situation also poses a challenge to the distinction, now part of anthropological orthodoxy, between voluntary possession or mediumship and involuntary possession or illness. I suggest that the distinction between possession/illness and mediumship lies not so much in the differences in possession behaviour or even in the role of possession within a historical trajectory but rather in the interpretation put upon such behaviour. Irvine has written that the meaning of possession depends upon 'active participation by an audience that collaborates in attributing meaning to the speaker's behaviour' (1982: 245). In the Mahanubhav case such negotiation over meaning is not successfully resolved and conflicting interpretations of the nature, causes and distribution of possession persist. These conflicting views rest upon inequalities between men and women which manifest themselves most sharply in mental affliction.

Acknowledgements

I am grateful to the British Academy for funding my second field trip to Maharashtra from July to September 1988. I am also grateful to colleagues who read and commented on the draft paper, Rohit Barot, Pam Constantinides, Roland Littlewood and Roy Willis. Above all I am indebted to my research assistant Mr Suresh Kakade.

Notes

1. The material on which this paper is based was originally presented in Venice in September 1988 at the 10th European Conference for Modern South Asian Studies. An earlier version of this paper will be included in the Proceedings of that conference, 'Gender, Caste, and Power in South Asia – Social Status and Mobility in Transitional Societies,' forthcoming, Manohar Publishers, New Delhi.
2. This equation was suggested by Pam Constantinides.
3. I owe this insight to Maxine Bemtsen with whom I discussed the fieldwork and who offered this precise formulation of the problem.

6

ANTHROPOLOGY AND PSYCHIATRY: THE UNEASY ALLIANCE

The subtitle 'the uneasy alliance' reflects the history of the relationship between psychiatry and anthropology. This chapter[1] explores some of the sources of that uneasiness and mutual suspicion. It consists of three parts. The first considers the history of ideas about 'primitive' mentalities and mental illness and the spur this has provided to the anthropological analysis of psychiatric beliefs and practices. The relativist assumptions of this position are examined. The second explores the divergent preoccupations of anthropologists and psychiatrists and the way in which differences in intellectual orientation have led to conflicting ideas as to what constitutes cross-cultural research. The third section shows how the legacy of history combined with current doubts about the validity of anthropological fieldwork have contributed to an uncertainty about the cross-cultural psychiatric enterprise and an over-preoccupation with the role of the researcher at the expense of the material to be studied.

To begin with, I want to argue that the present state of cross-cultural psychiatry can only be understood when set in terms of its historical development. Adam Kuper has recently looked at the history of anthropological thought regarding primitive society and concludes that 'the history of the theory of primitive society is the history of an illusion' (1988: 8). Nowhere is this illusion more in evidence than in speculations about primitive mentalities and the ensuing ideas about mental illness in primitive societies.

Another cause of the difficulties relates to the early history of psychiatric interest in primitive societies. Not only were many of the early anthropologists trained in medicine but virtually all the early psychoanalysts expressed an interest in 'primitive man'. The developmental and archaeological model of the psyche favoured by psychoanalysts lent itself particularly well to a search for homologous structures in society. The chronologically early, instinctual portions of the human psyche were, indeed, described as primitive and therefore the very vocabulary of psychoanalysis invited a comparison of the untamed potentially disruptive instinctual parts of the self with primitive societies. Common to all the psychoanalytic thinkers is the idea that the study of the psychology of primitive peoples is a useful adjunct to self-understanding. On the first page of *Totem and Taboo* Freud writes 'a comparison between the psychology of primitive peoples, as it is taught by social anthropology, and the psychology of neurotics, as it has been revealed by psychoanalysis, will be bound to show numerous points of agreement and will throw new light upon familiar facts in both sciences' (1950: 1). The alleged correspondence between the repressed and unconscious layers of civilized man's psyche and the mentality of primitive man led Jung to write of the dangers for civilized man of contact with primitive societies. He wrote 'Now what is more contagious than to live side by side with a rather primitive people? Go to Africa and see what happens. The inferior man exercises a tremendous pull upon civilized beings who are forced to live with him, because he fascinates the inferior layers of our psyche, which has lived through untold ages of similar conditions' (quoted in Fernando 1988: 20). So contact with primitive man is seen as disrupting the delicate balancing act required for civilized society because primitive man embodies the untrammelled expression of desires repressed in his civilized counterpart. One reason why such freedom of expression was thought to reign among primitives was because the social, moral and spiritual aspects of the psyche were thought to be poorly developed among them. Jung held that negroes are lacking a whole historical layer in the brain. Seligman wrote of the greater suggestibility, proneness to disassociation and extroversion of savages compared to North Europeans. Indeed, he went on to claim that 'superficially in certain reactions they resembled hysterics' (1924a: 15).

Another source of the difference between civilized and primitive man is held to lie in the ease with which unconscious factors permeate the thought processes of primitive man. Ernest Jones wrote that 'the conscious thinking of savages is more directly and extensively influenced by unconscious factors' and two consequences of this are that 'savages have held one another just as responsible for their intentions as for their deeds and also that they possess an acute capacity for divining those intentions as evidenced by the accuracy of witchcraft accusations' (1924a: 56). Small wonder then that Kraepelin (though not a psychoanalyst) thought that primitive societies were useful to Western man in providing 'natural laboratories for the study of insanity' (1974: 4). Both primitive societies and insanity were thought to represent earlier stages of mental evolution. The intellectual advantages of the comparison were seemingly not outweighed by the differences between civilized and primitive man. The moral inferiority of primitive man did not detract from the fascination of the comparison, although it did give rise to later extraordinary claims such as that there was an absence of depression in primitive man.

Nowadays these early psychiatric and psychoanalytic ideas are frequently mentioned and are judged to reveal more about the theorizers than about the societies which they purport to describe. They are perceived as gross fantasies nurtured by the social structures within which they have arisen. For example, the coupling of women's psyches with that of primitive man as equally excitable, suggestible and lacking in self-control could plausibly be analyzed as a reflection of the weakness of women's social position combined with the disruptive potential of their sexuality. Although much of the early psychoanalytic literature now inspires shame and ridicule, it yet provides an opportunity for demonstrating the anthropologists' analytical prowess.

The anthropological study of psychiatry has received a stimulus not only from an investigation of the recent past of both disciplines but also from the burgeoning of more wide-ranging research in the history of psychiatry and medicine. Proceeding from the investigation of isolated and startling facets of medical and psychiatric history the scope of the subject has been much enlarged. Earlier interest focused on episodes in medical history, often shameful and obviously instances in which the doctor had got it wrong. Szasz's (1971) presentation of Benjamin Rush's theory of negritude is a good example. Rush was persuaded that blackness was an illness and this idea was suggested to him by the case of Henry Moss, a negro slave who suffered from a rare skin condition called vitiligo in which the skin lost all pigmentation. This convinced Rush that Moss had undergone a spontaneous cure of the condition of blackness and that all negroes were afflicted with the congenital condition of blackness. The nature of the condition of negritude meant that negro slaves were passed as medically safe for work as domestic servants and yet the hereditary nature of the disease required their sexual segregation. It was, argued Szasz, the perfect medical category in that it served both the medical profession by expanding its legitimate area of competence and the interests of society which called for segregation and subordination of negroes. The medical condition of nostalgia suffered by soldiers during the First World War, drapetomania (the tendency of slaves to run away from their masters), and masturbational insanity are further examples which readily lend themselves to an anthropological analysis. It seems that the further removed we are from the social values and practices which nurtured such nosological categories, the easier it becomes to perceive the aptness of a sociological type of analysis. Hysteria retains a middle ground in this respect in that, although anthropological and feminist critiques of hysteria abound, psychiatrists have not altogether dispensed with the diagnosis. Its lingering hold on psychiatry suggests that we still share some of the values which encouraged its appearance. Whilst many of these examples are arresting they can sometimes be perceived as isolated instances of the psychiatrists' irrationality or of medicine losing its way. The same cannot be said of the more recent work in the history of medicine and psychiatry. Recent historians have avoided an emphasis on medical eccentricities but have instead sought to bring a more consistent and steady attention to bear upon the study of psychiatric ideas and institutions.

Much of this work has been deeply influenced by anthropology if not actually carried out by anthropologists or sociologists. Michael MacDonald, Keith Thomas and Roy Porter are historians profoundly and fruitfully influenced by anthropology. Andrew Scull and David Armstrong are sociologists both of whom have made a huge contribution to the history of psychiatry. The work of these historians is characterized by what could be described as an immanentist approach which seeks to make sense of allegedly symptomatic behaviour from within, thus demystifying it. MacDonald's book *Mystical Bedlam* (1981) looks at the practice of the astrologist Napier and through a meticulous examination of his notebooks is able to reconstruct for us the interior world of seventeenth-century men and women and link the fearsome role that insanity played in their minds to the outward features of their social life. The procedures for determining whether or not a man or woman is insane throw the social contours of the time into sharp relief. For example, MacDonald writes of people who 'to show that a person was insane examined his relations with his family with an intensity that mirrored the importance of those ties in their own life' (ibid.: 165). Much attention was also paid to the clothing of the insane. Again he writes: 'Nothing signalizes the rank of a person more plainly than dress and Tudor and Stuart observers paid inordinate attention to the clothes – or lack of them – of madmen. Nakedness was included among the symptoms of mania in ancient and medieval times' (ibid.: 129). MacDonald's acute presentation draws out both the individual's thoughts and feelings about insanity as well as the relationship of such individual attitudes to shared values regarding the family, property and social rank. In a truly Durkheimian analysis the characterization of madness is perceived as reflecting the public domain of institutions and values whilst at the same time providing an opportunity for their reaffirmation.

The work of the sociologists, on the other hand, has had a different emphasis. It has been concerned with questioning the independent scientific status of psychiatry. For example, Andrew Scull's (1989) analysis of the development of institutional psychiatry in the nineteenth century points to the interdependence of the supposedly pure and scientific aspects of psychiatric theory and the changing character of society. He examines the demographic shifts from country to town, the difficulty of maintaining idle or non-working family members in the new urban setting and the growth of specializations such as psychiatry within medicine. The consequence of these changes was the need to delimit an area of competence exclusive to psychiatry and this was achieved by developing an increasingly detailed system of psychiatric nosology and an asylum-based system of therapeutics. According to Scull modern psychiatry has grown out of the simultaneous *push* from society which now required an institutional solution to the problem of madness and the *pull* from doctors anxious to establish for themselves a distinctive medical specialization. Scull's analysis denies any independent intellectual status to psychiatry since the growth of this specialization and its characterization of the nature and treatment of mental illness are judged to be intimately linked to the industrialization of nineteenth century society. To the all-embracing eye of the social scientist psychiatric theory and practice are just pieces of a jigsaw which produce a meaningful picture only when joined to other pieces of the puzzle which form its context.

Armstrong is another sociologist who has developed an interest in the history of psychiatry. His book *The Political Anatomy of the Body* offers a discussion of the development of twentieth-century psychiatry in a language which owes much to Foucault. Armstrong describes anatomy as political because the way in which the body is perceived and described depends, he argues, upon 'certain mechanisms of power which, since the eighteenth century, have pervaded the body and continue to hold it in its grasp' (1983: 2).

But the more important part of his argument relates to the subtitle of the book, namely 'medical knowledge in the 20th century'. The argument which Armstrong pursues, with considerably more subtlety than my brief summary can convey, is that in this century a new way of seeing illness has emerged to which he gives the shorthand title of Dispensary. 'The Dispensary was a device, above all else, for making visible to constant surveillance the interaction between people, normal and abnormal, and thereby transforming the physical space between bodies into a social space traversed by power. At the beginning of the twentieth-century the "social" was born as an autonomous realm' (ibid.: 10). Thus the late-eighteenth-century clinical gaze which Foucault had described as concentrating on pathology contained within discrete and passive bodies was replaced by a new vision (1973: 3). By the early twentieth-century, health was seen as social and the dispensary as providing the appropriate techniques for its surveillance. In this new conceptualisation the policy was not essentially a static phenomenon to be localized to a specific point but was seen to travel through the social body appearing only intermittently. Whereas the nineteenth-century public health movement had seen the environment, both natural and socially created, as posing threats to individual health, the new approach perceived the dangers to lie in social relationships. Armstrong develops this theme by reviewing changes in the fields of psychiatry, paediatrics, geriatrics and general practice. A concomitant of this extension of the clinical gaze into the community and the monitoring of social relationships is that the hitherto unbroken boundary between normal and abnormal disappears. This has particular importance in the field of psychiatry where the fusing of distinct categories of sane and insane gives birth to a new concept – the neurosis. Armstrong argues that in the first half of the century psychiatric attention shifted from insanity to psychoneuroses and explains this in terms of an increasingly panoptic, disciplinarian vision. 'The diagnosis of insanity had been a ritual of exclusion. In contrast, the neuroses celebrated the ideal of a disciplined society in which all were analysed and distributed' (ibid.: 22).

The question which the book fails to address, and therefore to answer, concerns the ultimate nature and purpose of this hidden agenda: namely, what lies behind the will to control and coerce? Whilst the panoptic vision of the psychiatrist is presented as having a sinister effect if not intent, this is emulated by an even more panoptic sociological vision. Indeed, the fascination of the work of all three historians described could be said to reside in the panoptic vision which they offer and in the intellectual freedom opened up by this vision. Although MacDonald, Scull and Armstrong write from different theoretical perspectives (being influenced by Durkheim, Marx and Foucault respectively), each in a different way throws doubt on the intellectual purity of psychiatric ideas. Once underway, this intellectual exercise inevitably influences the perception of present-day psychiatric practice and of what should be involved in the study of cross-cultural psychiatry. This kind of vision is easier to exercise over societies far removed in time and space since the quality of alienness provides a spur to anthropological understanding. Thus the social roots of indigenous ideas of mental illness are more readily perceived. However, it also leads to a questioning of contemporary psychiatric practices. Why should Western psychiatry have acquired an intellectual immunity from its social surroundings? Historical studies of psychiatry insistently force this question upon our attention. Reading history books must reduce the confidence of practitioners in the theoretical framework of psychiatry.

Ethnocentrism has been as much a feature of anthropological as of psychiatric thought. Indeed, social anthropology has shared many of the ideas and attitudes of the early psychiatrists to the psychology of primitive man although the paths taken to arrive at this final position have been different. Lévy-Bruhl (1966) advocated a polarity between primitive and scientific thought, the former being characterized by a rejection of the law of contradiction and its replacement by mystical participation. This style of thought he named pre-logical. This distinction bears a remarkable resemblance to Freud's primary and secondary thought processes as characterized in *The Interpretation of Dreams* (1900: 588–621). Primary thought processes are concerned with instinctual gratification and are characterized by condensation (images are fused) and displacement (images readily replace one another) and are unconstrained by time and space. By contrast, secondary thought processes obey the laws of grammar and formal logic and are constrained by space, time and the demands of reality. In sum, Freud appears to be giving a detailed analysis of what Lévy-Bruhl later called pre-logical and scientific mentality. However, whereas Freud's account is biologically grounded Lévy-Bruhl's analysis is culturally grounded. Primitive mentality is held to arise from collective representations and not from primitive genetic endowment. Thus although the anthropological and psychoanalytic interpretation of mind is quite different, the final position is to all intents and purposes identical. The benefit of hindsight enables us to perceive both anthropological and psychoanalytic accounts as belonging to a common European tradition of attitudes towards primitive man and to pursue analyses which reveal their underlying ethnocentrism.

This ethnocentrism of the early psychiatric and anthropological theories has been condemned, in particular the misguidedness of imposing psychological or psychoanalytic theoretical constructs onto indigenous constructs and the behaviour which they mould. A phenomenological perspective is deployed to reveal the wrongness of imposing second-order constructs on a reality which is already ordered by beliefs about the human body, illness, suffering and madness. Whilst such a critique yields dividends in terms of the development of a sociology and history of psychiatry, the problems in dealing with the first-order constructs remain. Short of a thoroughgoing relativism, which exposes but does not explain, the problems of translating one culture in terms of another remain. The ethnomethodological approach provides one attempt to circumvent the problems of relativism. For example, Dorothy Smith (1978) produces a rich ethnographic account of the sub-texts of mental illness but does not escape from the orthodoxy of relativism. The detailed mapping of cognitive transformations from events into 'facts' about a college girl who comes to be recognized by her friends as mentally ill forms an important but incomplete part of an anthropological enterprise. Nichter's (1981) work on idioms of distress in South India provides another illustration of both the strengths and weaknesses of the relativists' position. His immersion in the culture provides an anthropologically informed 'narrative from within'. It does not provide a basis for comparison. The substitution of a non-medical word such as distress for disorder or illness does not solve the problem of understanding another culture. It is not dispelled by avoiding medical and psychiatric language, although the problem may be more readily visible in that context. For how can we be sure that we are not imposing a Western conception of distress on South Indian people? Simply using English as a medium of description already poses problems.

On the other hand, it is difficult to see what would constitute anthropo-logical explanation if it gave up all claims to translation of one culture into another and of comparison. Anthropological understanding is achieved not simply by immersion in the language and mores of a culture but by subjecting belief systems to the scrutiny of an alien conceptual framework. If anthropology is to remain a comparative discipline, as Radcliffe-Brown (1952) urged it should, then ethnomethodological description is not enough. We need both the richness and internal perspective provided by the ethnomethodological, or revised participant observer approach and also the intellectual opportunities opened up by second-order analysis consciously and explicitly pursued.

The uncovering of ethnocentrism, racism or whatever else in psychiatric theory in no way resolves the problems which it identifies. It simply superimposes a third-order analysis substituting sociological for medical and psychological concepts. Whilst the anthropological analysis may look convincing now, there is no guarantee that a later, broader and more sophisticated perspective may not produce yet a further fourth-order analysis and so on *ad infinitum*. Intellectual limitations may require us to put a halt to this imaginative exercise, but it should alert us to the logical contradictions involved in critical enterprises of this kind. The privileged access of anthropologists to the people they study derives from their Trojan-horse disguise and the fact that anthropological theoretical armamentaria lie hidden within. The implicit needs to be made explicit.

The problems common to psychiatry and anthropology are more difficult to perceive when it comes to the present. One source of the perceived division between the two disciplines and of the anthropologist's distrust of psychology (and by implication psychiatry) derives from Durkheim. Although Durkheim did not specifically address the subject of mental illness his writing has had enormous influence on cross-cultural psychiatry. More specifically his analysis of the social origins of religious thought (which for Durkheim was equated with the irrational) has been readily extended and elaborated to provide a fresh intellectual perspective on mental illness. The Durkheimian stance is best summarized in the famous edict: 'Every time a social phenomenon is directly explained by a psychological phenomenon we may be sure that the explanation is false' (Durkheim 1966: 104). Taken to heart by cross-cultural psychiatry the impact of this statement has been the reappraisal of concepts of mental health and illness as culturally grounded categories whose intelligibility depends upon a proper identification of their social roots rather than the identification of the behaviour to which they refer. Secondly, Durkheim's writing on crime has also been influential. He argues that it is the societal reaction rather than the intrinsic nature of the act which determines whether or not it is a crime. Moreover, crime is a universal feature of all societies because it performs a vital function: the social response to crime defines and reinforces social values. This analysis of crime has been transplanted to an analysis of concepts and attitudes concerned with mental health and illness.

With the exception of a few unreconstructed Freudians, twentieth-century medical anthropologists have maintained a tight grip on their Durkheimian hats. References such as Marvin Opler's to 'the trap of deriving cultural forms from psychodynamic processes' (1969: 91) have now become part of anthropological orthodoxy. The so-called 'new' cross-cultural psychiatry claims to have taken on board Durkheim's approach with seemingly little acknowledgement of its earlier influence. For example, W.H.R. Rivers had many years earlier stated 'it is only by the study of such social processes and institutions as mythology, language and religion that we can hope to understand the mental states in which these and all other forms of social activity have their ultimate source' (1916: 246). However, his dual training in medicine and anthropology must have left him rather confused because we also find him saying 'To me as to most students of the subject the final aim of the study of society is the explanation of social behaviour in terms of psychology' (ibid.: 234). Clearly he was not quite sure which hat he was supposed to be wearing.

However, the introduction of a Durkheimian perspective, whilst it emphasizes the importance of relativism for the concepts studied, can in no way exempt the cross-cultural psychiatrist or the medical anthropologist from that relativism. Both are tarred by their own brush. The writings of Lévy-Bruhl and Freud on primitive mentality and primary thought processes provide a concrete example of what Durkheim was affirming and it demonstrates how psychological as well as sociological theorizing is rooted in a social matrix. Thus whilst the anthropological perspective provides ammunition for a demolition job on the theoretical forays of earlier times and other disciplines (in particular of other disciplines in earlier times) it also throws uncertainty over anthropological theorizing as such. If such theories do, indeed, have social roots then their truth must be as short-lived as the forms of social life from which they emerge. According to Kleinman 'the chief failing of the "old transcultural psychiatry" is its total reliance on Western psychiatric categories which are applied by clinicians and epidemiologists as if they were independent of cultural bias, but which in fact are culture-specific categories' (1977: 4). Explaining the source of that bias and the social roots of conceptual (in this case diagnostic) categories becomes the chief task of the self-referential cross-cultural psychiatrist. The 'new' cross-cultural psychiatry combines anthropological and psychiatric research perspectives and thus it is claimed overcomes the ethnocentric pitfalls of earlier work. However, despite protestations to the contrary, Kleinman does not dispense with Western diagnosis. The innocent sounding claim 'My research assistants and I assembled a group of 25 patients with the depressive syndrome who presented consecutively at two of the daily psychiatric clinics' (ibid.: 5) hurriedly passes over the most momentous theoretical obstacles. How and why were these patients identified as suffering from the depressive syndrome? Twenty-two of these patients did not actually complain of depressive feelings. Ten never admitted to such feelings. What were the criteria used for identifying them if not those of Western psychiatric diagnostic categories? However much Kleinman may protest his sensitivity to cultural variations he has not dispensed with the intellectual outlook of the Western psychiatrist. It seems that he has retained a stealthy hold of Western nosology whilst publicly proclaiming the wrongness of so doing. As in the earlier case of Rivers, the dual training in psychiatry and anthropology, whilst it may temporarily mask problems, does not overcome them. The fact that any one individual is capable of wearing two hats does not remove the fact that those two hats sit on top of contradictory theoretical positions. Unless one concedes to anthropology a lowly under-worker role of identifying cultural influences on the presentation of illness taken to task by Littlewood (1985), anthropology reveals the radical role of culture in shaping categories of health and illness. Within this model there is little room for the psychiatrist and acquiring a second hat does nothing to ease the awkward fit of the first. Some might not have entered the alliance if they knew exactly what they were letting themselves in for.

The methodological problems of understanding and explaining which cross-cultural psychiatry poses are, of course, not unique to it, but an offshoot of anthropology's pervasive problems of relativism, rationality and interpretation. However, they surface most acutely and persistently in the interface between anthropology and psychiatry and can perhaps be put into perspective by considering some of the central issues raised by the rationality debate. These relate to such questions as: how, if at all, understanding across cultures is to be achieved, given that other cultures have radically different ways of addressing reality and organizing social life? Are cultures relative to particular types of men and women, social context, or – to use Wittgenstein's term – 'forms of life'? (2001: 23). Or is there a common core of rationality which transcends outward differences of beliefs and practices? Are there shared features which unite all human beings and all societies? Do different worlds have parts in common? Given the differences between people how can one culture be made intelligible to another? Does understanding involve an empathic leap into the dark, so to speak, or does it rest upon a cautious building up from a shared common core of assumptions? Is there an intrinsic indeterminacy regarding trans-lation from one culture to another as the philosopher Quine maintained? (1960) Or are different cultures simply incommensurable, such that their respective rules of thought have nothing in common and understanding between them is impossible? The indeterminacy thesis suggests that there are too many translations and no way of deciding which is the correct one, while the incommensurability thesis suggests that there are no translations at all.

These are problems which beset every practising anthropologist but they bedevil the anthropological study of psychiatry twice over. Not only are anthropologists faced with alien cultures, but they are faced with behaviours which alien cultures judge to be alien. The neat hermeneutic triangle of meaning, belief and action (see Newton-Smith 1982: 114) which most anthropologists aspire to and succeed in entering appears to break apart and splinter into a plurality of worlds.

The 'old' transcultural psychiatrists set about this problem by assessing the abnormality of behaviour against the yardstick of Western psychiatric diagnostic categories. The term itself implied that culture can be transcended. Where the behaviour did not readily fit these categories it was claimed that the culture had influenced the overt content of the illness, but that the underlying form was the same. More attention was paid to behaviour than beliefs. The Russian dolls model (Littlewood 1985) suggests that, if the outer layers are removed, hidden within lies a core of illness which is common to all people. This approach, whilst it is still widely held by most psychiatrists, has become very unfashionable amongst anthropologists. The 'new' cross-cultural psychiatry by contrast offers an anthropological investigation of indigenous disease categories. It castigates the 'old' transcultural psychiatry for its ethnocentric over reliance on Western psychiatric categories. These categories are not, they argued, free of cultural bias but are in fact culture-specific; specific, that is to the West. Disease categories must be analysed in terms of the indigenous culture's values and roles and the conflicts and contradictions which they generate.

How do the two positions, namely transcultural psychiatry and the new cross-cultural psychiatry, relate to the quarrel over rationality and to sociological theory? The most striking observation is that the argument between the transcultural and new cross-cultural psychiatrists has been conducted as though the rationality debate had never taken place. The new cross-cultural psychiatrists advocate a contextual analysis of indigenous disease categories and decry the importation of all Western categories. But how precisely is understanding of mental illness categories and the behaviour to which they relate arrived at? Why is a particular state of affairs or pattern of feeling and behaviour considered to fall under the category of 'mental illness' at all? The rationality debate opens up some of the problems inherent in both the old and the new approaches.

But if we accept relativism then how is interpretation possible? As Gellner (1982: 185) has said, no anthropologist has come back from a field trip where the people have been so strange that he has had to admit total failure of understanding. My psychiatrist colleagues on the other hand frequently admit to complete bafflement about their patients. Even the most ardent relativist holds that there is a common core of shared assumptions. Without some measure of agreement, disagreement becomes meaningless. But according to a relativist or coherence theory of truth such agreement as to what constitutes distress is impossible to account for. The shared common core remains in essence obscure. This unresolved issue presents particular problems for the new cross-cultural psychiatry. The very success of its approach, the fact that it has explanatory power, throws doubt on the relativism which it claims to espouse.

Before I move on to the next section a recapitulation of the main points of the argument may be useful. One of the reasons why relations between anthropologists and psychiatrists are not always easy stems from the early history of the psychoanalytic movement. Much psychoanalytic writing displayed what we now perceive to be racist attitudes to primitive peoples. Whilst anthropological analysis enables us to distance ourselves from such views, it also introduces the fearsome prospect of total relativism. Present day cross-cultural psychiatrists have attempted to eschew these earlier pitfalls by providing an internal perspective on disease categories. However, in practice this policy is not easy to follow and the anthropologist's or cross-cultural psychiatrist's own conceptual framework is brought to bear upon alien medical systems. Buttressing both the sociological analyses of earlier psychiatric writing and contemporary anthropological studies of psychiatric ideas and practices is the Durkheimian approach which explains psychological factors in terms of sociological ones. However, the Durkheimian approach also introduces an element of intellectual instability and uncertainty into the situation since the search for the social roots of belief systems undermines the claims to truth not only of the belief systems studied but also of the anthropological analysis itself and is potentially endless.

The last half of my chapter examines some crucial differences in the theoretical orientations of anthropology and psychiatry. In a classic essay Devereux (1956) asked what were the key concepts in psychiatry and anthropology and identified the concepts of normality and culture respectively. Although much of the rest of that essay (devoted to the question of the normality of the shaman) sounds dated, the importance given to normality and culture was surely right. Devereux argues that cross-cultural psychiatry must encompass both the concepts of normality/ abnormality and of culture within its theoretical embrace. But his own article attests to the difficulty of so doing. As a psychiatrist he is concerned with 'the determination of the exact locus of the boundary between normal and abnormal' (ibid.: 3). As an anthropologist his interest in normality should be less pragmatic and focused on its meaning within a particular culture. Much interdisciplinary conflict revolves around these two basic concepts. The concepts of norm, normality and abnormality central to psychiatric thought are, as the philosopher Peter Alexander (1973) reminds us, essentially statistical concepts and it is clear that despite his psychoanalytic terminology Devereux had a statistical notion in mind. Alexander argues that we only have a concept of the abnormal because we know how people usually behave. Any radical departure from the statistical norms of usual behaviour is recognized as deviance. This view does not ignore the subsidiary role of culture and values in moulding behaviour. However, it does deny the direct role of culture in shaping concepts of normality and abnormality. This statistical notion is, I would agree, deeply embedded in psychiatric thought, even though the statistical norms may be imaginary and out-dated and may have grafted upon them secondary value-based concepts of normality and abnormality. A third basic concept of empathy is shared by both disciplines but plays a different role in each. Where statistical notions of normality operate, empathy is limited to an understanding of the usual. Empathy is ineffective beyond the bounds of the usual. For example, Kraepelin argued that 'empathy is a very unsure process ... as a research method it can lead to the greatest self deception', and further, 'we should place little trust in the information we receive from mentally disturbed patients about the processes going on in their minds and about any coherent relationships between them' (1974: 10). Laing and his colleagues notwithstanding, this distrust of empathy as an intellectual tool, as opposed to a contribution towards the oiling of the doctor/patient interaction remains a dominant characteristic of psychiatric theory and practice.

Empathy on the other hand is central to the practice of fieldwork in social anthropology and to the understanding of culture. Geertz in *Works and Lives* writes, 'The ability of anthropologists to get us to take what they say seriously has less to do with either a factual look or an air of conceptual elegance than it has to do with their capacity to convince us that what they say is the result of their having actually penetrated (or, if you prefer, been penetrated by) another form of life, having one way or another, truly "been there"' (1988: 4). And he goes on to say that the anthropologist's chief task in writing is to persuade us that this 'off-stage miracle' has occurred (ibid.: 5). Whatever the qualms voiced by anthropologists themselves about participant observation, for example the lack of systematic training among British anthropologists and its misleading claims to complete authenticity, 'subjective soaking' still forms the ideological core of the anthropological enterprise and specifically the immanentist critique of psychiatry. This whole debate goes back to the *Methodenstreit* in the philosophy of the human sciences in nineteenth-century Germany.

In the context of the alliance between anthropology and psychiatry this has had certain consequences. Some time ago, Durkheim not withstanding, Victor Turner set modest limitations to the scope of anthropological competence, suggesting that 'the structure and properties of psyches' (1964: 5) be left to the psychoanalysts. Turner demarcates two poles for the understanding of ritual; the normative social pole and the sensory, individual pole, this latter being, he argued, beyond the limits of the anthropologist's legitimate field of competence. Most medical anthropologists and cross-cultural psychiatrists would now argue that he was beating too hasty a retreat, and that on the score of skills, both in fieldwork techniques and in theoretical analysis, they were uniquely equipped to give an account of the problems of individual psyches. The empathic skills required for participant observation are able to provide an internally coherent account of deviant behaviour which is then translated into the culture and language of the observer. The analytic skills of the observing anthropologist demonstrate the relationship between that behaviour and other aspects of the culture – in short its intelligibility.

This divergence of perspectives gives rise to inter-disciplinary problems. Whilst psychiatrists tend not to perceive themselves as being in short supply of empathy this is conceived as empathic concern contributing to recovery rather than intellectual understanding. The appropriation of empathy by anthropologists thus leaves the psychiatrist rather bewildered. Why should anthropologists be particularly good at it? The immanentist arguments provide a critique, but in no way guarantee the presence of that scarce commodity. There seems to be no good reason why it should be their exclusive preserve. Indeed, psychiatrists might plausibly argue that they have a greater opportunity to develop empathy because of the nature of their work. They could point to the continued contact with other human beings and their exposure to a wide spectrum of suffering. Moreover, the elevation of empathy to a research tool creates puzzlement among non-anthropologists, which finds expression in such questions as 'what exactly are you doing?' or 'I'm not quite clear as to what your objectives are' or 'what exactly is your methodology?' Often attempts at answers to these questions lead to more confusion rather than enlightenment. Thus whilst the presence of an anthropologist in a department of psychiatry or on a project may be perceived as a good thing in principle, in practice this may occasion puzzlement.

Moreover, the analytic and interpretative skills of the anthropologist as directed towards psychiatric problems frequently have the effect of dissolving the essence of what was conceived as a psychiatric problem and refashioning it as a social problem. Thus the introduction of anthropologists as part of a team may be perceived as a form of hijacking or an imperialist venture. Perhaps the more accurate term would be 'irredentism' suggested by Peter Sedgwick (1972). This term refers to the recovery of lost territory rather than the conquest of new territory. The new cross-cultural psychiatry and its practitioners no longer recognize the limits of naivety so carefully guarded by an earlier generation. The theoretical framework of Western psychiatry itself, such as the central concepts of mind/body duality and personality, as well as the system of psychiatric classification, have come under the scrutiny of the anthropological eye. Since Roland Littlewood and Maurice Lipsedge started writing (e.g. 1982), so called culture-bound syndromes are no longer perceived as the product of remote and exotic cultures.

The anthropological move in the direction of psychiatry is encouraged not only by this example of psychiatric history, but also by the need to find new pastures for anthropological investigation. The drying up of 'exemplary elsewheres' as Geertz (1988: 132) calls the societies studied by anthropologists has led to a search for the strange or alien within, namely psychiatric theory and practice – its patients and hospitals. Whilst anthropologists have developed an anxiety about the moral legitimacy of anthropological fieldwork in less developed societies such reservations have not been transferred to the study of psychiatric patients where the fieldworker is cast in the role of ally or victim.

The study of mental illness by psychiatrists is perceived as dehumanizing and morally insulting. The very terminology of psychiatry is, it is argued, morally loaded against the sufferer. Words like patient, case, illness and psychiatric diagnoses, engender a profound unease in the anthropologist. In short, not only does classification involve illegitimate cultural extrapolation, it is also equated with contempt for the actor's thoughts and feelings. However, the anthropologist is persuaded and must persuade that his or her approach does not do this. Geertz's (1988) 'pervasive nervousness' about the whole business of claiming to explain 'enigmatical others' comes to the fore here (ibid.: 137). The result is that the researcher and his or her subjective experience of research becomes the primary focus of attention if not the object of analysis. Goffman set the confessional tone in his introduction to *Asylums*. 'Unlike some patients I come to the hospital with no great respect for the discipline of psychiatry nor for the agencies content with its current practice' (1968: 8). Other writers feel called upon to emphasize the transformation wrought within themselves by the ethnographic experience. Sue Estroff (1981) in *Making It Crazy* describes the emotional scars left by the ethnographic experience.

It seems that cross-cultural anthropology has taken over where anti-psychiatry petered out. Whereas the anti-psychiatrists saw mental illness as convenient social fictions, the anthropologists see mental illness as nodules of conflict. In both there is in the final analysis a denial of a valid field of psychiatric activity. What role then is left for the fieldworker after the anthropological analysis of indigenous categories of mental illness has taken place? It has, I would suggest, not only removed the legitimate object of study of psychiatry but has also made the anthropological study of mental illness difficult. Hence, the growing emphasis on the researcher's role at the expense of the subjects studied. A west of England study on depression among Asian women tries, so it seems, to walk without touching the ground (Fenton and Sadiq-Sangster 1996). At a recent conference the two field workers described their involvement and attachment to the women studied. But the presentation of material about the depressed women was problematic. Whilst they claimed not to accept the category of depression they did accept the depth of feeling. What then were they studying? They were, they claimed, studying the kinds of feelings others would describe as depression.

I would like now to draw my discussion to a close by offering a few concluding remarks. One result of the growth of a history of psychiatry which has drawn upon a variety of theoretical sources in anthropology and sociology has been the encompassment of psychiatry within the sociology of knowledge. Whilst this has thrown the shadow of epistemological relativism over cross-cultural psychiatry it has also moved the subject to the centre stage where anthropology's perennial problems of theory and method meet. However, the new anthropological approach to psychiatry is neither so very new nor is it exempt from relativism. Its own arguments condemn it. We all know that self-reference can lead to problems, not least the problems of knowing when to stop (see, for example, Hollis 1982).

The second half of the chapter focused on certain incompatibilities of outlook between the two disciplines. The anthropological approach, by focusing on submersion in a culture and empathy as a method for understanding one's informants, aims to overcome these problems of relativism. The consequences for an interdisciplinary alliance are problematic. Some have attempted to solve these by joining both camps – only to find like Rivers that this does not lessen the theoretical confusion. Others clearly relish the tension on which the alliance is built. Perhaps, like all good alliances, that between anthropology and psychiatry contains a major theoretical paradox.

Notes

1. Based upon the Keynote Address at the 10th Annual Meeting of the Society for the Study of Psychiatry and Culture, Farnham Castle, England, October, 1989.

7

REMEMBERING AND FORGETTING: ANTHROPOLOGY AND PSYCHIATRY – THE CHANGING RELATIONSHIP

Those who are incapable of a science, write its history, discuss its methods or criticise its scope.

Marcel Mauss (1979: 10)

I propose in this chapter to look at the sources of solidarity and difference between anthropology and psychiatry. Historically there is more uniting than dividing the two disciplines. Differences are of recent origin and relate to the more radical role that anthropology has assumed towards memory and other psychological processes. This turn in anthropology is in line with postmodernist trends and leaves psychiatry outside. I want to explore the nature of this bifurcation by focusing on memory. Until relatively recently memory was the preserve of psychologists and psychiatrists. Its appropriation by social anthropologists and its very differently perceived status and function serve to highlight the nature of the rift that is opening up between the two disciplines.

Anthropologists bury their ancestors – and especially the unwanted ones – deep. But like certain New Guinea peoples they then feel called upon ritually to exhume them; the deeper the burial, the more fun the exhumation. I propose to look at some of anthropology's ancestors and kinship ties and to examine how and why its psychological relatives came to be unwanted.

But first, let us return to the similarities. Anthropology and psychiatry are children of the Enlightenment project: the optimistic commitment to human reason and its powers of penetrating and dispersing unreason. Nineteenth-century evolutionary anthropologists and psychiatrists were within this tradition. They were united by a certain evangelical interest in the primitive. Tylor's view of cultures was hierarchical, but like Tory self-perceptions ultimately democratic in the long run (1958). This contrasts with the early divisive view of culture of Lévy-Bruhl (1966). Civilization lay within the grasp of all peoples who joined the evolutionary master narrative. Freud's view of the conscious replacing the unconscious – where id was, ego shall be – is in this same tradition (1973: 50). Indeed, psycho-analytic theory succeeds in fusing individual and evolutionary time. The indebtedness was mutual. Nineteenth-century and early twentieth-century anthropologists borrowed ideas from contemporary psychologists and psychiatrists to explain primitive beliefs and rituals. Conversely, psychia-trists made free use of anthropological writings for their own ends. Thus, Malinowski made much use of Freud's ideas, while Freud himself relied heavily on (highly suspect and speculative) anthropology (Stocking 1986).

Anthropology has been defined as the study of the other. Roland Littlewood and Maurice Lipsedge (1997) in their justly celebrated book *Aliens and Alienists* draw our attention to the shared preoccupations of psychiatrists and anthropologists in this respect. Anthropology started life as the study of the exotic, providing Victorian society with a reverse image of itself and the barbaric conditions it had left behind. Psychiatry as an institutionalized set of practices is associated with the Enlightenment and the elevation of reason. Its object, the madman, provides the reverse image of humanity's most highly valued characteristic – reason.

There are other issues which draw the two disciplines together. The Socratic precept 'know thyself' has long been a core ingredient of psycho-analytic and psychotherapeutic practice. More recently this injunction has been adopted by some anthropological circles as orthodoxy. The imper-sonal voice and the timeless present of earlier ethnographic studies concealed interests that had little bearing on the scientific study of mankind. Tense and person, it is argued, create the spurious illusion of objectivity and moral impartiality, at the same time allowing the anthropo-logist to get away with unexamined prejudices. Such unreflexive practices promote the projection of stereotypes which in turn shape and sustain the anthropologist's own fragile identity. The emergence of a critical self-awareness has put the anthropologist under the microscopic gaze of profes-sional peers. If an anthropological monograph does not contain a personal or autobiographical statement of the author's position and involvement in their research it is sure to be highlighted by their critics. If we follow this road, we may end by asking: are we really studying ourselves? Has our preoccupation with our own involvement in the production of research come to interfere with our ability to recognize differences between others as Barth (1996) suggests? Or have anthropologists learnt from psychiatrists that self-knowledge contributes both to the ways in which we glean knowledge from others and how we subsequently represent it. My own view is that self-awareness and ethnography are mutually enriching. In Bakhtin's words, 'The listener becomes the speaker' (1986: 68) – but this very audibility of the silent listener promotes clarity and understanding. Ethnography is thus not negated but affirmed.

These issues of voice and the construction of knowledge bear on a related field of importance for both psychiatry and anthropology. I refer to the psychoanalytic theories of normal human development and pathology. One of Freud's greatest achievements was to break down the division between the normal and the pathological (1901). The abnormal or pathological does not inhabit a separate order of reality: it is merely a specific elaboration of it. We can describe Freud's achievement either as pathologizing the normal or as normalizing the pathological depending upon our interests and perspective. The paradigm shift entailed by such a perspective has, I believe, influenced anthropological thought. The idea that anthropology is *par excellence* the study of the other, and that the other is constructed as an alter ego and that anthropology is therefore ultimately the study of oneself, belongs to a unifying vision of humankind.

Psychoanalysis, as we all know, is the talking cure. Patients suffer from unsatisfactory stories of the past and the aim of psychoanalysis is to construct a coherent and satisfying account of the past from the fragments of reminiscences. Freud was involved with reconstructing the fragmentary past at the same time as Durkheim was developing the idea of anomie (1984). Psychoanalysis and talking therapies dealt with narratives long before they were of any anthropological interest. Meanwhile, anthropologists, particularly those investigating violence, are acknowledging that lack of coherence can make us ill. The present anthropological and sociological interest in narrative owes much to its ancestor discipline.

For both disciplines the emergence of narrative brings into sharp focus problems of truth and verification. Where does truth lie? On the surface or, as Popper thought, at the bottom of a well (1974)? Do language and narrative open a window on the self and the past or do they create their own densely opaque meanings? We might even argue, following in the footsteps of Freud and more recently of Foucault (2002), that language hides rather than reveals (not, of course, an implication of Popper's view of truth). Language never says exactly what it means. The fascination of narrative is that it both reaches out to reality and in the process creates a new social and personal reality which obscures it. Or does this argument, as Littlewood suggests, presuppose an artificial distinction between form and content (2000)? We may think we are dealing with an artichoke and working our way towards its precious heart, when in fact what we are left with is the humble onion.

Narrative theory, so central to recent theoretical debate in anthropology, suggests that truth lies in every phrase and gesture if only we are skilful and attentive listeners. Narrative form is not merely the gilt on the gingerbread but carries substantive meanings. This approach is surely heavily indebted to the psychoanalytic emphasis on meaning and its unifying role – as well, of course, as drawing upon linguistic and literary theory. One of Freud's principal achievements was to draw in seemingly odd and 'irrational' phenomena – dreams, slips of the tongue, involuntary behaviours – and show them to be potent carriers of meaning.

So far I have suggested that psychoanalysis and anthropology have a number of areas of common theoretical concern. The dual training and more importantly the continued professional involvement of several of the early ancestors of our two disciplines bear witness to their harmonious co-existence. As Adam Kuper has pointed out, 'For the first twenty years of the [twentieth] century British anthropology was very largely in the hands of psychologists and physiologists' (1991: 132). Charles Seligman, William Halse Rivers and A.C. Haddon are examples. 'Other leading psychologists – including Bartlett and McDougall – were active for a while in anthropological research' (ibid.). Although none of them made tremendous advances towards the integration of the two disciplines or, indeed, to theory at all, they promoted a respectful and harmonious coexistence. If anything, priority was given to the explanatory powers of psychology over those of sociology and anthropology. Indeed, Rivers considered sociology to be a descriptive and psychology an explanatory discipline: 'To me, as to most students of the subject, the final aim of the study of society is the explanation of social behaviour in terms of psychology' (1916: 2). This is not, of course, a view that Durkheim would have endorsed particularly when applied to primitive society: 'It may be said, and with special force where societies devoid of all written records are concerned, that the chief instrument for the study of past history is a knowledge of psychology; that only through the knowledge of man's mental processes can we hope to reconstruct the past, so that the study of these mental processes should be our first care' (Rivers, 1916: 3). Seligman acknowledged the importance of Freud's theories to his own understanding of the dreams of 'the non-European races' (1924b: 186). Even Marcel Mauss, Durkheim's nephew, felt no embarrassment about acknowledging his indebtedness to psychology. In his essay on sociology and psychology, in a rhetorical address to psychologists generally, he admitted: 'You know how to get the best out of us' (1979: 2) and 'our analysis of the facts of collective consciousness can indeed speak no other language than your own' (1979: 12). It is thus ironic that Rodney Needham's (1962) famous structuralist onslaught on psychologism, *Structure and Sentiment*, is dedicated to Marcel Mauss. These are not views which anthropologists, psychologists or indeed psychiatrists would echo today. What has happened in the meantime?

Far later these views came to be regarded as heresy. Adam Kuper argues that the divergence in thought came about not because of the influence of the Durkheimian paradigm in anthropology but because of 'political considerations, having to do with the professionalization of British psychology' (1991: 132). The result was a 'sharp recoil' of each from the other.

However, the recoil was not as sharp or as clean cut as Kuper suggests. Radcliffe-Brown, of course, had no truck with psychological explanation but Malinowski's fieldwork was heavily influenced by psychoanalysis. Despite the well-known disagreements over the universality of Oedipus complex, Malinowski was a revisionist Freudian. Instincts or needs, in particular libido, were central to Malinowski's functionalism and, indeed, to his experience of fieldwork, as his diary was to reveal. Malinowski did not challenge Freud's instinct theory outright but made the modest proposal that culture modified the expression of instinct and should, therefore, be taken into account. He did, however, persist in the belief that ultimate explanations rested with psychology. This theoretical allegiance is expressed in his review of *The Group Mind*: 'McDougall was one of the first clearly to appreciate that in problems of social belief, custom and behaviour it is sentiment and instinct which play a paramount part' (Malinowski 1921: 107).

Psychoanalysis is a theory of memory, or rather of forgetting. Indeed W.H.R. Rivers singled out active forgetting 'as the distinctive feature of Freud's system' (1917: 913) More recently Ian Hacking has put this more memorably: 'One feature of the modern sensibility is dazzling in its implausibility: the idea that what has been forgotten is what forms our character, our personality, our soul' (1996: 70). For Hacking the sciences of memory emerging in the nineteenth century enabled society to acquire knowledge, to expose and to discipline the soul. Proceeding hand in hand with 'anatomo-politics' of the human body and 'bio-politics' of human populations, 'memoro-politics' facilitated the shaping of large populations. 'The soul has been a way of internalizing the social order, of putting into myself those very virtues and cruelties that enable my society to survive' (ibid.: 73). Forgotten events offer more opportunity for the social reshaping of the past than those still remembered. Hacking's argument draws its power from his ideas on the indeterminacy of the past. By indeterminacy he means not only that we change our perspectives on the past but that indeterminacy is intrinsic to all human action. Any act can be presented under any number of descriptions:

> When new descriptions become available, when they come into circulation, or even when they become the sorts of things that it is all right to say, to think, then there are new things to choose to do. When new intentions become open to me, because new descriptions, new concepts, become available to me, I live in a new world of opportunities (ibid.: 236).

This type of argument illuminates the development of psychiatric diagnostic categories, in that new angles on human behaviour are discovered through new forms of description. Hacking focuses on multiple personality disorder which 'provided a new way to be an unhappy person' (ibid.: 236).

Hacking is a philosopher whose *Rewriting the Soul* is very influential among anthropologists, including Allan Young. Young's book (1995), as its subtitle *Inventing Post Traumatic Stress Disorder* suggests, is about the creation of diagnostic categories and medical knowledge. I must here, albeit apologetically, summarize this theoretically provocative and scholarly book in a few lines. Young argues that post-traumatic stress disorder (PTSD) is a way of medicalizing the past. Such medicalization and sanitization of the past enables collective traumas, such as war, for example, to be translated into individual problems, thereby alleviating collective responsibility and guilt. Kleinman's articles (1982, 1994) and his book *Writing at the Margins* (1997) also have as one of their central themes the translation of collective violence into individual illness. Now I do not wish to challenge the reality of such processes of medicalization. The astonishing expansion of the history of medicine provides ample evidence for such processes at work. I merely want to suggest that anthropology also has an interest in colonizing the past. It may be that in documenting the processes of medicalization and the politicisation of memory anthropology is seeking to expand its own empire. But to whom does the past belong? Whose empire is it anyway?

If psychoanalysis is a theory of forgetting, as Timpanaro (1976) suggests in *The Freudian Slip*, it does not account for the positive aspects of memory. Why we remember is as important a question as why we forget. On this question anthropologists have much to tell us. Maurice Halbwachs's *The Collective Memory* was translated into English in 1950. It lay dormant for some decades and has belatedly achieved the status of a classic. Halbwachs argues that although we may regard memory as quintessentially private it is, in fact, thoroughly social. Both the quality of experience and memory are determined by the frameworks given by society. Society directs our attention to some aspects of the past and not to others. It is because social frameworks are not yet in place that we remember so little of our childhoods. Halbwachs captures the essentially social nature of memory with the phrase 'We are never alone' (1981: 23). There are, of course, purely personal aspects of memory, but Halbwachs was surely right in questioning the dichotomy between a private world of memory and a public world of experience and perception. *The Collective Memory* has set in motion a series of anthropological and historical studies of memory. These studies pursue a number of different issues, most being a variation on a presentist theme – the idea that narrative and memory tell us more about the present than the past.

Elizabeth Tonkin (1995) has developed a powerful argument about genre in narrative along these lines. A 'genre' in the sense in which Tonkin uses the term 'provides a mode or code for people's transmission of experience, and, as well, by its own transmission, maintains a version of the past which people can use for their own ends' (ibid.: 114). Thus each recollection, be it an oral recitation or a publication, sets up a resonance with the personal experience of its listeners and readers as well as influencing later writers. The genre I am most familiar with is that of testimony, drawn from my study of Latvian memories of collectivization, deportation and exile. In common with all testimonies, these accounts are statements of social as much as of personal identity. In Latvia this genre focuses on the narrative development of a common ethnic identity. The hero of the story is the Latvian nation, and national character ensures survival. The narrative 'I' is sometimes fused with Latvian culture heroes (Skultans 1996, 1998a).

I described anthropological approaches to memory as presentist: versions of the past depend upon the narrator's present experience. However, the situation is yet more complex and its complexity escapes a straightforward presentist position. The testimonies I encountered are given in the present tense. They refer to experiences that have not yet been processed and laid to rest. Past experience of dispossession and dislocation is trapped in an arbitrary and capricious present which makes separation from them difficult and ensures their continued hold over the imagination. As Valentine Daniel writes so insightfully of the Tamils of Sri Lanka: 'When the present looms large in this manner, both memory and hope become either emaciated or bloated. In either case, it is the present that determines the past, making the past a mere simulacrum of the present' (1996: 106–7).

However, for philosophers from Augustine onwards the present has been the most perplexing aspect of time. We may be able to focus on the past and the future, but the present is more inscrutable and escapes our grasp in the very act of focusing on it. Extremes of experience, both joy and terror, transform the present. The presence of violence expands the present so that it has us in its grasp. Thus testimonies about past experience enable the testifier to escape both the past and the present and move towards the future. It is not so much the nature of the present which releases, as the hope and mapping out of a future which violence and the caprice of the present have erased.

Stories of the past therefore relate as much to the future as they do to the past. The programmatic statements of the Latvian Oral History Project make this point quite explicitly, by linking life histories with the quest for a common ethnic identity. Particular versions of the past give a desired shape to the future. Bakhtin's (1986: 68) arresting claim that the listener becomes the speaker is at work here. Listeners and speakers unite in the production of tales of destiny. Thus memory is shaped by the contexts in which it is told and the futures which communities plan for themselves. In focusing on the future – on the imaginative mapping out of the unknown – I am able to single out the specifically anthropological contribution to our understanding of the life of the mind.

Commemorative practices play an important role in the shaping of memory. Through commemorative ritual and architecture, the writing of children's history books and the retelling of stories within the family, a special kind of light is directed at a particular area of the past leaving other areas in darkness. Paul Connerton (1989) in *How Societies Remember* argues that social memory (by which I mean the shared social aspect of individual memory) and the memory of groups depend upon public commemorative practices. A prohibition on commemoration would, therefore, pose a threat to social memory. Connerton writes: 'What is horrifying in totalitarian regimes is not only the violation of human dignity but the fear that there might remain nobody who would ever again properly bear witness to the past' (ibid.: 15). However, this account of social memory does not explain the persistence of oppositional memory in the Baltic countries under Soviet rule. Commemorative practices were strictly censored and even within the family references to the past were for the most part suppressed. Yet individual memory in Latvia survived without the support of public commemoration. How long it could have continued to survive is another question. Do memories have a sell-by date, as Cathy Merridale (1996) so aptly asks? Or does their recycling depend upon a transition from the interior life of an individual (never, of course, entirely pure) to the public realm of ritual commemoration?

Public acknowledgement and commemoration of a past relate to questions about the audience and its readiness to listen. That audience may be the society or group of which the individual is a member or it may be the academic community which chooses to listen now but not at an earlier time. I have in mind here Arthur Kleinman's (1982) earlier work on somatization, neurasthenia and depression in China. Kleinman's fieldwork was carried out in the wake of the cultural revolution when many of his patients and their families must have been suffering devastating consequences of dispossession, displacement and the assault on their identity which these constituted. He must have had first-hand experience of this and yet there is hardly a suggestion of such experiences in his books. His approach to neurasthenia using quasi-clinical classificatory categories of pain and unhappiness makes it difficult to get a sense of the subjective meanings of illness for patients. I have only been able to find one narrative that connects in any way with the historical memory of the cultural revolution. It is 'case 4' of a 52-year-old woman who together with her husband and children had been subjected to political harassment and oppression. Here Kleinman offers us a paraphrase of this woman's spoken narrative:

> Suppose, she said, you were looking at the ground, you were climbing a mountain and the mountain was very steep and difficult to climb. To the right and to the left you could see people falling off the mountainside. Holding onto your neck and back were several family members so that if you fell so would they. For twenty years you climbed this mountain with your eyes fixed on the

handholds and footholds. You neither looked back nor ahead. Finally you reached the top of the mountain. Perhaps this is the first time you have looked backward and seen how much you have endured, how difficult your life and your family's situation has been, how blighted your hopes ... She ended by asking me if this was not a good enough reason to become depressed. (ibid.: 169)

I have quoted this at length because I feel it highlights a dimension missing from the rest of his earlier work. This case does not suggest an unwillingness to confront painful emotions. The paradox of Kleinman's position is that he attributes behaviour to his patients which he himself exemplifies. The theme of this early work is the inability of the Chinese to recognize and disclose painful emotions and their translation and perception of psychological distress as bodily symptoms. Kleinman's more recent writing on the ways in which the effects of state-induced violence and mass brutality are represented as individual weakness and vulnerability had to wait until the break-up of the Soviet Union and the public revelations about the extent of Communist violence before making an appearance in print in the 1990s.

I mention Kleinman not because I wish to make him a public scapegoat but because his case illustrates some important theoretical issues about active listening. The psychiatrists among our readers will be more familiar with this art. To anthropologists and others it is highly perplexing. Reception theorists tell us that it is easier to write a book than to read it. Similarly we could say that it is easier to talk than to listen. The art of active reconstruction lies with the reader or listener and is a highly complex and mysterious process. As my example indicates, it depends not only upon the qualities of the listener but also upon the social context and political climate in which they find themselves. Hacking's concept of semantic contagion or leaking is relevant here: the idea that our renaming of an experience has repercussions on the way in which we reassess the rest of our experience (1995: 255–59). Why is it that we are now more ready to hear the voices of victims of torture? Of sexually abused children? Those voices were surely there before but we were not ready to listen. Perhaps we were too busy paying attention to a different set of voices. So it is with Arthur Kleinman. Is he now remembering the faint voices of his Chinese patients across two decades, or is he listening to the more powerful and louder voices of his academic colleagues? I will leave you to look for the answers.

Paul Connerton (1989: 13) reminds us that each beginning, each act of forgetting involves recollection and preserves a memory of the old order. We might also say that remembering depends upon forgetting. So it is that memory and forgetting depend upon each other.

What does this brief review of the anthropological interest in memory tell us? Early anthropologists looked to psychoanalysis for an under-standing of culture. Theories of memory and forgetting provided the meeting ground between the instinctual life of individuals and their culture.

The recent work on memory attributes a more radical role to culture in the shaping of memory. The shape of memory may tell us how knowledge is constructed, but it does not tell us about the past. At this point I return to my original problem about the bifurcation of the two disciplines over the issue of memory.

Despite the recent interest in false memory psychiatry still holds to the Enlightenment project: it assumes there is a set of facts. False memory points away from the facts, true memory towards it. Anthropology has for the most part (with notable exceptions) abandoned the Enlightenment project. Memory is not studied as a road to truth but because it provides us with lessons in what Hacking describes as 'that overtilled country' (1996: 257) of the social construction of meanings.

Let me finish by returning again to Mauss: 'Our debt is great and I do not think we shall ever repay it. Perhaps we will only ever reward you with new usurpations' (1979: 19).

8

A HISTORICAL DISORDER: NEURASTHENIA AND THE TESTIMONY OF LIVES IN LATVIA

Neurasthenic illnesses in Latvia embody many of the contradictions and difficulties of life under Soviet rule.[1] In trying to understand the Latvian experience of neurasthenia I address two interrelated theoretical issues. First, I examine the implications of viewing autobiographies of illness as alternative histories. I look at the ways in which the medicalization enterprise is restricted if a whole life is brought into consideration. When life histories translate injury into collective trauma they succeed in hindering the transformation of planned state violence and terrorization into medical knowledge.[2] And second, if Latvian illness narratives are 'evocative transcripts' of resistance, where does this leave medical anthropology?[3] If Latvian informants succeed in dismantling and dismissing attempts to medicalize their pain, in what sense, if any, can its study be called medical? To address these questions I compare the Soviet psychiatric writing on neurasthenia with its implementation in everyday medical practice in Latvia. In particular, I focus on life stories, which are an important marker of difference between lay and medical understandings of suffering and illness.

Paul Calloway has claimed that 'neuroses have had a relatively low profile in Russian and Soviet psychiatry' (1992: 167). I would suggest that it was their ubiquity which rendered them invisible. A recent article on neurasthenia ends with the dramatic statement that 'Neurasthenia is extinct in the west because its cultural work is done' (Lutz 1995: 542). Neurasthenia was alive in Soviet Latvia because its cultural work was so widespread. However, the uncertain political allegiance of Latvians to the Soviet Union introduced ambivalence and cognitive dissonance to this work. Doctors and psychiatrists had the difficult task of bridging political and conceptual differences. Perhaps Latvian doctors were ready to diagnose themselves as suffering from neurasthenia for this very reason.

Everyday medical accounts of neurasthenia attempt to reconcile two contradictory perspectives: one focuses on individual inadequacy, the other on the difficult social circumstances and hardship of lives. In conversation doctors acknowledged the contribution to the development of neurasthenia of the impossible conditions under which lives are lived. Medical histories, on the other hand, scrutinize patients' past lives for signs of character weakness. However, informants themselves opened up the discussion of ill health by introducing yet another dimension, namely the historical and collective nature of their experience. My work rests on some sixty-three letters and thirty subsequent interviews with people responding to a newspaper advertisement calling for neurasthenia sufferers to write to me about their experience of illness. These autobiographies are transformed by a historical consciousness: individual injuries contribute and testify to a collective national trauma. The autobiographical narrative of one particular provincial doctor – Kristīna – illustrates the way in which a life history bridges the personal and collective and the two-way movement across this bridge. History frames Kristīna's life and explains the damage inflicted on her health: thus history both takes away and gives back meaning. However, Kristīna also uses her life story to construct an alternative history which challenges Soviet history. Clearly such uses were not anticipated by Soviet psychiatric theory.

Soviet Theories of Neuroses

Soviet psychiatry was charged with the heavy duty of explaining not only politically incorrect behaviour but also disaffection and discontent. Doctor/patient conflicts testify to the difficulties of explaining away the persistence of human unhappiness. Time and history – so important for dialectical theory – play no part in Soviet psychiatry: their inclusion would have undermined its ideological aspirations. Rather, Soviet psychiatric ideas occupy a timeless realm in which puppet characters shadow-box with society. However, the implementation of theory was constantly endangered by the unhappy voice of memory.

Official psychiatric pronouncements have a more optimistic ring: 'The formation of new socialistic consciousness is associated with the overcoming of the conflicts between personal and social-in the new socialistic understanding the individual and the social form a single entity' (Myasischev 1963: 50). The challenge of welding together social and indivi-dual interests was met by developing a diagnostic system with a strong emphasis on somatic character types. The work of Pavlov provides a theoretical basis for this enterprise. Myasischev's theory of four character

Table 8.1: The Theory of Four Character Types

Strength	Balance	Mobility	Humoural Type
+	+	+	Sanguine
+	+	−	Phlegmatic
+	−	?	Choleric
−	?	?	Melancholic

Source: Adapted from Myasischev (1963: 196).

types derives from Pavlov's tripartite description of the nervous system: strength, mobility and balance. These yield the classification of human types set out in Table 8.1.

The classical provenance of this classification – acknowledged by Myasischev himself – needs no emphasis. However, the fact that he does not bother to follow it through in a systematic way, leaving certain dimensions unaccounted for, suggests that there are other implicit but more important principles of categorization at work. Indeed, towards the end of the book we find a more basic dualistic typology which categorizes human character into the social versus the individualistic or egoistic (ibid.: 207). This accounts for why neurasthenia and hysteria, both characterized as typical of a weak nervous system, are not further differentiated in terms of mobility and balance. The simplified dichotomy is of more importance for psychiatric thinking and practice than the classification spelt out at greater length. It offered a means of translating political threat into psychiatric language.

One of the principal axes along which egoism and the commitment to the collectivity are measured is the attitude to work. 'Incapacity for work deprives individuals from earning a living but equally importantly excludes them from the working group' (ibid.: 12). Thus attitudes to work also play an important diagnostic role: 'We do not obtain proper criteria for assessment of the functional disturbances unless we consider the patient's attitudes towards his task and how this changes during work and in working conditions' (ibid.: 14).

Thus although a Pavlovian-derived typology provides the theoretical infrastructure for an overall theory of neurosis, it is the orientation of society towards the collectivity and the work collectivity in particular, which informs the exigencies of everyday psychiatric practice. The theoretical exegesis of neurotic disorders also rests upon pragmatic considerations concerning the individual's relationship to the collectivity rather than on a humoral-based typology. Myasischev has developed a schema which relates the type of neurosis to the locus of conflict. In this schema there are three categories of neuroses: neurasthenia, hysteria and obsessive-compulsive disorders. Each category is linked to a particular kind of conflict between the individual and society (see Table 8.2).

Table 8.2: Relation between Type of Neurosis and Locus of Conflict

NEUROTIC ILLNESS	LOCUS OF CONFLICT BETWEEN	AND
NEURASTHENIA	Individual's abilities	Social and self-imposed expectation
HYSTERIA	Individual wants	Social expectations
COMPULSIVE DISORDERS	Wants	Moral imperatives

As the table shows, in the case of neurasthenia the conflict and mismatch is between the individual's physical and psychological abilities and social and self-imposed expectations. The individual finds himself, or more often herself, unable to fulfil these expectations. The symptoms of neurasthenia are: 'Irritability, an unstable or depressed mood, a tendency to become fatigued or tired easily with complaints of headache, loss of memory and poor appetite' (ibid.: 192). Official Latvian psychiatric thought closely follows this account of the aetiology and symptomatology of neurasthenia. For example, Imants Eglītis writes of 'an exaggerated excitability and tendency to tire, emotional and somatic lability' (1989: 164).

Thus all neurotic disorders are perceived as conflicts whose source lies in a mismatch between social expectations and norms and the individual's abilities to meet those norms. They are situated at the interface between the individual and society. However, their power to monitor relations between individuals and the collectivity is restricted by the ancient language of somatic character types which deprive voices of their meaning.

The role of the psychiatrist as educator, one who teaches correct attitudes towards self and society, derives from this underlying dualistic typology. Indeed, Myasischev acknowledged that, 'The field of the struggle with the neuroses is a borderline field between education and medicine' (1963: 279). Soviet psychiatry has generally been acknowledged to be collectivist in orientation (Field 1967: 234). In keeping with this orientation, the task of Soviet psychiatrists was seen as one of restoring individual confidence (Ziferstein 1976: 165) but at the same time directing the patient towards socially required standards of behaviour (Ziferstein 1972: 599). Although the relationship between psychiatrist and patient was described as being more intimate and friendlier than in the West, the role of the psychiatrist was also described as active and educative (Ziferstein 1976: 440). Dispensaries rather than hospitals were thought to be more appropriate for the monitoring of psychiatric illness (Lebensohn 1962: 297; Kolb 1966: 433–44). Dispensaries were also thought to be more effective in restoring patients to full social functioning. Soviet psychiatry was characterized by the relatively large numbers of psychiatrists and small numbers of hospital beds (Lebensohn 1962: 298; Field 1967: 154). All these features contributed to the powerful role of Soviet psychiatry in 'educating' its peoples.

Latvian Psychiatric Practice

Psychiatric practice in Latvia diverges in some ways from Soviet psychiatric principles in that hospital treatment and community care are given equal importance. There are ten psychiatric hospitals in Latvia providing a total of some 6,000 beds. This yields approximately 2.5 beds per thousand inhabitants, an extraordinarily high ratio by any standards.[4] The ratio of psychiatrists per head of population is also high, but particularly so in the capital. Psychoneurological departments attached to polyclinics also treat psychiatric disorders. There are twenty-five such psychoneurological units in Latvia and each unit is responsible for some 300,000 people. Within Riga there is the City Psychoneurological Dispensary with thirty psychiatrists each allocated responsibility for a designated area of the city with some 30,000 inhabitants (Velmers 1992). In addition, there are ten emergency ambulance centres in Riga, each of which has a psychoneurological brigade. It appears then that Latvia is well provided for in terms of both in-patient and out-patient psychiatric facilities. No doubt this was related to its socially educative role, particularly important in a country where political allegiance could not be counted upon.

In Latvia the diagnosis of neurasthenia is elusive and paradoxical. Prior to my research I had been assured by psychiatrists and doctors of its ubiquity: it was, I was told, the most commonly used diagnosis. Yet in the course of my fieldwork I found it exceptionally difficult to pin down. This elusiveness appeared in the letters which I received early in 1992. Of the 63 letters only a few discussed their author's illness. The diagnosis of neurasthenia meant little to them and most were not sure whether it was what they were suffering from. For example, a letter from Liepāja begins, 'It is difficult for me to judge whether I am suffering from neurasthenia-I will leave that for you to decide'. People's focus on the past and on their life histories rather than their illness experience makes any such decision difficult. I found commonalities of history and memory rather than of symptoms and illness categories. Informants did complain of anxiety and fear. Some spoke of an inner fever. For many these feelings were particularly strong at night when they would wake terrified, feeling suffocated and with hearts racing. Common phrases were 'I am short of air', 'I don't have enough air' or 'My heart is on strike'. These expressions of distress have strong political resonances and pay little regard to the medical specificities of the neurasthenic experience.

Neurasthenia is equally elusive in psychiatric hospitals and clinics, not being considered sufficiently serious to warrant psychiatric treatment. The diagnosis appears to have been used principally within general medicine and particularly within the psychoneurological specialisms of community health clinics or polyclinics. Here neurasthenia accounts for about a third of all diagnoses. It also figures significantly in the work of the emergency services, which I shall discuss later. However, literature on neurasthenia is sparse. The standard psychiatric textbook devotes an incomplete paragraph to it. Arthur Kleinman found something very similar in China and he writes of 'the limited space devoted to neurasthenia in current Chinese textbooks of medicine' (1982: 178) attributing this reluctance to a professional anxiety about its scientific status.

A Local History

The semantic complexity of neurasthenia reflects Latvian history. Its sedimented layers of meaning have been deposited by successive occupying powers and cultural hegemonies. Neurasthenia was a common diagnosis in the early part of the century, as witnessed by one of my narrators born in 1910:

> In 1929 I volunteered for the army in the hope that I would be sent to Riga, where I would be able to go to night school. Instead, I was sent to Gulbene [a small provincial town in north-east Vidzeme] and on top of that I got a very strict sergeant. Before enrolling I wondered how I would feel, because I needed a lot of sleep, but in the army I didn't suffer from lack of sleep, but still I didn't feel well. I went to the doctor, he couldn't find anything wrong. He drew a cross on my chest with his stethoscope and left a red 'wound' as though drawn with a knife. The doctor was amazed – a country boy and he feels unwell. 'You have neurasthenia.' He wrote out a prescription for some drops – strychnine. I said, 'but that's a poison'. He said, 'Yes, but it should be drunk in small measure'. He gave me three days off. After a while I went back again and got five days off. My companions were surprised – a neurasthenic. Returning from the doctor I gave my records to the medical assistant. She said, 'Well, yes, neurasthenia has been dragged over here from America.' 'Is it catching?' I asked. 'No', the assistant replied. Later I was transferred to another division and then felt better.

Ernest's recollections illustrate many of the features attributed to neurasthenia in the nineteenth century: it is associated with study and city life. For example, the doctor evinces surprise that despite being a country boy he is yet so sensitive. Neurasthenia has a certain cachet. The American provenance of the illness is very clearly recognized. This American-derived layer of meaning informs Ernest's letter and it is also evident in the illness of other older informants.[5]

Neurasthenia continued to be a common diagnosis during the independence period. It is described as 'One of the most commonly encountered illnesses of the nerves, which belongs to the functional group, that is those whose occurrence is not reflected in organic or perceptible changes, but whose essence consists in weakness in the functioning of nervous processes. The chief characteristic of neurasthenia is increased irritability of the nervous system and weakened endurance for work' (Švābe, Būmanis and Dišlers 1937: 28850). However, Harijs Buduls, a well-known psychiatrist of the independence period, devotes very little of his writing to neurasthenia – a mere paragraph. He discusses neurasthenia in the course of a short chapter on the psychopathic personality. 'Many psychopaths have many characteristics of the neurasthenic with an exaggerated sensitivity, quickness to tire, lack of direction and some other disturbances of somatic and psychic function. Psychopathy has many points of contact particularly with a form of neurasthenia which has psychological manifestations and which is called psychic asthenia' (1928: 125–26). The link with a particular type of asocial personality and the limited prospects of cure or indeed improvement provide an important bridge with later Soviet ideas.

In Latvia, Soviet psychiatry thus met ground that was already well worked and one might have supposed it to have been receptive to it. The Soviet neuropsychiatric version of neurasthenia was not that different from the older Latvian versions. Why was it not superimposed unobtrusively onto existing ideas? Moreover, in Soviet Latvia all psychiatrists received postgraduate specialist training in Russia, principally in Moscow but also in Leningrad. They were, therefore, well versed in Soviet psychiatric theory.[6] And yet Soviet ideas about neurasthenia did not take root in Latvia and lost what ground they had hitherto occupied. The reasons for the paradoxical status of neurasthenia – its simultaneous omnipresence and invisibility – lie outside the realms of psychiatry.

Everyday Resistance of Medicalization

Lay thought in Latvia attributes the breakdown of health to history and the burden of historical consciousness and memory. A recurring phrase refers to 'all these mad times' and 'all these chaotic times'. The impact of such times on health is perceived as direct, brutal and inevitable. People use a language of physical assault and violence to describe their experience of health and illness. They talk of health being spoiled, damaged, destroyed and beaten. The heart and the head are often singled out as sites of violence. Events can only be resisted up to a point, before health finally succumbs to their impact. The relentless grip of memory is also thought to make people ill. Thus lay accounts rework psychiatric theory, reinterpreting the nature of the conflict between individual and society. Rather than recognizing individual inadequacy they turn the medical account on its head and lay the blame for illness at the doors of society and history. Latvian history shapes lives and with it health and illness. Latvian doctors have the difficult task of mediating between these opposed interpretations of illness and finding a common ground between lay and psychiatric language.

Doctors share with ordinary people the belief in collective damage to health. In conversation doctors and psychiatrists admit that the majority of Latvians are suffering from neurasthenia. The estimates of neurasthenia sufferers varied from 60 per cent to 90 per cent. Some even claimed that it was a universal condition:

> In principle virtually everyone suffers from these problems of neurasthenia. Either these or related problems, because all these social circumstances leave a heavy imprint on people (Dr I.A., Riga, August 1992).

It seems that lay ideas about the universality of neurasthenia have also been assimilated by the medical profession and that they are responsible for the sweepingly high estimates of neurasthenia prevalence. A paradoxical corollary of this is that doctors tend to avoid the diagnosis and to have a generally pessimistic view of the prognosis (Skultans 1995: 16).

Although Latvian doctors are aware of the difficult circumstances of people's lives and of their histories, they operate with a model of psychoneurotic illness which focuses on individual inadequacies. Social factors play an ambivalent role within medical and psychiatric practice. Although in conversation about their work and their patients doctors and psychiatrists make constant references to social circumstances, these are not incorporated into official categories. Indeed it is the acknowledged ubiquity of a distressing past and stressful present circumstances which help to create a feeling of helplessness; nothing can be done:

> Of course, of course. Many people cannot be helped either then, or now. There are people who've lived all their lives in a communal flat. We can't give them a flat. There are people who live three or four to a room. There is no way we can help them. You will ask me about drugs. We have no drugs. Very often we have no antibiotics. O.K. We have no psychotropic drugs, nobody will die because of that, but at present we do not even have antibiotics; that's how far it's got (Dr I.E., March 1993).

Such attitudes are reinforced by the fact that many doctors have lived through and continue to live in circumstances which are similar to those of their patients. This casts them in the role of mediators. The crucial role of psychiatrists in instilling Soviet ideological goals and political conformity is well documented (Podrabinek 1980; Bloch and Reddaway 1977). Their role as mediators between ideological practice and the miseries of daily life is even more important and less well known. Thus the multiple meanings and ambiguity of neurasthenia permit idiosyncrasy in diagnostic practice and promote the social work of neurasthenia.

At the outset of my research I had wanted to exclude the overtly political dimensions of psychiatry. However, I found as the work proceeded that I had to change my position about this at the insistence of my narrators. First, narratives constructed illness in political terms; second, perceptions of the everyday practice of psychiatry were inevitably coloured by its political involvement. Most people were aware of the way in which compulsory psychiatric treatment had been used against dissenting political figures such as Pēteris Lazda and Ģederts Melngailis. Psychiatrists could recount many such incidents. For example, Dr Kiršentāls, director of the City Psychoneurological Dispensary, described the way in which political dissidents would be rounded up in ambulances and confined to a psychiatric hospital before any state celebrations. Certainly all psychiatrists were aware of the reputation of their profession. I asked Dr A.S. how she felt about the earlier political role of psychiatry:

> *I will tell you straight: I am ashamed to be a psychiatrist. Although I like my work, I am ashamed that my colleagues can do something so base and dishonest. Because I think to exploit this specialism for dishonest purposes, where it is so difficult to prove anything objectively. ... In surgery it is not so difficult to see that a bone is broken by making an X-ray, but here it is impossible to prove whether a person is speaking the truth or whether he is making it up and therefore I simply have nothing to say. I am ashamed.*

However, not only were the dissenting words and behaviour of major political figures treated as psychiatric problems, but smaller acts of rebellion and criticism of everyday practices could be met with a psychiatric response. For example, Dainis found that his exasperation at not being able to find a flat and his accusation that the executive committee were taking bribes led to his forced psychiatric hospitalization. Nīna, who worked in a state bank, found that her complaints about dishonest practices at work gave rise to compulsory psychiatric treatment. Her letter complained that 'In our society, nervous people are often made out to be mad'. Dzintra, a history teacher, found that her lessons were perceived as anti-Soviet and she also was compulsorily confined. I could give more examples. The rights and wrongs of any one case cannot be established in retrospect, but these examples demonstrate the general reputation of psychiatry. As one psychiatrist discussing the reluctance of people to consult her profession put it, 'The old imprint is still there'.

Among my original sample of sixty-three letter writers there were five doctors who wrote about themselves rather than in a professional capacity.[7] One consequence of this readiness for self-disclosure is that there is far less of a professional distance between doctors and their patients than there is in Britain (Skultans 1995: 14–18). This greater intimacy puts doctors in a difficult role. Doctors use both medical and lay ideas of neurasthenia: as an illustration, the doctors who replied to the neurasthenia advertisement wrote about themselves and their accounts were similar to lay people's. For example, Anna is a psychiatrist who offered to talk about her own neurasthenia. She spoke about her life and emphasized its commonality with others:

> *I don't for a moment think that I am the only one who hasn't succeeded. No. I've always told myself that I'm not the only one like that, the whole Latvian nation is like that.*

Illness narratives offer a political critique in parallel with descriptions of personal injury. There is a shared language of damage, injury and exploitation which is applied to society as well as to individuals. The principal complaints were of dishonesty, disorder and unpredictability.

> *I feel I'm being strangled. I cannot stand all the irregularities. There are no rules.*

> *I feel like a taut bow the whole time. There are irregularities at work. All the corners of the heavens have been spoilt.*

> *It is an unfulfilled life. Everywhere everything is dishonest, dirty.*

> *I cannot bring any order into my life.*

> *All that disorder is eating away at me. My son is stealing, but is there anyone in this society who isn't stealing?*

> *That's been imported here [i.e. from Russia]. No contract can be made. Everything is through bribes. There is no clarity. We are like meat in a mincing machine.*

Nina's narrative makes a direct connection between dishonesty at work and the erosion of health:

> *I worked in the state bank as an inspector. That was a thankless sort of profession. I came into contact with all sorts of dishonest people as you know in our Soviet period. I had to sort out the irregularities but the system wouldn't allow that. And that's why I had the conflicts at the bank. They simply took revenge on me so that I wouldn't be able to poke my nose there and even today they dislike me. Dealers, you know, were speculating, they were carrying out all sorts of malpractices and the appropriation of state funds took place before my very eyes, but I wasn't allowed to identify it. Well, that traumatized me the whole time ... I want to work honestly, but we weren't allowed to work honestly. You're probably familiar with these things? You read the Latvian press don't you? All that wears down the nervous system.*

Underpinning these extracts from letters and subsequent interviews is a sociohistorical model of illness, which draws upon life histories to explain the erosion of health.

A Doctor's Life Story

Kristīna is a doctor whose accounts of her illness, her life and her understanding of history are inseparable. Her life story is offered as testimony. In
her letter she wrote, 'Perhaps you will be able to use my life story' and I
would like to do so. Her life story is unique to her and yet at one and the
same time records both a shared history and a collective experience and
memory.

Like many older narrators, Kristīna's life story is dichotomized by the
Second World War into a before and after period. Her account of her pre-
war childhood is typical in its emphasis on books and unchanging spiritual
values:

> I lived nearly four years in independent Latvia. I don't remember much. But I
> remember those years as very sunny. Those early years are linked to my father's
> shop, to books. I imbibed a love of books that is still with me ... I'm so tired in
> the evenings but I definitely have to read something. That's stayed with me all
> my life. So those first four years were very happy. My parents cared for us,
> brought us up properly.

Kristīna singles out a birthday to mark the boundary between the
Latvian period and the Soviet occupation. Her emphasis on family
celebrations and rituals is typical of many narratives which contrast a
sacred, cyclical time with disorder and unpredictability. The following
incident with the dough and the hens emphasizes the disorder and
wastefulness of events.

> When the Russians came in I remember that our parents were very frightened.
> And it happened like this, that the deportations were on 14 June 1941 and my
> mother's birthday is on 14 June. And the day before we had moved. ... And we
> moved on 13 June. And the next day, 14 June, was my mother's birthday and we
> were planning a small family celebration, nobody could foresee. ... We'd asked
> some very close friends. And I just remember that in the morning while we were
> still sleeping my mother ran somewhere very anxiously. She came running back
> very alarmed and was crying ... I still remember what she looked like with untidy
> hair. She grabbed her head and said 'Rich, everything is lost there won't be any
> celebration, all our friends have been taken and deported'. She mentioned the
> Zīlnieks family in particular. Then in her panic she took the dough which she'd
> prepared for the pīrāgi and poured it out for the hens. Father shouted, 'What are
> you doing? You could have baked the pīrāgi and taken them to the station to
> those unfortunate people.' As I remember it, there was tragedy in the move to
> that house and also life developed in a tragic way. My mother said that she built
> the house with enormous care and effort, but that she didn't spend one happy
> day there.

Kristīna dates her ill-health from the time of her father's imprisonment:

> He was six years in prison. He sat out his sentence to the last day, until 1951. ...
> He was in Ventspils prison, after that he was in Riga prison, and after that he

was sent to the Archangel district in Voisk. He was there for about four years. And then he was released on 30 April 1951. And he returned to Ventspils on condition that he did not register in Ventspils, or live there or work there. He was considered a criminal and Ventspils – being a port – he was not allowed to register there or work there. Well, that period of time destroyed my nervous system [Latvian sagrāva, *literally crumbled or ate away]. My father was really intelligent, he didn't know how to do farm work. My mother had lived in the country with her foster parents, she was different. She could cope with any situation, but father wasn't like that. And then when he returned from deportation, he wasn't given any work. And then at one time he worked in Zura agricultural school as a horse groom. But he didn't get on well because he didn't know how to ... [she trails off]*

... And then I remember that my mother used to go there specially to show him how to harness a horse. He said, 'Yes, yes, It's all clear'. But when mother left he harnessed the horse and the horse unharnessed itself. Quite simply he was unhappy because he wasn't allowed to work where he wanted to work. Then I think he was probably made redundant ... .

An episode during the German occupation involving a soldier and his dog is held responsible for her contracting meningitis.

Well, and then in the autumn of 1944 I fell ill with infectious meningitis. Well, I don't know what the cause was, but a few weeks earlier I was learning the piano with a private teacher and I went to her for lessons. And I had a red dress, bright red, with little white spots. And I was going with my notes to the piano teacher and I remember it as though it were today: there was a German officer lying in the grass and next to him a big alsatian dog was eating from a tin. And suddenly he attacked me. He did shout at the dog in his own language but he didn't come to my help, until my mother ran out. My dress was torn. He hadn't bitten me, only scratched me, but I was terribly frightened. And it turned out. ... Well, every army has its policy, it turned out that he'd been specially trained to attack the colour red. And he saw me with the red dress and that upset him and that's why he attacked. Later the officer apologized to my mother, so she recounted. I was terribly frightened and two weeks later I fell ill with meningitis. And I was very ill and I remember that my father went on his bike to some German first aid post for brontusil. And he brought it home and with its help I got better. And then soon after my father was arrested and then there was all that uncertainty about my father and my mother was floundering about. She was left without means and with four small children. I was nine, my brothers were seven and five and my little sister was two and she had no means of livelihood. I was the oldest and I was exceptionally emotional. And all my mother's troubles, all her anxieties about how to feed the family, I took upon myself even though I was still a small child. And I remember the following episode at school. ... The teacher comes up to me and calls me. She calls me once, she calls me twice and I don't hear her and then she starts shaking me. ... What am I thinking about. ... And I was so startled as though from a sleep and I say to the teacher: 'I'm sorry but I'm thinking about where to get hay for my mother's cow.' And I wasn't listening to the lesson, I was living in my own world. And the teacher wanted to scold me but when I told her she wasn't cross with me, she understood.

But then I remember after the meningitis I had terrible headaches and I was terribly anxious and my period of convalescence coincided with all those terrible events when my father was arrested. ... And then I remember that I often had headaches and the stuttering started.[8] *... And it became especially bad during the period that my father was arrested, when I was just going to school. I started going to school during the German period; I finished the first class, but after the war I was in the second and third class and those were the most terrible. And I wrote to you in my letter about that episode. ... They were terrible times. ... They were our very own Latvians. I have to say there is a category of people that know how to adapt to whatever government is in power. And there was a teacher there, her name was Trāge; by the way she was my father's childhood friend, they had gone to school together. They knew each other well but she knew how to adapt to those in power. And then there was another teacher Kupče, who was also known to my father, because my father was the director of the bookshop. Everybody knew him as an intelligent man but the new government despised him as an enemy of the state and his children had to be despised too. And I remember, there was a Russian language lesson and there was a little poem. ... Well, I hadn't heard the Russian language and as a child I didn't know its accents and I said it wrong. ... And the teacher grabbed me ... I had a plait in a doorknocker and two bows.*[9] *... And I remember, it as though it were today, how she caught me by that plait and dragged me along the corridor to the staff room and said 'You criminal's child. You won't cripple the Russian language'. And then she didn't take me inside the class room, but made me stand in the corner near the door. And then all the children went past and laughed and each called me different names. And that was a terrible trauma for me, for the whole of my life. To this day I see myself standing there and relive what I was feeling at that moment. At that moment I wanted to die and I thought, if only something would happen which would stop me from having to live in this terrible world.*

And during that period of study what tormented me most was a neurocircular dystonia of a cardiovascular type ... that's the so-called heart neurosis. And by the way that started when I was just eleven years old, when I was in school. At the time when all the teachers were calling me a criminal's child, terrorizing me, that's when the heart neurosis started. And it manifested itself in a stenocardial fashion, I had a severe pain in the region of the heart being just thirteen years old.

My mother worked in a hospital and her wages were 310 rubles in old money, in today's money that would be 31 rubles.[10] *And my mother – so that we four children would not die of hunger – kept a cow, some pigs, and then during the summer we would grow vegetables, pick nettles, mother would boil them and add a handful of bran and gave them to the pig and the cow, so that we could survive. And I was the oldest and I saw and understood all that.*

Although I asked Kristīna for her medical history hers is not a narrative of health and illness. Rather illness is introduced in her autobiography for rhetorical purposes to lend weight to her perspective and evaluation of past events. Illness makes its first appearance at the beginning of the second period of Soviet occupation. Her father's arrest and his being branded as a criminal reverses the earlier order in which he was a respectable bookseller. Kristīna describes her health as disintegrating in a way which mirrors the disintegration of society. Kristīna's memory of the German occupation is set in a military and violent context. Her illness – meningitis – is equally dramatic and violent.

The problems of the early Soviet period – the fatherless families, the shortage of food and the difficulties which many Latvians encountered in learning to speak Russian – were long term and they led to chronic health problems, namely headaches. However, the humiliation experienced in the Russian lesson finds a precise symbolic equivalent in stuttering. Like many children whose parents were imprisoned or deported Kristīna was taunted by teachers and children alike. The common jeer that she was a criminal's child strikes at the heart and she describes herself as suffering from a cardiac neurosis.

All these difficulties and problems are heightened by Kristīna's own understanding and perceptiveness. However, not all her memories are of repression and violence. She recalls episodes which speak of accommodation and the overcoming of difficulties.

> *Well what I remember from my childhood is that we survived mostly on fish – Ventspils being a port – and milk. We got the milk in this way. My mother's foster-mother's sister turned out to be a communist. ... And when the* kolkhozi *[collective farms] were founded she said ... I still remember her words: 'Latvian* kolkhozi *won't suffer if I give away one cow to some poor children.' And then she gave us a cow from her byre, which was to have been handed over to the communal farm in a week's time. She gave us a cow. And you could write a whole story of how we brought the cow from Piebalga. First of all we took it by lorry to Tukums, then on foot. And then in Tukums my mother agreed with some railway workers that the cow would be loaded onto an old carriage. There were some old carriages there for transporting timber for the sawmills in Ventspils and ... That was in 1946. At that time I was not quite ten. And I was with her and we were all so tired that we all fell asleep. Even the cow stopped fretting and we woke up when the train was already being uncoupled and the carriage was lifted from the rails and taken to the saw mill. And I remember that two men went to receive the carriages and one of them called out: 'Hey, there's a cow here, and a woman and a child!' Then we went on foot from the saw mill – it's some four of five kilometers. And then the children were very happy.*

Kristīna's autobiographical and illness narrative can almost be read as a political allegory. Her personal memories share many common elements with other narratives. For example, there is the reference to a 'sunny' pre-war childhood, inferred rather than remembered, and the coming together of personal and national destinies on 14 June 1941, being a birthday and the day of deportations. The arbitrariness and unfairness of her father's arrest and deportation are described. There is the moral chaos following the Russian occupation when even respectable, established firms like the Rapa bookshop do not keep their word. In the immediate post-war years there is the threat of famine felt particularly acutely by her mother, but also through empathy by Kristīna. For her father there is the difficulty of finding a place for himself after his return to the homeland and for Kristīna there is the trauma of finding herself called a criminal's child. Kristīna dates the origins of her nervous ill health to that early period in her childhood and the chaotic times the family were going through. She is very ready to attribute neurasthenia to herself, but she does not talk directly about illness. Instead what she gives me is a social history of the past fifty years as it is filtered through her personal experience and memory.

I felt I must have missed out on some of the illness-related aspects of her account and asked Kristīna to tell me more about her symptoms. This was her reply:

I don't feel exhaustion. On the contrary by nature I am very energetic despite the fact that I have a heavy load at work. I have three gardens. I grow sugar beet, but I manage everything on my own: work, cleaning the house, the gardens ... I grow potatoes, sugar beet, I also grow some vegetables to sell because it's quite hard for three people to survive on one salary. So I don't think that I'm suffering from nervous exhaustion. I have quite the opposite, a kind of tension and anxiety. About my work conditions. The work situation is such that there are a lot of difficulties with transport. We have one ambulance and it very often goes wrong, there are no spare parts. But we still have to get to the patients, children fall ill regardless. Often there is no petrol. And particularly in the winter there are enormous problems, when the parents telephone and call you to the patient but you have no transport. Earlier people used to come themselves to fetch you, the kolkhoz *where they worked would help; there used to be a rule that the collective where the parent worked had to provide transport when a child was ill. Now we all have such petrol difficulties and there is a petrol famine, that the* kolkhoz *can't supply it either. And that's why we're all so anxious and nervous about what's going to happen tomorrow, what the future will be like.*

Kristīna succeeds in turning what was intended to be a medical discussion into one about problems at work and lack of petrol, almost as though the existence of neurasthenia could be inferred from the existence of such problems and social injustices.

The practice of medicine in Soviet Latvia disclosed the uneasy fit between ideology and reality. Neurasthenia, positioned on the meeting ground between individual and society, exemplifies this uncertain relationship. In conceptualizing and situating neurasthenia in this way, Soviet psychiatry paved the way for the metamorphosis of neurasthenia to fit Latvian experience. Thus, where there is a mismatch between individual resources and social expectations, the argument can be developed in one of two directions: one can either question the adequacy of individual resources or one can question the legitimacy of historical happenings and social expectations.

How do these findings relate to the theoretical agenda set out at the beginning of this chapter? What effect do life stories have on the creation of medical knowledge? Latvian resistance to Soviet occupation was embodied in evocative transcripts of ill health. Evocation is a most appropriate term because it emphasizes the universality of the experience of ill health and yet acknowledges the rich potential for ambiguity in the language of illness. However, the narratives themselves are not primarily about illness. Rather the polyphony of the narrative 'I' enables the most commanding voice – that of collective experience – to call the others to its bidding. Thus the voice of personal distress and certainly the medical voice are subservient to the grand historical narrative: the distressed voice of the individual is enlisted to promote the collective narrative. Illness is used to flesh out and give weight and meaning to historical events. The spirit of testimony points to the social and collective nature of these narratives.[11] Their anxiety is as much about collective as about individual survival. So where does this leave the medical anthropology enterprise? The answer must be that it leaves it initially perplexed but ultimately enriched. Anthropologists, although this may not be how they would view it, have concentrated on medicine's success stories. An example that is particularly relevant to my concerns is Allan Young's study of post-traumatic stress disorder: he displays psychiatry's successful colonization and medicalization of past time (1995: 7). This road was blocked to Soviet psychiatry by its insecure hold on the historical past. Failures to establish medical knowledge are less easy to identify and document. Only by listening closely to our informants, by entering into dialogue with them as well as our colleagues, can we acknowledge such failure and move on to the wide pastures which lie beyond the confines of medical anthropology as it is currently conceived.

Acknowledgements

I am grateful to the British Academy and to the ESRC for funding the fieldwork on which this paper is based.

Notes

1. I use the present tense advisedly because although Soviet rule ended formally with the declaration of Independence in 1991 its legacy in terms of personal suffering remains. Diagnostic practices also have yet to change. Any uncertainty over tense reflects the indeterminacy of social change.
2. The planned use of terror falls into three periods. During the first year of Soviet occupation in 1940–41 some 15,000 people were arrested and killed. They were for the most part people in senior positions. During the post-war period arbitrary arrests continued. Partisans and anyone suspected of aiding them were targeted. On 25 March 1949 one-tenth of all farmers were departed to Siberia thus paving the way for the collectivization of farming. For a history of these events, see Plakans (1995).
3. I borrow the term 'evocative transcript' from Caroline Humphrey who reworks Scott's thesis on hidden transcripts in the context of the Soviet Union. She argues that the social circumstances for the production of hidden transcripts were not to be found in Socialist Mongolia. In particular, there was no sharing of a social space by an enduring group. The production of a hidden transcript was subverted 'by the knowledge that virtually everyone had a double life' (1994: 25). The term 'evocative' simultaneously captures the universality and ambiguity of these transcripts. Medicine in Latvia makes extensive use of such evocative transcripts.

4. The comparable Bristol, UK figure is 0.20 beds per thousand inhabitants.
5. George Beard's study of neurasthenia was published in 1880. The symptoms of neurasthenia derived from the inadequate workings of the nervous system rather than any pathological changes in its structure. Neurasthenia was thus a disease with a physiological base which although associated with the stress of modern life and overwork was nevertheless distinct from modern mental illness. It affected women rather than men and bed rest was advocated as a cure. It affected upper class women and, therefore, had a certain social cachet.
6. Arthur Kleinman has documented a similar process influencing Chinese psychiatry and refers to 'the importation of a tripartite Russian classification of neurosis in which neurasthenia figured importantly along with hysteria and obsessive compulsive disorders' (1986: 33).
7. Kleinman found a similar over-representation of health professionals in his clinic sample of one hundred neurasthenia patients (1982: 138).
8. In Latvia stuttering is usually classified as a form of neurosis.
9. Although officially there was no one state language – the constitution (c1.36) refers explicitly to the right to use one's native tongue – in practice there was pressure to use Russian and, in particular, to conduct official business in Russian. Russian was introduced as the language of clerical, administrative and business affairs as early as 1940. For example, the Communist party in Jelgava used Latvian in 1940, but by the beginning of 1941 it was Russian. Throughout the Soviet period all major congresses and official ceremonies of the Communist party both at national and district levels were held in Russian. In May 1947 the Ministry of Education of LSSR ordered the introduction of the Russian language in all schools. In March 1950 further instructions for the expansion and improvement of Russian language teaching were introduced. See L. Zile (1991).
10. Currency devaluation took place in 1961.
11. For a discussion of the way in which different cultural groups use testimony see Wieviorka (1994).

9

NARRATIVES OF THE BODY AND HISTORY: ILLNESS IN JUDGEMENT ON THE SOVIET PAST

We have to swim with the current of the time. If you don't swim with the current destiny destroys you.

Māra, 15 March 1993, Drusti, Latvia.

Introduction

This chapter examines the ways in which resistance to authority in Soviet Latvia has come to be experienced as illness, and how narratives of the body and its sufferings are used to articulate a political critique of history and society. The research project started out as a study of neurasthenia. My initial sample consisted of more than sixty letter writers who responded to two newspaper advertisements inviting them to write to me about their illness. Most wrote about their past lives, of which illness was seen as the logical outcome. Illness was intertwined with the life course yet seldom singled out for separate attention.

Autobiographical and Fieldwork Background

My interest in Latvian illness narratives was, in large part, the outcome of my own personal narrative. Born in Riga, the child of Latvian parents, my family fled Latvia in October 1944 along with tens of thousands of other refugees. As part of a small exile community in Britain, Latvian children were groomed for a homecoming – delayed in my case until my research following the break-up of the Soviet Union. This early preparation meant that I was bilingual and was particularly attuned to words and their nuances. It also meant that as an identified exile – the local term was 'foreigner' or 'Latvian from abroad' – certain categories of people, namely those closely involved with the Soviet power structure in Latvia, were almost, though not altogether, absent from my sample. I expected to encounter resistances in discussing experiences which spoke of collaboration with the Soviet system. In the event, such collaboration was presented as an inevitable part of the narrator's autobiography.

In the summer of 1992 I was able to visit these letter writers in their homes. They in turn introduced me to their friends and relatives. Three-quarters of my informants were women. Most were elderly. The total sample snowballed to over 100. About a third of my informants had themselves experienced deportation or imprisonment. All had had experience of relatives being deported. However, this chapter will concentrate on the narrative of one informant, Māra, who first wrote to me in February 1992 having read my advertisement. Māra is a countrywoman from the parish of Drusti in the province of Vidzeme in north-east Latvia. She was born in 1924 and grew up during the Ulmanis period. Kārlis Ulmanis was president of Latvia between 1925 and 1926, during 1931 and between 1934 and 1940. However, the entire independence period between 1918 and 1940 is loosely referred to as the Ulmanis period by older Latvians. She was an adolescent during the Second World War and a young married woman and mother during the post-war period and the setting up of the collective farms. In interweaving her account of her own and her family's health with her experience of Soviet occupation and policy in Latvia, her story can stand for many others. Illness and bodily experience have the role of a sounding board which Māra uses to measure the rationality of governments and history.

Autobiography as Testimony

My justification for presenting a single life story rests with its claims to testify. Testimony is a judicial term which carries with it special claims to truth. As Felman and Laub (1992: 6) point out testimony has become a dominant genre of history writing. In historical testimony the individual experience is recalled only because it stands for the experience of a much larger group. A single life is also better able to convey the nature of narrative construction. Narrative encompasses the actor who lived through the experiences recounted and the author telling the story. It is selective and recasts the past in terms of present concerns and values. Personal narratives differ from medical accounts in that they are 'selective snapshots from an individual's own past' (Williams and Wood, 1986: 1436). These snapshots are selected not only because of their past impact on a life but because they are of use in making certain sorts of connections, certain meanings and a particular kind of story.

Medical historians remind us how the ways of the body have 'proved immensely resilient against indoctrination and infiltration from above' (Porter 1991: 219) and that to understand the history of the body we must examine the 'interplay' between the body as 'a biological given' and its representations. In Soviet Latvia the body was the site of competing lay and medical narratives. I want to examine the conflicting heterogeneity of these representations, their historical and social roots and their different purposes. In the process I shall re-examine the collapse of the old dualism which opposes body and mind and resuscitate the dualism of body and society and explore their local meanings. My case study will also reinvest the loosely and individually defined term 'resistance' with shared meanings and political purpose. Turner's brilliant critique of Foucault highlights my divergence from current Foucauldian usages:

> Foucault treats the body ... as 'resisting' power, not to be sure in collective political alliance with other bodies, but through private acts of 'deviance' or 'perversion' in which its innate capacity for pleasures find expression in ways at variance from the normative forms of desire enjoined by the disciplines of power... In being thus depoliticised and desocialized Foucault's 'resistance' thus ironically becomes, in effect, a category of transcendental subjectivity situated in the body (1994: 38).

I argue that in Soviet Latvia, bodily resistance, rather than being a private act of deviance, was constitutive of the patriotic body.

Historical Context

In order to understand the micro-narratives of the body I must introduce some macro-historical narratives. Lying as it does on the eastern shores of the Baltic, Latvia's geography has contributed in large measure to its turbulent and bloody history. The ice-free port of Liepāja and the thousand navigable kilometres of the River Daugava made the Baltic lands worth fighting for, and the openness of the terrain made it easy. For Peter the Great, who incorporated much of present day Latvia into the Russian empire in 1721, it provided a window on the West. Swedes, Russians, Poles, Baltic Germans and latterly Soviets have fought over this land.

Latvia, along with Lithuania and Estonia, was first occupied by the Soviets in 1939 thus bringing to an end the twenty-year period of independence. The first occupation has come to be remembered as 'the terrible year'. Arbitrary arrests and deportations of senior people took place throughout the year culminating in the arrest of 15,000 people on the night of 15 June.

German occupation followed from 1941 to 1944 and with it the destruction of the Jewish population. The Soviets returned in 1944 and their occupation lasted until the disintegration of the Soviet Union in 1991. Arbitrary arrests were widespread throughout the 1940s and 50s. The hunting of forest partisans throughout the countryside created the feeling that the war was not yet over. All able-bodied country people were required to provide large quotas of timber for state use. Impossibly heavy taxes and levies on farm produce in 1947 and 1948 paved the way for the collectivization of farming. This is what Māra has to say:

> *Those levies were obligatory. They were imposed. Whether you wanted them or not you had to do it ... And the same with anyone who had land or a horse. And they said, 'If you don't do it we'll take your horse away and give the horse to someone else'. Then you were obliged to do it.*

However, it was the co-ordinated deportation of one-tenth of all farmers throughout the three Baltic states on 25 March 1949 which precipitated the movement from private to collective farms. It also created an opportunity for the further arrests of townspeople. The establishment of *kolkhozi* was reinforced by legislation which restricted the amount of land and number of animals which could be owned.[1] These restrictions changed, however, as Māra's narrative testifies. These dates are now days of ritual commemoration and national mourning. Huge losses of the native population through death and deportation were compensated for by a policy of settling Russian workers in the three Baltic countries. Latvia's population changes were the largest. Throughout the Soviet period political allegiance was most problematic in the three Baltic countries, and all three saw greater openness in public affairs as an opportunity to move towards independence. This was formally recognized in May 1991. However, informants wanted to talk about the Second World War and its aftermath rather than these later developments.

The Interplay of Individual and Collective Narratives

In Soviet Latvia there was and still is an intense identification of narratives of the body and the self with macro-narratives of history. Indeed, certain historical events such as deportations, collectivization and changes in housing policy have had a profound influence on both medical and lay thinking about the body and illness. Le Roy Ladurie (1979: 130) writes of a creative event – the *événement créatrice* – which destroys traditional structures and brings about new structures. The Soviet occupation of the Baltic states and its aftermath could with a certain irony be termed such creative events which called for a radical restructuring of medical thinking about the body. The anthropologist Sahlins writes of the way categories are put at risk each time they are used to interpret a changing world (quoted in Burke 1991: 245). Medical categories are put at risk in each medical encounter where Latvian patients measure the adequacy of medical diagnoses against their life stories and experience.

From a comparative perspective Soviet Latvia was well provided for in terms of numbers of doctors per head of population and hospital beds, although this was not the lay perception. However, notwithstanding the generosity of medical provision the arena of health and illness was riven with conflicting perceptions and expectations. Diagnostic categories might be termed 'split symbols' reflecting political cleavages and carrying systematically opposed meanings for doctors and lay people (see Chapter 11, this volume). Whereas Latvians have a thoroughly historicized view of illness, Soviet medicine attempted to somatize history and psychological distress. Although perceptions about the real nature and causes of illness diverged, patients did receive medical attention.[2]

My research findings provide a Soviet variation of the clash between lay and medical interpretations of illness and, in interpreting them, I draw upon Williams's (1984) prescient article on chronic illness and narrative reconstruction. Williams applies the concepts of genesis and narrative reconstruction to the illness narratives of sufferers from rheumatoid arthritis. For Williams, illness narratives are directed towards the problem of genesis – the mode of formation of the illness – and the answers are sought in the relationship between the body, self and society (1987: 179). Such narratives are teleological in the sense that, like all autobiographical accounts, they involve a backward reading of events from the present. In the course of their construction, ends and beginnings are brought together and purposes and meanings bridge the two. Williams's three case studies show how 'the body is defined in its relationship to a world of social action' (ibid.: 182). The articulation of this relationship opens up the possibility of a critique of power, inequality and injustice. Bill, for example, 'linked his own demise with that of others, transcended the particulars of his own illness, and redefined his personal trouble as a public issue' (ibid.: 187).

So too, Latvian narrators define their individual illness histories in relation to the social world. In particular, autobiographies of illness are shaped by major turning points in Soviet history with their inevitable social and individual consequences. Like Bill, Māra redefines her own and her family's health in relation to the events which followed the Soviet occupation. Illness is the mode in which Latvians articulate their relationship to history and in doing so transfer it from the private to the public domain. This perspective is far removed from the emphatically somatic orientation of Soviet medicine. However, whereas in the West, as Scheper-Hughes and Lock (1987: 10) note, the distinction between disease and illness has led to a medical appropriation of illness, this did not occur in Soviet Latvia. The experience and narrativization of illness is deeply politicized and collectivized. The generous provision of medical diagnoses as well as medical care has to be seen in the light of a highly politicized and historicized lay perspective on illness.

Medical Practice in Soviet Latvia

Soviet Latvia was well provided for in terms of medical and psychiatric care, as measured by the numbers of doctors per head of population and hospital beds. Two features stand out as characteristic of medical provision. First, there was an absence of generalist or family practitioners and, as a consequence, patients were able to exercise a considerable degree of autonomy in defining the nature of their medical problem and determining the specialist treatment which they required. Secondly, Soviet medical practice encompassed a large number of diagnoses which, from a Western perspective, we would class as psychosomatic. However, whereas in Western medical thinking the direction of causation is primarily from psyche to soma, in Soviet medical thinking the direction is from soma to psyche. On the Jamesian model disturbed emotions are attributed to bodily malfunction. In this respect Soviet medicine is generous in its dispensation of medical diagnoses and protects patients against experiences of felt transitory stigma so characteristic of British general practice. Diagnoses such as cardiac and vegetativa neurosis and neurasthenia put an emphasis on physical symptoms and malfunctioning, and these have an inevitable impact on the person's psychological state. One of my informants, who had taken on board a somatic and depersonalized medical language, spoke of having an anxious person's heart. However, most of my letter writers found that official medical categories were unable to contain the meanings at the core of their illness experience. Meanings were constructed through a dramatized dialogue between the embodied present and memory of the past. In the process, narratives invariably reached out to the society of which they had been and continued to be a part.

Māra's Story

Māra's narrative, both written and oral, illustrates the social embeddedness of illness and its inescapably historical dimension. Māra was born into a farming family in 1924 in the parish of Drusti. She was fifteen at the time of the first Soviet occupation and a young woman of twenty at the time of the second occupation. Her memories from infancy onwards are of hard work.

> *I started my working life at the age of five and a half, because my parents at the time were building on inherited land. They started on a bare hillside. During the first summer starting from 23rd April (St. George's Day) we lived in a newly built shed without heating. Food for the family, craftsmen and house builders was prepared in a little timber hut. My duty was to herd three or four cows and small animals (letter dated 17 February 1992).*

However, it is not the hard work but the arbitrariness and unreason-ableness of events which she singles out in her later life. Illness is interwoven with historical events and seen as their logical outcome. Māra's auto-biographical narrative locates illness in the oppressive relationship between the individual and the state. Illnesses identify the points of greatest historical and social tension. Narratives of the genesis and development of illness are inseparable from the history of Soviet Latvia. Māra's account documents the effects of a reduced labour force on expectations of women's work in the years following the Second World War: work took priority over reproduction and childrearing. She describes the moves preceding and the consequences of collectivization. Farmers were driven from outlying farmsteads to the parish centre by indirect means as well as by brute force. Expropriation of horses meant that farm roads were no longer used and outlying farmsteads rapidly became inaccessible. Arbitrary and rapidly changing regulations, restricting the area of land and the number of farm animals which could be owned, reduced the ability of farmers to make adequate provision for their families. The communal organization of work in so-called brigades and the widespread custom of payment for special favours in vodka is held responsible for excessively high rates of male alcoholism. Military service is held responsible for nervous exhaustion both in the soldiers themselves and in their mothers. Public events and their repercussions on personal health are linked by an inexorable chain of consequences.

Like British narratives of chronic illness, Latvian lay accounts constitute a moral critique of society, but of a more absolute and uncompromising nature. Unlike Mrs Fields whose pursuit of virtue, though directed towards the enactment of a cohesive moral identity (Williams 1993: 99), is nevertheless rooted in the historical values of the society to which she belongs, no such overlap is to be found in Latvian illness narratives. Similarly, Bury's (1982) account of illness creating biographical disruption needs to be reversed in the context of Soviet Latvia: it is biographical disruption which causes illness. The genesis of illness is to be found in society and history but the illness narrative does not draw upon the values of that society in order to manage the illness. The story is one of stark conflict.

Childbirth and Forestry Work

Māra's account of pregnancy and childbirth focuses on tensions in the post-war period between Soviet expectations of women as workers and women as reproducers of workers. She places her account in the context of forestry work which was compulsory for all country people.[3] Her husband was away felling timber for weeks at a time in Trapāne near the Estonian border. But women were not excluded from supplying a specified quota of felled timber.

> *But I was required to fulfil the same quota. But I ... I was lucky ... at that time ... it was 1951 and I was pregnant ... I was expecting a child, he was born in February. But somehow they didn't believe me. They ... how shall I put it ... the director of the executive committee arrived at the house and he'd brought the doctor with him. He wanted to check. He thought that I was just lying and deceitful. Well I could have shown him my doctor's certificate but they didn't ask for it and it wasn't shown. And they arrived in such a deep winter and examined me. And I had to go to the maternity hospital any minute and I said, 'What on earth shall I do?' Well the eldest boy – how old was he. He was two or two-and-a-half years old. Well there was just my mother and I. And we'd all had our horses taken away. And the horse farm was about two kilometres away and the snow was terribly thick then. And what would happen if I suddenly had to leave in the night. And we didn't have any roads because we didn't have any horses. And somehow my husband got to the farm on skis and there was no track to the main road either, none at all. And so they just made off as quickly as possible. But somehow that husband of mine managed to stay at home and then it was quite lucky that he didn't have to stay long. He wasn't allowed to stay long at home. Then I was taken away ... At that time ... Yes.*

At the heart of this story is a sustained sense of victimhood and a plea for the listener to acknowledge the unreasonable situation in which she was put. Compulsory forest work was a universal requirement of all able bodied men and women in post-war Soviet Latvia. Sickness and pregnancy provided grounds for exemption but, as this episode illustrates, both were reluctantly recognized.

Māra uses her medical biography to highlight the cruelty of government requirements. The fulfilment of quotas is put above individual needs and differences. Her difficulty in reaching the maternity hospital is linked to the Soviet policy of destroying isolated farmsteads typical of the Latvian countryside and driving the inhabitants into centralized villages. The destruction of roads played a major role in this process. This is what Māra has to say on the subject:

> *Well those roads were destroyed while we were ... ah ... well before the kolkhozi. Then we were three houses together and we each had a horse and there was a road and we could ... But with joining the kolkhozi the horses were taken away from everybody and we were left without roads. Well and my husband's work place was about three kilometres away and completely without roads. He could only move with skis in the winter. Well and in the summer there was dew again and so on. Then there were no roads. That's how it was. We were forced. And during the summers the tractors would destroy all the tracks. We were forced to move somewhere nearer the road, the main road.*

Her anxiety-ridden pregnancy is linked to the mechanisms used to implement collectivization and a drive from the periphery to the centre. It also provides a potent vehicle of social criticism.

The Difficulties of Childrearing

Māra's children were born during the turbulent and impoverished post war period. Her three sons were born in 1948, 1951 and 1954. She experienced great difficulties in feeding her sons during their weaning period and uses those difficulties to mount a powerful critique of Soviet attitudes towards women with young children.

> *It was hard. It was very hard. We had to make do with more basic things. It was during the difficult times. At one point we couldn't get any semolina or white flour or any such things you need when a child goes on to solids … The semolina, we managed to get a little ration of a kilogram a month. Bread was on rations too. And then I used to say as a joke that those children were like enemies of the state. Because adults got a ration, being workers, but not the children. Now children receive a state benefit but at that time there wasn't any benefit … A woman with a child cannot work but that wasn't taken into account at all. It wasn't taken into account. I used to say 'But they are going to be the workers of the future' and that the whole of society should help. But that wasn't taken into account.*

Husband's Drinking and Collectivization

Māra has been widowed since 1980. In recalling her husband's life and health she takes the opportunity to link his health problems and indeed his death to aspects of collective farming, and to contrast this unfavourably with an earlier state of affairs.

> *Well on the whole he was really strong and healthy … but finally … finally he died of the liver. Just yesterday evening I was talking about it with my son … Well, he worked just nearby in the farm. And there were these friends who went there … Well and he'd got into the habit, he couldn't manage without drinking a couple of bottles of wine a day. That cheap wine called bumbas or bombas, whatever it was. And it seems that lately he brewed some sort of ale. I don't know the ins and outs of it but then suddenly he became quite yellow so that he was taken to hospital and that's where he stayed.*

I wanted to know whether Māra knew that he was drinking.

> *Well, yes, I did know. How could I not know? I could tell just from his voice and his behaviour. But that's how it was. His friends were always around. And that's how he'd got into the habit. He liked the taste of the wine. Well, when he wasn't drinking he was good. And then he was hardworking. But when he was drunk he behaved as drunks do. But I have to say if we lived in a private house, a farmstead where we were separate and didn't have connections with others then it wouldn't have come to this but now … But I have to say that it's a disease of the times (laikmeta vaina) where the men are altogether and then they start …*

I asked whether Māra's own health was affected by diseases of the time.

Well in just the same way ... There is a nervousness the whole time.

Military Service and Nervousness

They wanted to send my son away again. The same one who's here at home who was serving in the peninsula of Novaja Zemla. He was doing his military service on Novaja Zemla and at that time he wasn't allowed to say that they were destroying atomic weapons there. And he himself says that after the military service he feels a constant tiredness ... that there is tiredness. And then when he returned home again it was someone local. He was a military inspector (virsdienests) or whatever the name is. He'd already done his military service. And he's been promised, he'd been told that he would be given lighter work because his health had been affected and that they wouldn't be bothered any more. But here the war commission wouldn't recognize that and he was called to all sorts of ... well, every two months ... They were local but they even wanted to send him to Chernobyl. For two whole years. That was a terrible anxiety and how could it not affect the nerves? All of life has gone by in a turmoil. There hasn't been any peaceful life.

There was widespread resistance throughout the Soviet Union particularly on the part of mothers to the military drafting of their sons. High mortality rates were the experience of ethnic minorities even when not involved in active warfare. Māra recalls her son's military service in terms of its health consequences both for him and for herself.

Collectivization of 1949 and Māra's Health

Well yes ... it got taken away ... We didn't have a lot of land ... We only had ten hectares and that husband of mine had got it into his head that he would never join the kolkhoz. And the larger farmers they didn't sow rye or anything anymore, they understood that they wouldn't be able to ... well, pay the taxes and hand over the levies.[4] But we sowed a large area of rye and it was beautiful rye and we had clover when we had to hand over those large animals and horses ... We had two horses, we gave them away. Well then, during the Khrushchev period things were difficult because they wanted to destroy the private farms and they took away the land. When we were working in the kolkhoz we had half a hectare of land. But finally it changed so that everything had to be given to the Soviet enterprise, everything had to go to the sovhoz.[5] It was the same around our house. We were just left with half a hectare. And during the Khrushchev period ... Khrushchev had a programme to make everyone work in that ... He took the half hectare and left even less. They measured around the house. Our house was on a little hill, we'd planted all around it ... well, it was a Latvian farmstead ... We were just left so much ... And then we dug up all the fruit bushes and what have you with a spade so that we could plant potatoes or some such. And we couldn't mow the hay until it hadn't been mowed for the collective. The hay could only be mown in cold September and by that time the rains had started. It was very difficult with the hay. Then we could only keep one cow and one pig ... That was towards the end of Khrushchev's government, I don't remember the year any more. It was towards the end of Khrushchev's period and we were six people: the two of us with my husband, there was my mother and three children that makes six people. And they took the pig away, the pig was taken away. It was taken away as tax and the land was taken away and the cow.

I wanted to know how much land they were left.

I think it was about 0.15 hectares. And they also wanted to destroy the cow so that one would only work for the collective so that one would make do with work for the collective. But because my husband was the only worker, there was me and three children and my mother was old, we couldn't survive on that. We couldn't manage with one person's wage ... Where would we get more? we didn't get it anywhere. We didn't get it anywhere. But I just know that we had to take that pig and we were left with one and even that we had to give away for very little money. We sold a large pig and that autumn it seems that Khrushchev was no more so that that autumn we were suddenly allowed to keep as many animals as wanted... We were allowed to keep many piglets. And so it turned out that in place of that large pig we got a small piglet. The piglets were so expensive we could just get one piglet. And then I remember in the market my husband saying 'We must buy two piglets. We must buy two piglets.' But I said 'No. What's the point? We'll raise a fat pig and then have to give it away again.' He said: 'No, no. One is not enough.' And so we bought two after all. And then things were different again. We could keep more.[6]

This narrative of the drive into collective farms and the impact it had on families emphasizes the arbitrariness and constantly changing character of legislation. So much so that any planning or providing for the future came to seem pointless. Māra feels robbed of any sense of agency. Indeed, she links her ill health, particularly her asthma, to the regulations imposed in order to achieve collectivization of the Latvian countryside.

Well, I began to be ill when I was about twenty. When the children started going to school at that time I was ill with asthma. I had asthma. If I worked harder or washed clothes or got hot then I would suffocate terribly. Well, and we lived far from the road so I couldn't call the doctor just at that time. So I would wait a little until it was over and then they would think I was putting it on or something ... We didn't have electricity there, we weren't allowed to install it. We were all driven into the villages. Then I started washing the clothes in a machine and then I didn't get hot ... and then it started getting better ... Of course my heart had been affected and I got tired easily. So I can't say that my health has been good. And with regard to my nerves, well ... it's clear that my nerves suffered along with these events. They suffer from all of that.

Discussion

This case study illustrates the 'thickness' of medical narratives: Māra's medical autobiography reaches out to encompass events and structures in the political arena. Her medical history bears the signature of a public history. However, although historical events have left their mark on the structure of both lay and medical ideas about illness, the mode of their incorporation is different. Whereas lay thought makes explicit reference to such events, medical reference is allusive and implicit. For this reason medical encounters frequently turn into social dramas of the kind described by Victor Turner: concealed conflicts in which opposing interpretations of the past and present emerge in the course of the medical encounter (Turner 1974). Patients challenge existing structures in the light of their individual experience (see Chapter 7, this volume). Māra's account of the doctor's visit to her farmstead during her second pregnancy constitutes such a social drama in which the conflicting needs of childbirth and the state's demands for timber are pitted against each other. In a society short of labour power due to war deaths and deportations the role of the doctor in declaring people sick role was particularly fraught and accusations of malingering were common. The folk wisdom on this issue is summed up in an anecdote which Māra recounted to me.

> *Everyone, men and women, had to work. The women even if they had small children. One was only let off work with a doctor's certificate. But the doctors were hesitant: everyone feared deportation. Even the sick couldn't get a certificate and often they died working. In hospitals they used the word malingerer* (simulants) *or rogue. Let me give you an anecdote. In the morning the doctor asks the duty nurse 'What's new?' She answers, 'Nothing much, only the malingerer has died!'* (quoted in Skultans 1997b: 21).

However, this challenge is not issued on a private or *ad hoc* basis. Rather, the experience of illness and its emotional reverberations provide a principal mechanism for transforming private memory into public or social memory. In the course of this transformation the body and its historical experience are invested with a rationality and wisdom of their own. This cultural configuration reverses certain other powerful and common stereotypes such as, 'a deep-seated cultural stereotype ... which pictures the body as an anarch, a lord of misrule, emblematic of excess in food, drink, sex, violence – the embodiment of the principle which Freud later intellectualised as the "id" ' (Porter 1991: 217).

Medical practice provides an important arena in which the convergence and divergence of collective and individual experience can be examined. Frank's (1995) perceptive exploration of Western illness narratives shows the interpenetration of medical and philosophical thought in the shaping of individual stories of illness. Illness as political critique and resistance is not among the paradigms which he discusses in the North American context. However, anthropological studies can provide us with many examples of this classic paradigm first articulated by Lewis (1966). For example, Ong sees spirit possession as disclosing the anguish and resistance of young Malay women factory workers (1987: 195–213). Women use their possessed bodies to defy the punitive discipline imposed upon them in situations where they are deprived of a voice.

Before we look at the symbolic and communicative dimensions of illness, it is worth reminding ourselves that totalitarian societies can have very direct and brutal effects on health. Poor living conditions, not to speak of exile, imprisonment and years in labour camps, leave visible marks on people's bodies. The signs of physical violation point to past repression even before informants have incorporated their feelings of exhaustion, dizziness and anxiety into a personal voice. While Kleinman's Chinese patients emphasized the somatic aspects of their illness, Latvians were more concerned with worn-down nerves and painful feelings both of which were unambiguously attributed to historical events which they had experienced (Kleinman 1988; Skultans 1998a). Thus history is both experienced in and represented by the body. Bodies are both sign and symbols. Such representations take a common shape, and interactions between patients and doctors drew, to a certain extent, upon a shared language. And yet what was exchanged was a common form and not a common meaning. Whilst patients had a deeply historicized and social view of health and illness, doctors interpreted psychological symptoms in physiological terms. Common forms enabled the interaction to proceed, but conflicting meanings meant that patients felt that problems were never fully addressed. Soviet medicine appropriated historical suffering and renamed it to suit itself.[7]

And yet this transformation is never complete. Memory belongs to the world of shared meanings and language but it also belongs to a private world of experience. Thomson's work on Anzac memories highlights the difficult relationship between public and private memories:

> *In one sense we 'compose' or construct memories using the public language and meanings of our culture. In another sense we 'compose' memories which help us to feel relatively comfortable with our lives, which give us a feeling of composure … One key theoretical connection, and the link between the two senses of composure, is that the apparently private processes of composing safe memories is in fact very public. Our memories are risky and painful if they do not conform with the public norms or versions of the past* (1998: 300–1).

What is implied by the narrator may be at odds with the public memories and meanings which are the subject of the narrative. Just as anthropologists and sociologists have 'socialized' memory, so too they have 'socialized' emotion: 'Emotion arises from or inheres in the structural relations of society' (Barbalet 1992: 161). Emotions always have an object which connects the individual experience with the world of shared meanings and structures. But the nature of that connection can promote integration or division. It can make the individual feel protected by a larger whole or rejected and alone (Kemper 1984: 374). As Rosaldo has so movingly written, we have a need to exaggerate the power of social institutions and ritual to tame negative and painful emotions such as grief (1993: 20). Emotions of anger and grief are not easy to integrate into society, even less so when, as in Soviet Latvia, there was no common consensus around the object (in this case the historical past) which gave rise to such negative feelings. Indeed, as Jenkins found in El Salvador, the very expression of distress or negative feelings may be interpreted as a politically subversive act (1991: 154).

The life story which Māra recounts does not give her a feeling of composure. Indeed, she attributes her lack of composure to the course which her life has taken. The experience of illness is both the outcome of a life such as hers and provides the conceptual tools for criticizing the events she has endured. A critical review of her life opens up an ever-widening rift between medical (or state) constructions of the problem and her own grounded experience. Indeed, important aspects of her life history are marked out by conflicts with the medical profession: narratives of pregnancy, childbirth and married life are constructed around the opposed needs of the body and the demands of doctors. The historical critique furnished by her life and medical history has much in common with other narratives which I listened to: the same historical events were incorporated into many other narratives and the same appeal was made to a common culture and identity under threat. It is in this sense that I speak of individual narratives contributing to a common narrative which constructs a patriotic body. My analysis of this narrative is indebted to the theoretical agenda which Scheper-Hughes and Lock (1987) set out in their literature review of the body. They propose three levels of analysis or three discursive perspectives on the body: the individual, the social, and the political. The individual body is characterized by lived experience, the social body by exchanges of meaning, and the political body by control and surveillance. In proposing this tripartite approach they challenge the reigning medical dualisms which relegate individual and social experience to the margins.

Latvian illness narratives do not fit easily with the tri-partite categorisation of the body proposed by Scheper-Hughes and Lock (ibid.). They set out three distinctive perspectives on the body: the phenomenally experienced body-self, the social body which provides a rich source of symbols for thinking about society, and the political body which is the target of discipline and control. The individual body is experienced as subject, the social and political body as object. In a tantalizingly brief addendum the authors propose emotion as the mediating link between the three bodies, thus imposing a heavy explanatory load upon what is a highly contested theoretical area. Scheper-Hughes and Lock endorse a constructionist account of the emotions. However, this does not enable the emotions to perform their mediating function. Only an essentialist account can do this, to which the authors clearly do not wish to subscribe. However, what has been separated needs to be put together and we are, therefore, offered a composite account which combines feeling with its cultural expression 'capable of bridging mind and body, individual, society, and body politic' (ibid.: 29). I would argue that the three bodies may be useful as a heuristic exercise or a way of organizing a review of the literature. However, as a more far reaching conceptual device for accessing varieties of corporeal experience, it unwittingly sets up boundaries which problematize the recognition and subjective appropriation of the experiences of the political and social body. Latvian illness narratives suggest that the three bodies are not simply three theoretical perspectives on the body, but three deeply interpenetrating ways of experiencing the body. Thus, the social body is not just a way of thinking about the body but also a way of experiencing it. The political body is not simply a way of disciplining the individual body, but also a way of actively using the body to register protest.

Scheper-Hughes (1992) has given an intensely moving account of illness and death among the poor of Brazil. She describes the material embeddedness of hunger and disease. However, she also asks how hunger and political exploitation come to be medicalized.

> How have these people come to see themselves primarily as nervous and only secondarily as hungry? How is it that mortally tired cane cutters and washer-women define themselves as weak rather than as exploited? Worse, when overwork and exploitation *are* recognized, how in the world do these get reinterpreted as an illness, *nervos de trabalhar muito*, for which the appropriate cure is a tonic, vitamin A, or a sugar injection? Finally how does it happen that chronically hungry people 'eat' medicines while going without food? (ibid.: 177).

My answer to these rhetorical questions is that hunger, overwork and illness are not reinterpreted as illnesses but are experienced as such. The answer which Scheper-Hughes gives is that illness is a kind of incomplete narrative and that the body is used to register a muted form of protest: 'To raise one's voice in active political protest is impossible and wildly dangerous. To be totally silenced, however, is intolerable. Into "impossible" situations such as these, the nervous, shaking, agitated, angry body may be enlisted to keep alive the perception that a real "state of emergency" exists' (ibid.: 187). However, this reading of the situation prioritizes the political over the phenomenological body.

These shared political narratives of the body do not altogether encompass the entire person. Narratology emphasizes the difference between the act of narration and narrative or between the person and the story. These differences create a space for silence as well as a diversity of voices. Gergen has argued persuasively that, 'Narratives of the self are not personal impulses made social, but social processes realized on the site of the personal' (1994: 210). Similarly, Gergen argues that emotion is not a personal property of the individual but comes into being through relationships: 'Emotional discourse gains its meaning not by virtue of its relationship to an inner world (of experience, disposition or biology), but by the way it figures in patterns of cultural relationship. Communities generate conventional modes of relating; patterns of action within these relationships are often given labels. Some forms of action – by current western standards – are said to indicate emotions' (ibid.: 222). And yet the site of the personal can never be fully colonized by the social, particularly where the social is itself fragmented and calls for conflicting allegiances. Māra's emotional discourse gains meaning through its relationship to the past and yet that relationship is not fully realized in narrative. For her as for many others emotion as relationship remains a potentiality rather than an actuality. Māra's physical presence, the timbre of her voice – lost in transcription – is a reminder of the bodily base and inescapably private dimension of emotional experience. This means that her experience can never be fully captured in words, especially in a culture which sets great store by self-control (cf. Gerber 1985: 121). This position finds support in phrases such as 'only those who have lived through the past can understand it', or 'that can't be put into words'. The illness narrative may make connections with a shared history but the illness experience remains a source of private pain. There are connections to be made with the literature on the Holocaust and the problems of representing experience which lies beyond the limits of imagination (Lang 1992: 304). It is impossible to give narrative shape to experience which destroys the goals of the self because the destruction of those goals will impair the powers of narrative memory. Langer writes of 'the uneasy feeling of the literary transforming the real in away that obscures even as it seeks to enlighten' (1991: 19). However, the residues of such experience find a ready home in the body.

Kleinman and Kleinman's recent interest in the idea of social suffering, or the question 'To what uses are experiences of suffering put?' (1996: 3), is especially worth asking in the context of accelerated social change and reassessments of the past experienced by the Baltic states and the former Soviet Union. Their earlier essay on bodily memory explores the relationship between history and physiology in terms of the question, 'How do political processes of terror (and resistance) cross over from public space to traumatize (or reanimate) inner space and then cross back as collective experience?' (1994: 711). Although their writing is richly suggestive they do not succeed, as they set out to do, in formulating the necessary concepts for this new field of study. The failure of analysis to which they allude is about 'a story of the prodigality of interpretation [and] ... a story of the aridity of methods – the study of the processes that mediate and transform the bodily forms of social experience has yet to be written' (ibid.: 711). Their own writing contributes further to such interpretations but not to the methods. We cannot follow the movement from public to inner space, even if we knew where to look for this space. Instead, we can listen to collective and individual narratives. My argument is that the linked questions posed by the Kleinmans can only be answered by concentrated attention to and detailed analysis of the narratives which arise from the experience of historical suffering, and which in turn give it shape. If we do so, I believe we will find that collective and individual memory are not so thoroughly interconnected as Connerton (1989) has suggested, but that they are involved in continual processes of coming together and moving apart over time. When they move apart we must look for traces of the individual's experience in the body.

Notes

1. *Kolkhoz* is a Russian term for a collective farm where workers are paid in produce.
2. This is no longer the case as a large category of diagnoses such as neurasthenia, cardiac neurosis and *vegetatīvā neiroze* are being abruptly discarded. Thus patients who have grown accustomed to living with a particular medical version of their problems are suddenly being forced to accept an alternative medical history, often one which fails to recognize their problems in any shape or form. Not least, the privatisation of medicine creates further problems of access.
3. Obligatory forestry work was widespread between 1945 and 1949, 1946 and 1947 being particularly bad years. The rules were issued by the Council of People's Commissariat for timber felling, transmitted to the Latvian government and then to local executives. These local officials decided on the requirements from particular individuals. Country people were forced to sign contracts promising to deliver stipulated amounts of timber. Availability of transport was not taken into account.
4. In 1947 taxes were 40 per cent of estimated revenue; in 1948 they rose to 75 per cent.
5. *Sovhoz* is Russian for a state owned farm where workers receive a stipulated wage.
6. According to the 1935 agricultural statutes of Soviet Russia, applied to Latvia under Soviet occupation, each household could have one cow, two young calves, one sow with piglet (or two piglets without the sow), ten sheep and goats and 20 beehives. In Khrushchev's time the rules were tightened. From 1971 onwards permission had to be sought from the *kolkhoz*.
7. The post-Soviet reorganization of the medical diagnostic system and medical practice has thrown forms and meanings into the air. There is a problem not only about conflicting meanings, but the linguistic forms which held these conflicts together no longer carry authority and have become unavailable.

10

FROM DAMAGED NERVES TO MASKED DEPRESSION: INEVITABILITY AND HOPE IN LATVIAN PSYCHIATRIC NARRATIVES

❧

Introduction

Rapid changes in Latvian psychiatric thinking and practice over the last decade raise questions about the nature of distress, of mental illness, its relationship to changes in styles of psychiatric reasoning and to political and economic changes in society. Social differentiation in Latvian society has led to a proliferation of narratives and the transformation of subjectivities. This chapter explores the movement from a somatic to a psychological language of distress and considers the ways in which these changes link with ideas of agency, victimhood and shared versus private articulations of pain. This chapter then lies between three domains and three sets of polarities and seeks to find their interconnections. The first domain concerns changing social and economic conditions. The second domain concerns ideas and beliefs in popular culture about illness and distress. The third domain concerns changing psychiatric ideas and practices. In seeking to understand changes within these domains and their interconnections I make use of three sets of polarities: that between individual and social as well as historical accounts of illness; that between the individual as agent versus passive victim, and that between somatic and psychological thinking about illness. These polarities do not map onto each other in a straightforward way.

Let me start by outlining my ethnographic credentials and the fieldwork upon which this chapter draws. Since 1992 I have spent some twenty-four months on fieldwork projects in Latvia, most recently 6 months in 2001 exploring changes in psychiatric ideas and practice. As part of this project I sat in on psychiatric consultations in two urban and four provincial polyclinics and a private clinic in Riga. Altogether some three hundred consultations were tape-recorded and these have been transcribed into over a thousand typed pages. I also interviewed some fifteen or so psycho-therapists, psychiatrists and neurologists, sometimes by formal arrange-ment but more often through more casual conversation squeezed in between consultations, during a short break or a hasty lunch of coffee and *pirāgi*. My own psychotherapeutic cum ethnographic interviews of around thirty-five patients in a polyclinic in north-east Vidzeme constituted the eighth clinical setting. I also organized focus groups and interviews with psychotherapists, psychiatrists and neurologists. I attended several con-ferences organized by pharmaceutical companies on the subject of depres-sion, anxiety and panic attacks. These conferences take place at least once a month and are attended by several hundred psychiatrists and psycho-neurologists. As a result unanimity in the theory and practice of psychiatry is promoted throughout Latvia. The siting of the research in several settings helped to identify the multiple influences shaping languages of distress arising both from within the profession of psychiatry and more broadly from within society.

Changing Social and Economic Conditions

Before embarking on a discussion of popular and psychiatric beliefs in Latvia let me give an outline of the first domain. In the early 1990s the Baltic states were most keen to sever their ties with the Soviet Union and played a key role in the dissolution of the Soviet Union. Latvian independence was declared following the unsuccessful Moscow putsch in August 1991. Since then Latvia has embarked on a rapid programme of decollectivization, the introduction of a market economy and the restruc-turing of the health service. Some people have benefited from these changes but for many others living conditions have deteriorated. Vulnerable categories include the old, lone women with children and the disabled and chronically sick. But everyone suffers from an increased sense of the unpredictability and precariousness of life. A recent report on social conditions in Latvia emphasizes the high rates of unemployment and the precariousness of working conditions (*Latvijas Republikas Labklājības Ministrija* 2000). Surveys of poverty suggest that some 75 per cent of the population think they are worse off now than they were ten years ago (Gassmann and de Neubourg 2000: 27).

At the same time the influx of Western television programmes, films and advertising holds out the promise of infinite possibilities for those who have the right personal qualities and aspirations. Removal of external restraints, the invisibility of barriers to economic success, the high visibility of some successful individuals and the greater increased presence of social and economic inequalities all combine to promote a culture of shame and guilt. Self-control and self-reliance have been features of Latvian culture for a long time and they are now being reinforced by the extreme capitalist ethic. One consequence of this ethic is that individuals suffering from physical and psychological disabilities are ashamed of their problems and reluctant to share them with others. This represents a change from Soviet times when problems tended to bring people together.

Despite fear and distrust of the state under communism individuals were integrated in many intimate ways with the *kolektīvs*, the collective group, and they now feel on their own and cast adrift. My perception differs from some other views. For example, the Polish sociologist Nowak argues that there was a social vacuum at the heart of communist society (summarized in Wedel 1992: 1–21). However, anthropologists such as Verdery (1996: 298) acknowledge the importance of close social networks, particularly as they relate to the pervasive split between public and private. In particular, vast differences in economic status have made people ashamed of their poverty and the problems associated with it. For example, public rituals such as school leaving ceremonies, traditionally associated with considerable expenditure, have now become huge sources of stress. The Baltic states, together with the Russian Federation and Belarus, have the highest suicide rates in the world. It is a commonplace that civic structures that have been associated with the best features of Western society have barely had a chance to develop in the countries of the former Soviet Union. Robert Putnam (2000: 326–35) and others have argued that the absence of social capital is associated with increased rates of depression and suicide in America. The absence of social capital, of social connectedness and trust play similar powerful roles in the Baltic states.

A paradoxical feature of a social philosophy that places increased emphasis on freedom of choice is that people now have less autonomy in the management of health and illness. Health care in Soviet Latvia was organized around the polyclinics staffed by a group of specialists including neurologists and psychiatrists. The system accorded the individual a considerable amount of autonomy in choosing specialist treatment and in access to their medical history and notes. Government policy after independence has been premised on the view that Latvians were over doctored and that there was a wasteful duplication of resources. For this reason the number of specialists has been reduced, family practitioners acting as gatekeepers to specialist treatment have been introduced and in the process the autonomy of the patient has been systematically eroded. In particular, the number of neurologists and psychiatrists has decreased more than the other specialists. In 1992 there were 301 neurologists in 2001 there were 236. The number of psychiatrists has also decreased by 14 per cent.

Meanwhile the number of family practitioners has increased from 43 in 1992 to 996 in the year 2000. Every inhabitant in Latvia is required to be registered with a family practitioner. Medical treatment is no longer free and patients are required to pay 50 santimes (around fifty pence) per consultation. The reduction in the number of psychiatrists and neurologists has been accompanied by a growth in the number of private psycho-therapists. The Association for Psychotherapists was founded in 1991 and now has sixty-four members. Psychotherapists emphasize the importance of strength of character and promise choice precisely at a time when, for many, life choices have narrowed and life seems most arbitrary.

Ideas about Illness and Distress in Popular Culture

Let me now move on to my second domain, namely, changing beliefs about illness and distress in popular culture. Traditional values advocate stoicism and contentment with one's lot. The folkloristic view of the self as the author of its emotions has never been fully laid to rest. However, the language of illness and distress has been thoroughly penetrated by Latvian history over the second half of the twentieth century. The language of *nervi* has become commonplace and suggests that to suffer from *nervi* (nerves) is an inevitable consequence of having lived under Soviet rule. *Nervi* formed the connective tissue between individuals both in lay discourse and in medical consultations. The discourse of *nervi* sets patients in the context of a shared past history and social circumstances. By contrast, independence and westernization have introduced a range of hitherto unrecognized syndromes and illnesses, foremost among them masked depression. However, rather than connecting them with others, depression, as I shall show, establishes a relationship with a hitherto, unknown abstract entity – an illness.

To ask about a person's *nervi* was, and still is, to invite a life story. Conversely, in speaking of *nervi* people emphasize temporal and social dimensions of the self. The state of one's *nervi* gives an indication of the course of one's life and singles out the relationship of the self, be it fraught or harmonious, to passing events and the passage of time. The verbs used in conjunction with *nervi* all have a temporal dimension and take an indirect object. Thus, to speak about *nervi* is to put one's life in a social and historical context. People spoke of what their *nervi* had been through (*izdzīvojuši*) and experienced or survived (*pārdzīvojuši*). The common stem in these words is *dzīve* or life. They also referred to what their *nervi* had endured (*pārcietuši*) and suffered (*cietuši*). Talk of *nervi*, therefore, points simultaneously in two directions: it points outwards, offering a way of understanding the world and its subjective importance and it points reflexively towards the speaking self, disclosing its particular nature and values. Rather like Ilongot talk about 'hearts', there is in Latvian discourse about *nervi* 'a sense of dialectic or dynamic tension between a state of sociality and one of opposition and withdrawal, between a self at ease with its environment and one that stands apart' (M.Z. Rosaldo 1980: 44).

However, while the discourse of *nervi* is still powerful, another discourse that emphasizes personal control is increasingly making itself heard. The move from somatic to psychological disorders, and depression in particular, represents the internalization of a heightened sense of accountability and responsibility for one's life circumstances despite the fact that few opportunities for changing those circumstances exist.

The ways of describing and accounting for distress in the eight clinical settings I observed represent not only changing diagnostic practices but also the changed nature of the individual's engagement with society. Indeed, I will argue that it is the individual's relationship to society that determines both the acceptance of new diagnoses and the experience of distress.

By way of example let me describe a recurring paradigm that underpins patients' accounts of distress in a polyclinic in Vidzeme. In seven clinical settings I was a relatively passive observer sitting in a corner of the psychiatrist's consulting room and tape-recording the consultation. However, before I was able to negotiate this privileged position I was given the opportunity to talk to patients directly. The director of one polyclinic that was without a psychotherapist or psychiatrist invited me to see patients in a psychotherapeutic capacity. A notice was placed in the local newspaper offering no-payment psychotherapy on particular dates. In this eighth clinical setting I was alone with the patients but for the presence of a tape recorder. All recordings were subsequently transcribed. Of the thirty-five patients who consulted me two-thirds began their narrative by complaining that they could not put themselves in order or that they seemed to have lost control of their lives. They used phrases such as 'I can't cope with myself' (*Es netieku galā ar sevi*), 'I can't cultivate myself' (*Es nevaru sakopt sevi*) or 'I can't put myself in order' (*Es nevaru savākt sevi*) or 'I overstep the limit' (*Es izeju no rāmjiem*) or, literally, 'I step outside the frame'. In each case there is a deep regret and anxiety that self-control has been lacking or inadequate and that the individual is responsible in important ways for the circumstances of their lives. I give some illustrations from my own psychotherapeutic interviews:

> *Ingrīda is twenty-nine years old, married and with a nine-year-old daughter. She feels she is lucky to have a husband who does not drink, a job she likes as a shop assistant, a self-contained two roomed flat and enough money to get by. She knows her circumstances are better than those of many of her neighbours. And yet, although she evaluates her life as one that should bring about satisfaction and happiness, she finds that she cannot contain her anger and exude the calmness that she would like. When pressed to give an illustration of her failure to live up to cultural ideals she describes coming home from work at 11 o'clock at night after a 15 hour shift and losing her temper because the dishes have been*

left unwashed and the flat is in a mess. The interesting point relates to the fact that Ingrīda blames herself and not her long working hours for her anger. Indeed, she pointed out that she did not have to walk home but that her husband collected her in the family car.

Anta is thirty-eight, widowed some twelve years ago with two teenage daughters aged sixteen and eighteen. She works as a supervisor in a sewing factory. Her younger daughter is getting very low marks at school. Her poor performance may be related to prematurity, low birth weight and some physical impairment. Anta knows that her daughter's chances of any kind of employment are non-existent if she fails to pass her exams and yet there is no school in the town that can meet her daughter's needs. Anta has a good relationship with her daughter and recognizes her daughter's physical and educational problems as well as the social and occupational limitations that these will entail. Mother and daughter are in a no-win situation. However, Anta formulates her problems not in terms of the shortcomings of the educational system or unequal employment opportunities but in terms of her inability to stay calm when questioning her daughter about her schoolwork.

The same constellation of lack of self-control and self-blame is found in varying, but always extremely difficult, social circumstances. It represents a curious inversion in earlier loci of control where disorder and lack of predictability appeared to be attributed to society (see Chapter 9, this volume). As the narrative structure of these accounts of distress makes plain, many of the inhabitants of this provincial town have internalized the values of the enterprise culture and the responsibility for personal failure that goes with it. The experience, expression and explanation of personal distress have all been shaped by the introduction of market principles in public life. And yet they also evoke resonances with earlier traditional values. There is at present no psychotherapist or fulltime psychiatrist working here. One inhabitant explained that she had no previous experience of meeting with a psychotherapist and that her experience was confined to seeing psychotherapy sessions portrayed in films. However, if and when a psychotherapist comes to work in this town he will find a client population well prepared and ready to embrace the individualistic ethic of Latvian psychotherapy.

Thus, several conceptual frames are available to try to make sense of people's experience of illness and distress. The experience of inevitability, contingency and limited choice which has been the experience of most middle-aged and elderly Latvians is more completely expressed through narratives of *nervi* which are compatible with Soviet diagnoses such as *vegetatīvā distonija* or dysfunction of the autonomic nervous system. On the other hand, younger people have taken on board the philosophy of possibility even though their own lives are narrowly circumscribed. Under these circumstances their own lack of agency is explained in terms of illness. Agency is confined to taking proper care of the illness and economizing and budgeting the monthly budget so as be able to afford the intake of the half dozen or so daily psychotropic medicines. As Shweder et al. have written, agency is transferred from the patient to the illness: 'The sufferer is a victim, under "attack" from natural forces devoid of intentionality. Suffering is decontextualized and separated from the narrative structure of human life. It is viewed as a kind of "noise", an accidental interference with the life drama of the sufferer. It is as though suffering had no intelligible relation to any plot, except as a chaotic interruption"' (1997: 159). We have, therefore, a theory of human distress and illness that draws upon several historical layers of meaning. Indeed, there may be advantages in using multiple and sometimes opposed discourses to represent the complex areas of human experience with which psychiatry deals. As Shweder et al. suggest, 'There is no reason that one must select one and only one discourse to represent an area of experience' (ibid.: 140).

I turn now to the third domain that is concerned with changes in psychiatric beliefs and practices.

Changing Psychiatric Beliefs and Practices

The appearance and explanation of distress, its nomenclature and its treatment have taken on a bewildering variety of new meanings since the collapse of communism and the advent of Latvian independence. The transience of social structures has given prominence to what Hacking (1999: 100) terms transient mental illnesses. Indeed, a review of the last few decades reveals the transience of much Latvian psychiatric theory and practice: many of the terms which were routinely used for diagnosing psychological and somatic distress are now becoming part of psychiatric history. For example, the handbook issued by the Ministry of Health of the Republic of Latvia entitled Standards of Quality for Medical Care outlines appropriate medical intervention for some 269 conditions (Latvijas Republikas Veselības Aizsardzības Ministrija 1991). We find there what is in essence an eighteenth-century view of the neuroses given a twentieth-century dress with reference to Pavlov. Neuroses are explained in terms of Pavlov's stimulus/response theories: unpredictable and over rapid stimuli lead to pathological responses. Thus somatoform disorders, including neurasthenia, appear in the neurological section. Neurasthenia, which is characterized by heightened anxiety, is similarly linked not to overwork and exhaustion, as in Western psychiatric teaching, but to unpredictable circumstances and conditions of work. An inability to plan or organize one's workload was thought to lie at the heart of neurasthenia (Hacking 1999: 20). Depression only figures as manic depressive psychosis but not as non-psychotic depression. An earlier handbook Nervu Slimības un to Profilakse (Nervous Illnesses and their Prophylaxes) has a section devoted to neuroses and one to neurasthenia (Penciks 1967). We find over a couple of decades radical changes both in the nomenclature of psychiatric illnesses and in the understanding of their nature.

These changes have been accelerated by the translation of ICD 10 (The International Classification of Diseases) into Latvian and by the several courses offered by Swedish and French psychiatrists and psychotherapists most of whom have been of a psychodynamic and psychoanalytic persuasion. Until the translation of ICD 10 as SSK 10 (*Starptautiskā Slimību Klasifikācija*) in 1997, Russian versions of ICD 7, 8 and 9 were in circulation, which were to a greater or lesser extent 'adapted to local circumstances'. Most of these adaptations concerned the sections dealing with psychiatric and neurological disorders. Psychoneurotic conditions occupied relatively little space in the Soviet version compared to the original Western templates. For example, depression only appears in the Soviet version of ICD 7 under the heading of Diseases of Old Age. However, there was a large category of somatoform disorders included in the neurology sector, which western psychiatrists would consider as properly belonging within the province of psychiatry. These are classified under the heading of 'Disorders of the Autonomic Nervous System' and include angiospasms, nerve tension, nerve asthenia, anxiety, neurasthenia and the Latvian term *vegetativā distonija* which resists easy translation but could be described as a kind of overwrought state of the autonomic nervous system. In the current Latvian version of ICD 10 these diagnoses have indeed been renamed and moved to the section on psychiatric disorders. Many of these conditions would now be considered to be signs of depression. *Vegetativā distonija* is now classified as acute panic disorder. But in the process of translation many of the rich semantic nuances and the insights it opened up on the individual and his or her social environment have been lost.

The reclassification of these disorders has been accompanied by changes in the numbers of different medical specialists, as noted earlier, and considerable tension between psychiatrists and neurologists. For example, one psychiatrist commenting on the neurologists' desire to hang on to the old diagnoses said: 'They are short of bread, they are trying to take our bread, our diagnoses'. Thus, Latvian contemporary psychiatric practice appears to have made considerable changes in diagnostic practice because of the influence of ICD 10.

However, the proselytizing activities of two pharmaceutical companies Solvay Pharma and Lundbeck have also shaped psychiatric beliefs and prescriptive practices. Both firms are actively engaged in the education of psychiatrists and family doctors through the organization of regular conferences on conditions such as masked depression, phobias and panic attacks. Patients are educated to recognize their conditions with the help of educative literature in the form of glossy brochures. Indeed, I have heard patients discussing their problems using the language of the pharmaceutical literature: 'I no longer see the colour of flowers'. There are clearly parallels here with the work of Healy (1997) who argues that the pharmaceutical companies in the West played a key role in the 'discovery' of depression. Healy documents the transformation of depression from a general feature of human experience to a medical category. He writes: 'In many respects the discovery of anti-depressants has been the invention and marketing of depression' (ibid.: 1997:5).

In many ways the expansion of available psychotropic medicines has come to epitomize the relationship of the individual to the market. The possibilities for well-being are measured in terms of the patient's financial assets. Most psychiatrists know how much their patients can afford to spend on drugs and adapt their prescriptions accordingly. Sometimes they will check whether circumstances have changed and whether the patient can still afford the 12 lats (around £15 in 2001) per month, for example. Psychiatric patients are prescribed an average of five psychotropic drugs in various combinations of fragments of a tablet. This drug regime and its adaptation to individual financial and emotional circumstances is sometimes referred to as an opera or more often as a bouquet, perhaps the single luxury item that Latvians most frequently buy. Psychiatrists use phrases such as 'Let's change a fragment of the opera' or 'Let's rearrange the bouquet'.

These three domains of economic and social change, changing popular beliefs about illness and distress, and changing psychiatric beliefs and practices are criss-crossed in unexpected ways by the polarities introduced at the beginning, of individual versus social/collective, agency versus passivity, and somatic versus psychological.

Individual Versus Social/Historical Accounts of Illness

A number of writers from different disciplines – among them Good (1994), Mishler (1985) and Waitzkin (1991) – have argued that medical interviews involve the systematic elimination of social context and subjectivity. Luhrmann by contrast characterizes American psychodynamic psychiatry as 'the naked encounter of two souls, these souls are imagined wrestling in a mud pit' (2000: 147) a powerful metaphor that emphasizes both the recognition of subjectivity and the social mud that patients bring to clinical encounters. However, Good argues that medical education teaches students how to eliminate context from the clinical interview (1994). For Waitzkin this process of contextual elimination is not about interviewing incompetence but is 'a fundamental feature of medical language, a feature that is linked with ideology and social control' (1991: 26). It represents a deliberately missed opportunity to do something about difficult social circumstances and the technologizing and medicalizing of troublesome emotions. It is more likely to take place where doctors come from more privileged social backgrounds than their patients. For Waitzkin the medical consultation is a 'micropolitical situation, in which the control of information reinforces power relations that parallel those in the broader society' (ibid.: 54).

In Latvia the situation is somewhat different. Doctors and psychiatrists are very much aware of the difficult social circumstances in which many of their patients live. During the gaps between consultations doctors sought my views on their patients but also gave me the opportunity to ask more personal questions. Frequently, the tape recorder was left running at such times. Many doctors emphasize that their own living and life circumstances are equally oppressive. In the context of talking about the social problems in Latvia one psychiatrist said:

> *By the way, we live in circumstances that are just as terrible. Our circumstances are even worse. We have studied, we have sacrificed maybe ten years of our personal lives. I was fanatically concerned with my studies and my patients. But as a result I had to walk without boots in the winter. But I knew I couldn't take a business job, although I had various offers. I knew I would receive those humiliating 20 lats a month but I wouldn't leave medicine. I knew that I couldn't improve my material and social circumstances, so I started working on myself, on my inner life. Quite simply I set myself in order more. This no-win situation forced me to put my soul in order which, of course, served me very well later in my work.*

Insufficient money and crowded living conditions are problems that many Latvian doctors share with many of their patients, and doctors see no reason to hide their personal problems from their patients. For example, doctors regularly take personal telephone calls during a consultation and often such calls concern some domestic crisis to do with food or money.

Nevertheless, despite the awareness of social problems and their powerful effect on the personal lives of doctors themselves, many psychiatrists systematically eliminate social context from the psychiatric interview. In order to explore the role that psychiatrists assign to social context in the development of psychiatric problems a focus group was set up with about forty members of the Association of Psychotherapists meeting in the Department of Psychotherapy at the University of Latvia. The discussions in this group were also tape-recorded. The transcribed recordings reveal a highly individualistic view of psychiatric problems and a reluctance to make any concessions to the part played by social problems and fragmentation. Having briefly outlined my interest in changing diagnostic practices and conceptualizations of distress I raised the question of whether some of the problems seen by psychiatrists and psychotherapists did not have a cultural rather than an individual source. Bewildered looks indicated that some examples were called for.

Take the problem of alcoholism, I said, which in some rural provinces such as Latgale affected 80 per cent of all male inhabitants. But the consensus response was that 20 per cent of Latgalian men did not drink.

And someone else added that these indeed took up prominent positions in Riga. A highly atomistic view of society and an individualistic view of peoples' problems prevented these clinicians from recognizing that if the only way to stay sober was for a man to move to Riga then this surely spoke of problems common to Latgalian society rather than to individual inhabitants. Indeed, official unemployment figures in Rēzekne, a region of Latgale, were the highest in the country in 1999 standing at 27.2 per cent (*Latvijas Republikas Labklājibas Ministrija* 2000: 12).

My other example was of a distant relative who had become depressed since losing her job as cultural secretary in VEF, a light engineering firm renowned for its radios and cameras. Aija had earned well, and enjoyed her job and responsibilities hugely. After independence the factory had closed down, since the internal market to Russia and the other Soviet republics dried up and its products came to be considered obsolete. Now in her mid fifties she was lucky to move to another company with a greatly diminished work force and a salary of 30 lats (about £35 pounds). My relative also has an unemployed husband and has had to move to a smaller one-roomed flat. Since the death of her younger brother from alcohol-related problems she has become seriously depressed. I gave this case study because it seemed to me to represent so many others: it was so deeply implicated in the economic reorganization which Latvia is undergoing and as a result so many middle-aged men and women have become economically and socially marginalized. Unemployment for women is almost twice as high as it is for men (ibid.: 13). Those without specialist qualifications are especially at risk. This problem was again approached in an individualistic way. Had she had previous episodes of depression that might give some insight into the vulnerable areas of her psyche? Could she not move to another part of the country where appropriate work was available? An individual solution could always be found, so they thought. The many social ties that might prevent a middle-aged woman from moving were not considered. No questions were raised about elderly parents, adolescent children, or grand-parenting duties.

In the course of a few years since independence the perception of disorder and responsibility for psychological distress and illness has shifted from society to the individual. The shape of psychiatric consultations, their seemingly polite, initial attention to narrative form and yet the ultimate exclusion of narrative from clinical concerns, can be understood as a response to the doctors' feelings of powerlessness in difficult social circumstances. In informal talk psychiatrists give a rich account which links acutely difficult social circumstances through an agreed-upon narrative logic to emotional distress and illness. However, this broad approach is not used in talking to patients. Psychiatric consultations are concerned with the construction of disease entities and demarcating the individual's relationship and responsibilities towards these entities. For this reason consultations move quickly away from particular events, circumstances and feelings to feelings and problems in the abstract. The movement is away from process and context to categories; from verbs to nouns. As the philosopher Sokolowski has written: 'Verbs, since they name a manifestation, are tied to a particular context and try to reconstitute it by accumulating many of its details' (1978: 37).

Let me give some examples of the strategies psychiatrists use to decontextualize distress. My short-hand term for these psychiatrists is Platonists. Individual distress is understood in relation to the diagnostic category conceived as 'an eternal form'. The following consultation took place in the psychiatric section of a polyclinic in Riga. I was sitting in a consulting room about 8 by 12 feet that was occupied by the psychiatrist, the psychiatric nurse, a patient seeing the nurse about their medication, a patient consulting the psychiatrist and more often than not another patient standing in the doorway with some query about their medication. I am aware of the enormous generosity and tolerance of everyone concerned in allowing me to tape-record proceedings under such cramped and stressful conditions. In this instance the patient was a 35-year-old man, the thirteenth patient seen that day by the psychiatrist. His consultation lasted about 15 minutes. The psychiatrist inquired about his headaches and his epileptic fits. The headaches continue he replied and he has had two fits this year. But then the patient tried to direct the conversation:

> Patient: 'The trouble is I get these fits of anger.'
> Doctor: 'Without provocation?'
> Patient: 'My mother provokes me.'
> Doctor (changing the subject): 'What would you like?'
> Patient: 'I'm not sure. Firstly, I'd like to know what's wrong with me.'

Interestingly, the doctor did not follow up the patient's pressing need to talk about the anger his mother provokes. Secondly, she managed to veer the conversation back towards his illness and to re-awaken an interest in his diagnosis.

The conversation continued:

> Patient: 'It seems ... I've a feeling that everything expires, that everything dies down.'
> Doctor: 'What bothers you exactly?'
> Patient: 'That I'm spare. That I'm not wanted.'
> Doctor: 'I can write you out some anti-depressants, but will you be able to buy them?'

In this segment the doctor asks a question but she does not follow up the answer. Rather, she uses the answer to introduce the issue of medication and to move on to the larger subject of looking after one's illness appropriately: in other words patient compliance. All the leads in this dialogue draw the listener into the context and particularities of the patient's narrative. They are deftly avoided by the psychiatrist who redefines the agenda of the dialogue as being about illness and its appropriate care and medication.

In some cases special techniques need to be used to establish the presence of the illness. The following extract is drawn from the psychiatric department of a provincial polyclinic. The patient was a healthy-looking 45-year-old country-woman. As she entered and sat down near the psychiatrist the dialogue opened:

> Doctor: 'How are we today?'
> Patient: 'Well. I'm really well. I don't even want any medicines.'
> Doctor: Says nothing, but takes out her blood pressure monitor and feels for the patient's pulse.

As it happens this particular patient has an alcohol problem, and high blood pressure can be an indicator of recent excessive drinking. However, I use this particular extract not to raise questions about the accuracy or relevance of the diagnosis to this patient, but simply to note the way in which medical equipment can be used to bring to a halt a narrative of well-being and optimism. Instead of exploring the sources of her well-being, and their potential for her future, the framework of the consultation is provided by emphasizing the relationship between the patient and the illness.

Another way of decontextualizing is by referring to patients as categories. Latvian psychiatric terms can be used both as adjectives and as nouns. Whereas 'endogenous' is used as an adjective describing types of mental illness in English, in Latvian *endogēns* can be used for a type of person, rather like the term hysteric. *Orgāniķis* is a relatively new term that can be translated as somatizer. Abstraction and decontextualization is one way in which the harsh realities of social life can be ignored.

Individual as Agent versus Passive Victim

The polar concepts of agency versus passivity are threaded throughout psychiatric and lay thought about distress and illness. During the Soviet period people described themselves as experiencing the full brunt of political oppression on their minds, feelings and bodies and used the term *nervi* as a short-hand term for this connection. But whilst they clearly saw themselves as victims – indeed, the word often used to describe the situation of Latvians under Soviet rule was slaves – in important areas to do with making judgements about evil, justice and fairness Latvians retained the sense of themselves as agents. Agency was to do with hanging on to one's ability to distinguish between right and wrong and to cultivate the self. Of course, the emphasis on individual power to control emotions of anger, bitterness and sorrow are not recent Western imports, but have deep cul-tural roots. Kirmayer (1988) has argued that mind and body are metaphors for the voluntary and involuntary aspects of human experience and this certainly accords with thinking in Soviet Latvia. However, the language of mental illness imported with ICD 10 and with the pharmaceutical companies has paradoxically contributed to the shrinking of belief in agency. Dr Irena, who runs a 'depression club' in Riga, talks about people being programmed to succumb to certain illnesses. In discussing a woman suffering from severe depression she has this to say: 'Vieda, now you understand how many people appear to be living a normal life, a pseudo-normal life, and some acute stress comes along and all sorts of chasms open up in the personality. Life changes and the gene makes itself felt. Perhaps, if circumstances had been more favourable, our patient would have reached the end of her life without mishap.' Agency in these cases is restricted to taking appropriate medication and learning about one's condition from popular literature and from the psychiatrist. The patient becomes 'a case of', an exemplification of a diagnostic category.

Somatic versus Psychological Thinking about Illness

And yet, although the perception of disorder has shifted from society to the individual changing idioms of distress do not support a simple mind/body dualism. Although during the Soviet period distress was expressed with reference to damage to the nerves (Latvian *nervi*) or sometimes nervous system (*nervu sistēma*), these concepts cut across a simple mind/body divide. To argue that somatization involves a repression of thought and feeling as Kleinman (1977) does in his early work is to present an artificially narrow view of somatic concepts of distress. By contrast, the Latvian view of *nervi* is more in tune with a phenomenological understanding of embodiment: 'Our own body is in the world as the heart is in the organism: it keeps the visible spectacle alive, it breathes life into it and sustains it inwardly, and with it forms a system' (Merleau-Ponty 1989: 203).

Somatic concepts do not exclude feeling; rather they depend upon them. Let me give an illustration. Anta, whose problems were alluded to above, consulted me in a psychotherapeutic capacity in the polyclinic where we met for about an hour in an oversized consulting room. She dated her difficulties with *nervi* from the time of her husband's death. Anta was 26 at the time of her husband's untimely death from a heart attack. She spent the next year crying and this, she feels, undoubtedly damaged her nerves. As Anta's case shows, there is no suggestion that somatic terms exclude a recognition of emotion. Indeed, the opposite appears to be the case.

A somatic approach to patients' illness does not necessarily involve social decontextualization. Provincial psychiatrists are more likely to recognize and take account of the social and economic constraints under which their patients live than their city counterparts. Nor do all psychiatrists feel it their duty to explain the illness to the patient. For example, a doctor from Kurzeme had this to say:

> *I do not like the patient to come to recognize that he has an illness at all or that his perspective is the name of the illness. And I always make the point that the word for the illness has been created by human beings. Human beings have created all words. And it should make no difference whether the name of the illness is schizophrenia or whether the name of the illness is lilac or whether the name of the illness is episode or some other word. Everybody is different and we cannot all feel the same. Your feelings are as they are and your feelings are unique. And there are days when you feel well and there are days when you feel different and there are days when you might even feel in a bad state. But nothing is eternal and I try to accept and remind him of those feelings that he has when he is well. And I always remind patients that human beings invent language. And I say 'Don't use the word schizophrenia. You are a human being with different feelings and experiences than us. But which feelings are normal who can tell? Perhaps, precisely your feelings are normal and our feelings are not the right ones.' I think then that the patient finds it easier.*

Some psychiatrists, rather than seeking to establish a relationship between the patient and their illness, seek to find a common language with which to describe the patient's distress. This particular doctor did this in a very concrete body-centred language:

> *Doctor: 'Where is your anxiety?'*
> *Patient: 'In my stomach.'*
> *Doctor: 'How long does it take to travel from your stomach to your face?'*
> *Patient: 'I don't know.'*
> *Doctor: Let your anxiety find another home'*

Here, the doctor was talking to Mãra, a retired nurse suffering from recurrent depression.

> *Doctor: 'Mãrite [diminutive], how do you feel? What does your body say? Where is the restlessness? Where does it live?'*
> *Patient: 'I can't say.'*
> *Doctor: 'Its place of habitation is not known.'*

Rather than denying emotion recognizing the bodily manifestations of emotion is a way for psychiatrists to affirm their solidarity with the patient and the patient's experience. As Csordas has written: 'Somatic modes of attention are culturally elaborated ways of attending to and with one's body in surroundings that include the embodied presence of others' (1993: 138).

Description leads on to a consideration of the context in which disturbing feelings arise and the narrative shape of the experience. Ilga is 50 years old, the daughter of a Lutheran pastor now deceased, unmarried and living with her mother. Her life is plagued by the sense of her sinfulness and her inability to control behaviour that in turn consolidates her view of herself as evil. In answer to a question about what has been going on in her life recently she recounts how she felt compelled to interrupt the parson by yelling obscenities at him during the Sunday sermon. The doctor takes her hand and asks how else she might have behaved during that Sunday service. Ilga replies that she does not know and the doctor straightens one finger at a time to register three narrative alternatives. One, she could have uttered the words silently to herself. Two, she could have whispered them to her mother. And three, she could have quietly left the church. The doctor asks Ilga to repeat the alternative narratives, thus acknowledging them as real possibilities. In this way the psychiatrist opens up the patient's single restrictive narrative and widens the horizon of narrative possibility. She asks the patient to subscribe to these possibilities by repeating them. And finally the psychiatrist turns to the patient's habitual practices. Shame at ineptitude and laziness is challenged by the reminder that the patient did manage to weed the vegetable garden, she did manage to help her mother cook and she did manage to bottle the cherries. The doctor reminds Ilga that she felt better, and rightly so, for having completed these tasks. Thus, during the consultations the doctor confirms the patient's feelings and daily achievements but introduces small yet highly significant changes in narrative outcome.

Discussion

I have shown how the experience of somato-psychological distress belongs to three separate domains. Traditional popular beliefs, changing psychiatric beliefs and practices, and the economic and social changes in everyday life brought about during the post-independence decade all contribute to the contemporary Latvian experience of distress. These three domains are not linked in any straightforward way with the conceptual polarities of individual versus social, agent versus patient, and mind versus body. For example, a socio-historical perspective does not necessarily preclude agency. Conversely, a psychological view of illness does not confer agency.

A well-known historian of medicine has written: 'When the doctors' ideas of "legitimate" disease changes, the patients' idea changes as well' (Shorter 1992: 67). Perhaps so, but these changes are not always harmoniously synchronized and certainly not so in Latvia. Wessely, writing about the demise of neurasthenia, suggests that: 'It disappeared because it has ceased to be "useful to the doctor" (Lancet 1912) – when it failed to allow sufferers to receive sympathetic treatment without the stigma of psychiatry' (1994a: 195). Of course, doctors play a very important part in bringing about diagnostic change and shaping the experience of psychological distress. However, the move from somatoform to psychological disorders, and depression in particular, represents the internalisation of a heightened sense of accountability and responsibility for one's life circumstances, albeit with limited opportunities for changing those circumstances. Thus, changing subjectivities are not simply a response to changing concepts but reflect the experience of a different kind of social world. My position here is that of a critical realist (Bhaskar 1993).

The important changes are not so much from a psychiatry of the body to one of the mind. Rather, as Sullivan (1986: 332) argues in the context of modern medicine, a more important dualism is between disease and illness. Or, as Kirmayer puts it, 'between the physician as active knower and the patient as passive known' (1988: 59). This model is increasingly relevant to post-Soviet Latvia. Soviet medicine extended considerable autonomy to the patient. Patients were in a sense experts on their health and illness. For example, patients could choose which specialist to consult without having to depend upon the judgement of a family practitioner. The medical consensus was that anyone over the age of 35 would be the bearer of some illness or other. The doctor's duty, therefore, was to interpret the patient's symptoms correctly and to identify the relevant illness. Recent changes in treatment and diagnostic practices have made this more difficult. As one doctor commenting on these changes put it: 'How can the patient suffer from a syndrome?' The idea of a cure is foreign to this kind of medical philosophy. There is a Latvian saying, 'One should not spit in God's eyes' (*Nevajag Dievam acīs splaut*) meaning that one should be grateful for what one is given and not ask for more. On being asked by a patient whether she would be cured of her depression the Riga psychiatrist replied, 'We should not spit in God's eyes. We can treat but we cannot cure' (*Var ārstēt, bet nevar izārstēt*). On the other hand, some doctors held opposite views and asked, 'Why do Latvian doctors want their patients to be ill?' The medical view under communism was that we are all ill. Under capitalism this has changed to a view where some of us are unlucky carriers of a gene that predisposes us to psychiatric disease. There are several paradoxes here: a Soviet disease-oriented medical practice had allowed considerable room both for the patient's narrative and for patient decision making. A society which places increasing emphasis on the individual's powers to shape their own life course is offering an increasingly restrictive and passive patient role and a disease model for psychiatric illness. The exception, of course, is private psychotherapy which is private in a double sense of privately paid for and inaccessible to outside observers.

It has been argued within the rhetoric of psychosomatic medicine that 'The body stands in relationship to the mind as the child to a parent' (Kirmayer 1988: 62). However, there are different varieties of psycho-somatic medicine. Soviet psychosomatic medicine at its best embraced the total human experience in its bodily feeling and behavioural expression. By contrast some contemporary Latvian psychiatrists use the general category *orgānikis*, or somatizer, thus turning embodied experience into an abstract generalization which then becomes treatable through imported drugs.

These structural and diagnostic changes in the delivery of psycho-neurological health care are part of the concerted effort to become more Westernised. Western psychiatry is held to be more scientific and to have a special purchase on reality, in this case the reality of human distress. This view is held by many, though not all, Latvian psychiatrists and certainly informs government policy. The idea developed by Jadhav (2000) that depression may be part of an ethnopsychiatry with deep local roots is totally foreign to this position. Rorty has stated with epigrammatic verve that the world does not have 'a preferred description of itself' (1989: 21). Or, that 'the world does not speak, only we do' (ibid.: 6). Silverstein (1998: 292) refers to this idea as 'referential cleanliness': the idea that certain ways of thinking are able to get closer to reality than others. When a particular language or dialogue is given higher status and prioritized, 'language acquires a "thinginess" such that the properties language takes on are continuous with other objects in the culture' (ibid.: 290). I have argued that the new terminology of depression, in particular the idea of masked depression, promotes the status of psychiatric diagnoses as things. If some-thing is masked its ontological status is consolidated – it is there despite not being seen. It exists independently of perception. Certainly, psychiatry in our culture speaks a dominant language and a number of clinicians would argue that the world does have a preferred description of itself and that it is theirs.

The experience of distress is both shaped by and on occasion resists descriptions of itself. New psychiatric descriptions must correspond to the totality of psychosomatic experience. They must be able to make room for the particularities of autobiographical and social context. For this reason questions about feelings rather than states are more appropriate. Verbs rather than nouns are more helpful in capturing psychological reality. Because the verb names a manifestation, it always connotes a context. Something appears at a certain time and with a particular mixture of circumstances. This is why Aristotle claims that verbs differ from nouns by involving time in what they signify: not only do they differ from nouns by involving time in what they signify and not only do they name a way of appearing, they imply a time when this appearance takes place (Sokolowski 1978: 12–13). This is why the idea of masked depression as a kind of transcendental medical object cannot stand. Psychiatric diagnoses such as depression are 'interactive kinds' to borrow Hacking's (1999: 193) useful term. The consultation process teaches distressed patients the meaning of depression and its appropriate behaviour. This is not to deny the reality of psychological distress and its many connections with the realities of social life. It is simply to acknowledge its openness to human intention and cultural shaping.

Acknowledgements

I wish to thank the ESRC for financing the fieldwork. Earlier versions of this chapter were given to the Department of Sociology and the Centre for the History of Medicine at the University of Warwick and to the Committee on Human Development at the University of Chicago. I am indebted to both audiences for clarification of my thoughts. Anja Timms read the paper at very short notice and provided useful references. I also wish to thank the helpful comments of the anonymous reviewers for Social Science and Medicine.

11

LOOKING FOR A SUBJECT: LATVIAN MEMORY AND NARRATIVE

Latvia lost about one fifth of its population during and after the Second World War. In addition to immediate killings this loss was made up of deaths resulting from deportations and imprisonment in labour camps. The scale of deaths means that there are few Latvian families without personal knowledge of such killings. Indeed, deportation has come to occupy a central place in the construction of national identity.

However, as Roberts Ķilis (1996) has noted, there is relatively little historical research which engages with this phase of the past, despite its central importance for Latvian consciousness. Such writing as there is tends to base its authority on earlier studies. For example, Andrejs Plakans in his recent history of Latvia (1995: 147) relies on the earlier history by Misiunas and Taagepera (1993: 41–47). Although certain events, such as the shooting of 500 army officers at Litene, have become emblems of national destiny, we do not have precise statistics about the numbers of men, women and children who were sent to different categories of camp or into exile. Nor do we know the ethnicity of those arrested and deported. The list of names of people killed in 1941, for example, excludes Jews (*These Names Accuse*, 1982).

The memory of witnesses has been called on to fill this gap in history. Since 1990 there has been a steady stream of publications of survivors' memories. These memoirs are one channel whereby personal memory is transformed into collective memory. They are a response to the need to consolidate national identity and they make their own important contribution to it. Published accounts mould private memory, inducing forgetfulness and endowing with significance certain aspects of the past. As a result, these memoirs come across as formulaic. I personally find them difficult to read for this reason, although I know that mine is not a representative reaction. By and large they are written by educated, articulate people. They strive to heighten pathos and this, of course, increases their power to shape readers' own memories. Many accounts concentrate on episodes which exemplify differences in cultural capital. The actual period spent in labour camps is often left unaccounted for.

In 1987 the first public anti-Soviet protest was also a commemoration of the deportations of 14 June 1941. Since 1990 that day and certain others have been inscribed in the Latvian calendar as days of commemoration. Each 25 March commemorates the deportations of 1949 which smoothed the way for collectivization. Each 27 August commemorates the signing of the Molotov-Ribbentrop pact. All shops and offices are required by law to fly a Latvian flag on those days. Thus deportation is made a constituent of national identity.

The Fieldwork Context

My own anthropological work was carried out between 1992 and 1993. It was concerned with personal memory, recorded on tape and subsequently transcribed by typists in Riga. In this way I recorded the memories of more than 100 informants. About a third had had personal experience of imprisonment and deportation. I too have found that what Steve Buckler (1996: 3–4) describes as 'unmediated accounts' are very different from published accounts, although the narratives I listened to could not be described as unmediated. They were, however, compelling in a way that written accounts were not. Latvian narratives record violence and dislocation both physical and moral.

Despite the fact that my narratives were clearly rooted in personal experience, that they were unrehearsed in any obvious sense, and that many narrators had not read the published accounts of deportees' experiences, they already incorporated elements of collective memory. Clearly, the euphoria which reigned throughout the Baltic states as the Soviet Union began to disintegrate had a part to play in giving a certain unity of feeling to the narratives. That euphoria affected me too. The research enabled me to overcome the contradictions between family memory and the accepted British line on the Baltic states. For example, the 15th edition of the *Encyclopaedia Britannica* makes no reference to deportations or, indeed, to any political oppression in the Baltic. School history books typically use phrases such as, 'swallowed up' or 'disappeared' to describe the fate of the Baltic states during the Second World War. The Baltic states reappeared in 1989 as suddenly and unexpectedly as they had disappeared.

Narratives also wove personal experience around fragments of history and fiction. As Stephen Jones (1994: 150) reminds us, the fragmentation of national histories gives them an enhanced status in the reconstruction of counter-histories. In Latvia such cultural fragments have acquired great emotive power: a few notes of a folk song, the embroidered sleeve of a peasant woman's costume, or a phrase from a poem can alter the register of dialogue or set people weeping. Latvian narrators incorporate these highly charged cultural fragments into their accounts of a personal past. And, of course, the form of the story itself is drawn from a collective literary tradition. Autobiographies require fitting endings which are not supplied by the ending of life. Thus the demarcation lines between the personal and the collective have been blurred even before the mechanisms for translating a personal past into a collective history start to work.

The problems associated with polarization of the personal and the collective take many forms. There is Hegel's (1997) dichotomy between *Erinnerung* and *Gedächtnis* (recollection and memory) and Ricoeur's (2004) between *Vorstellung* and *Vertretung* (presentation and representation.) They can be illustrated by looking at witnessing. There is in witnessing a claim to a fusion and an inseparability between subject and experience, from which derives the authority of the memory. Such claims have been contested: psychologists question the reliability of witnessing; historians its impartiality. Its immediacy has not been questioned. Indeed, Dori Laub makes out a case for the recollection of trauma as being experienced for the first time, as it were (Laub 1992: 57). I too found that memories reported in the witnessing mode supported this view, but witnessing embodied other ambivalences.

Nearly all my narrators resorted to the witnessing mode and they announced that they were doing so either by switching to the present tense or by framing what they were about to say with a truth-claim phrase: for example, 'And this is how it really was' or 'I saw it with my own eyes.' However, the recollection of the past to which they thus laid claim was in no sense 'rawer' than their other memories. Indeed, it seems that Latvian narrators chose to bear witness to those events in which cultural and experiential truth met. Events are singled out for witnessing not simply because the narrator has experienced them, but because of the cultural meanings with which the experience is invested.

In the course of constructing a narrative, informants draw selectively upon the cultural capital of the past. In doing so they reposition themselves from what James Fernandez calls 'peripheral loneliness' or even beyond the periphery to a 'centred sociality' (1995: 37). The narratives of all former deportees dwell on the long journey to Siberia, the chaos of the transit points and the vastness and emptiness of the landscape on arrival. They convey the feeling of being meaningless figures on the outside of human society in an inverted, unnatural landscape. Narrators initially position themselves on the margins and beyond. However, this is surely an untenable position, and the life story charts the narrator's progression from the cultural periphery to the centre.

The Narrator

These themes are found in most narratives, but I have chosen to construct my chapter around a single paradigmatic life-story: that of Uldis Vērsis, whom I met in April 1993. I had wanted to talk to Uldis because of his extensive experience of special hospitals as well of strict regime labour camps.

A throwaway remark suggests that he too has a polarized vision of experience and representation. There are, he tells us, many synonyms, many ways of talking about his personal experience:

> *I think I told you I have been through fifty-four concentration camps, you could call them colonies, settlements, zones (there are many synonyms) and about fourteen prisons. That's altogether, including transit points.*

At the time of our encounter Uldis was 59 years old. A broken nose and limp added to his tough and masculine aura of a lone survivor. He recounted his extraordinary life without hesitation or emotion. At the time I was struck by his apparent fearlessness and hardiness. On listening to the recorded interview and transcribing it much later I was struck by the absence of a constant grammatical subject in his narrative. Instead, distinct periods of his life belong to different subjects and each section of the narrative is attributed to different grammatical subjects. Of course, all natural speech is grouped around different pronouns. However, Uldis's mastery of this dramatic strategy serves to highlight the way in which the grammar of pronouns may reveal the speaker's allegiances and sources of personal identity. What I am referring to is a pronominal sequence in the narrative which moves between *we, I, they, he, you,* and rests with *they.* In Jakobson's terminology, these words are shifters: what they signify depends upon the context of speech (1971). Here I am not proposing to substitute a lexical analysis for the task of interpretation, but rather to enlist it to further the hermeneutic enterprise. In the present context, these pronouns reveal the narrator's varied relationship with the past. There are some segments of the past of which Uldis feels personally in command; other areas of his experience can be referred to only in the third person and commented on as a historical system; and yet others can be approached only jointly, drawing the listener in as the imaginary subject of the story.

The early part of Uldis's life story starts with a collective subject and then moves between the singular and collective.

Uldis opens his narrative in the plural by delineating his collective roots:

> *My roots, the clan of Vērsis, comes from the direction of Kurzeme. We come from the region of Kuldiga. For example, in Kuldiga there is a bridge built of bricks, constructed. It's one of the oldest in Europe. That was built in its time by my grandfather's father – Indriķis Vērsis.*

However, he soon moves to I and draws a distinction between collective and personal origins:

> *We come from Kurzeme, but I personally was born in Riga on 11 May 1934. Well, without a doubt, I was energetic, how shall I put it – too lively, probably too inquisitive. I always recount in an ironic and humorous way that I was born on 11 May and I looked around and saw that there wasn't any order after all and then I ordered Kārlis Ulmanis to carry out a coup on 15 May [laughing]. And that's what he did.*[1]

His childhood memories shift between a collective and singular subject. Dangerous situations are remembered by a collective *we*:

> *And then the war started and even during the war period in 1941, when the front line was drawing near, I wasn't aware that I could be shot. We were a little group of boys, my contemporaries, six-, seven-, eight-year-olds, we wandered around without fear of bullets or bombing even in old Riga where there was street fighting. We saw exactly how the street fighting took place. Because we thought that nobody would touch us children. Well, that was more or less our understanding.*

But certain spectacular events are witnessed by the singular *I*:

> *In 1941 I was present when the steeple of Saint Peter's Church crashed. I saw which direction it fell in and how it fell. The floors were burning inside the church. The pastors fled from their beds. They had been living there.*

Uldis includes details which authorize his entitlement to speak, but these personal details are required precisely because the event being described is of such monumental cultural importance. Saint Peter's Church in old Riga had the highest wooden steeple of any church in Europe. It gave to the old city its characteristic skyline.

By weaving his tale between a plural and singular subject Uldis sets up an antiphony between the collective and the individual, between structure and event, and between permanence and transience. Uldis uses *we* to embed himself in a landscape and to lay claim to European roots – his great-grandfather built one of the oldest bridges in Europe. When Uldis speaks in the *I* mode, however, it is about events rather than structures. The coup in the year of his birth epitomizes change. Uldis talks about the children's gangs and their impermeability to danger in the we mode. However, when he witnesses the destruction of Saint. Peter's Church he is back in the *I* mode. But it is not the act of witnessing which demands the first person singular subject – as we shall see later – but the involvement in risk and danger.

For Uldis, the construction of a narrative subject is possible only in what Bakhtin has described as adventure time:

> 'Suddenly' and 'at just that moment' best characterize this type of time, for this time usually has its origins and comes into its own in just those places where the normal, pragmatic and premeditated course of events is interrupted – and provides an opening for sheer chance, which has its own specific logic. This logic is one of random contingency, which is to say, chance simultaneity (meetings) and chance rupture (non-meetings), that is, a logic of random disjunctions as well (Bakhtin 1992: 92).

Indeed, as the subject of adventure narratives Uldis is undoubtedly a hero of grand proportions. However, the heroic *I* is counterpoised against later impersonal segments of narrative where no subject is discernible. Uldis has spent as much of his life in prison and prison camps as outside. But Uldis's first encounter with Siberia is recounted in the established literary tradition of romantic adventures, completely refashioning the notion of the Siberian exile or prisoner. His account is set in adventure time and starts in the context of the deportations of others. Narrative involves, of course, the temporal sequencing of events. However, time itself can become the object of narrative and carry its own meanings. It involves what Bakhtin describes as time expanding and taking on flesh. We find this in many narratives including this one. Uldis is able to represent himself as a subject, to reclaim his life, only in adventure time. This quality of time is essential for his sense of himself in the same way as developing fluid is essential for the capturing of a photographic image.

The Screen Memory

Uldis gives an account of what we might, following Freud (1899), call a screen memory. Its value as a memory lies not in its own content but in its relation to other later memories. In 1945 Uldis's grandfather, cousin and godmother were deported to Siberia; in 1949 his other godmother was deported. Uldis's own first experience of Siberia dramatically reverses the later order of events. The initial account substitutes for later experiences which he is unable to reclaim. It is emblematic of the identity which he wishes to project.

> *I had dreams, I read like all my contemporaries in those years – Mayne Reid and Cooper and Jack London[2] – I badly wanted to see Africa, America, Indians, parrots, elephants and monkeys [laughing]. Like all such boys. But then the war ended in 1945. In 1945 I joined the street fighting, I witnessed all that. ... In 1945 the swift deportations started. Especially local deportations. From our family my godmother, my cousin, my grandfather Ansis Vērsis, son of Indrikis, they were all deported in 1941. He had been a shoemaker, a craftsman, and he too was taken. As a* budžis *(a rich peasant) just because he was living at the time*

with his daughter. He'd come up from the country to stay with his daughter for a while. He too was taken. And look in 1949, my father's other sister, my second godmother, was taken, she was deported straight from Kabile as farmer-landowners, although they only had 30 hectares. Well, let's return to the theme. As I said, I badly wanted to see America and Africa. I thought about it a lot. I thought about running away. I started walking around Andrej docks, export docks, to see if I could sneak on to a boat. I was prepared. But then a word started circulating among local inhabitants which has as its synonym fear, a fearful word – Siberia. Siberia was pronounced by many people almost in a whisper, in a half-voice and always looking back over their shoulder. Well of course I as an adolescent – how old was I then? I was about eleven, twelve years old then. It started to interest me. What is this Siberia? Why is it mentioned in this way? And the opinion was around that people did not return from Siberia. Those who go to Siberia stay there and perish. And then I exchanged Africa and America for Siberia. I took more of an interest in Siberia. Because in queues ... wherever people met ... Siberia was mentioned. And particularly among us, when relatives or friends or colleagues visited, frequently conversations ended not as now with traffic accidents or illness or sex but with Siberia. And many people recounted extraordinary things about Siberia. I listened to all that quietly. And you see if there had been a good pedagogue around he might have noticed that something was happening to me. But my family didn't notice it. And so I decided I had to exchange Africa and America for Siberia. What was it? I decided that I had to see it with my own eyes.

And so in 1947, when I had turned thirteen, I had no money at all, nor any documents, I only took a little cup of sugar with me – I had a little white cup – and a loaf of bread. And I tried to sneak on to the Moscow train, the Riga-Moscow train. ... And so I succeeded and reached Moscow. ... Well, of course I was very dazed at first – I'd never seen such a large city. And besides I was very hungry. I had no money and no documents. And my spirit sagged. And then what? Then I remembered Annele, I remembered our Brigadere, I remembered Sprīdītis, because at one time I myself had played the part of Sprīdītis at school and also in the drama theatre when there was a children's production. I myself played Sprīdītis. Because Sprīdītis had tremendous courage when he was allowed to recuperate a tiny bit. And I had taken some postcards with me with views of Riga to cheer up my godmother and remind her of Riga and her homeland. And so I decided that perhaps I could trade the postcards. ... And I sold them and then I could get something to eat again. And then I got back my spirit just like Sprīdītis. And then I thought, 'No, I have to continue my journey.'

Literary Companions

Many of the narratives have a pronounced literary and biblical feel to them. In some, as in this instance, there is an explicit reference to a literary figure, and Uldis acknowledges the way in which his own life follows fiction. In other cases, segments of recognizable literary text are appropriated by the personal narrative. In Uldis's case, the textual and personal are so intertwined in memory that it is difficult to prise them apart. Uldis is very much aware of modelling his narrative on literary sources, initially foreign, but as his story becomes more tense he draws upon *Sprīdītis*, a local literary hero. Indeed, many narratives of Siberia model themselves consciously or unconsciously on *Sprīdītis*. Why is it so helpful in structuring these narratives? Why not Lācplēsis, the bear-slayer, a more imposing, powerful and publicly commemorated culture hero of the nineteenth century? The answers lie in the particular resonances which these two culture heroes evoke in contemporary narrators. Anna Brigadere wrote the fairytale play *Sprīdītis* in 1905. It is set in a typical lone farmstead. The hero, *Sprīdītis*, is a young boy whose mother dies and whose father remarries. His stepmother is not only cruel but also a snob, with two pampered daughters of her own. *Sprīdītis* is banished from the farm and enters the forest. He is given a magic whistle and a magic stick by the spirits of the forest. With the help of these he manages to defeat the devil, who holds the king's daughter in captivity. As a reward he is offered the princess in marriage. However, he turns his back on the princess and on palatial life and chooses instead to live in the farmstead. The play is structured around the two icons central to Latvian ethnic identity: namely, the farmstead and the forest. Indeed, it is a morality play around Latvian ethnic identity and social mobility. Rather than marry the princess, *Sprīdītis* chooses to return to the farmstead. The play ends with a celebratory homecoming, with the branches of trees reaching out to welcome him back. It has as its subtext concerns about the association of peasant social mobility with Germanicization. Brigadere is following in the tradition of the early nationalists and issuing a challenge to this association. At the same time she draws upon peasant traditions to construct a pastoral identity for Latvians. Why do so many personal narratives of exile and imprisonment draw upon this story? It has a number of obvious elements which lend themselves to appropriation. There is the fact of being an orphan and of banishment. But there is also the magical power which comes to *Sprīdītis* from the forest deities and finally the exultant homecoming to the farmstead. The play, therefore, reflects both destitution and magical power and promise, and it does this in the context of ethnic belonging.

The narrative *I* represents a fusion of voices: among them, the battered old man and the fearless twelve-year-old adventure seeker. Uldis finds himself

> *in a real Siberian house with horizontal timbers and little square windows where there are flowers. And then they all climbed on to the most real Russian stove of the kind that we now see in films. I was put on the floor on some sort of mattress. And when they fell asleep and started to snore and the wind was howling outside, then I was overcome with a great feeling of poetry that at last I was in Siberia, in a real Siberian house, with real Siberians, with a real Siberian stove. You could even say that I'd almost fulfilled my mission. And this romantic – I could even describe it as a euphoric – moment has settled in my blood in such a way that it will probably remain with me for the rest of my life. I gained my first victory.*

The victory was important to the twelve-year-old adventurer, but it has, I feel, come to be even more important to the older man and author. It serves as a screen for other memories which cannot be ordered in such a way as to offer an acceptable identity. However, the singular *I* seems to be underwritten by a collective identity as in the following passage:

> *I was unlucky. I fell ill with a very serious illness, with malaria, with Siberian malaria. I don't know how it happened, I can't explain it and nobody else can either. There were terrible mosquitoes! There were no medicines. And you understand that there was no food either. I was destined for nothingness. Nothing could save me any more. The fits of fever were terrible, with very high temperatures. My godmother was already sending telegrams. But that didn't help. And then my godmother brought a* feldscher,[3] *an exile, not a doctor but a feldscher, but with extensive medical experience to our* zemnīca – *our hole.*[4] *And he said – and his words were almost sacramental – that I could only be saved by a change of climate. If I were to return to my homeland, to my climate, then the malaria would recede. And you see that's how I returned, only this time it was much more difficult.*

The polarization of illness/exile/nothingness and health/the sacramental homeland/survival hardly needs emphasizing. Although there is a personal *I* in this narrative it is precarious and it cannot survive for long in isolation from the homeland.

After his return Uldis became rather a celebrity in Riga, with his house being treated as an information bureau:

> *And they brought sweets just to make me tell them what life was like there. And … I can say that I was one of the first to give real information to Latvians about the circumstances of the deportees in Siberia.*

At this high point the *I* as a contributor to the direction and meaning of the narrative all but disappears. Instead information is structured around a generalized prisoner. *He* or *they* become the subjects of the narrative.

The Sovietologist

> *Prisoners know much more about what is happening in the world outside than free people. After all, a free person is isolated. He's in his family and workplace – work, home, family, the theatre. But he's very far from daily or nightly events. All those events are concentrated in prisons, whether they're political or criminal. And you see, a great many people's destinies flow together here – collide. How they behave, happenings. And in places of imprisonment people are very truthful. He can be dishonest for a month or two, but he won't last longer. He has to be honest because otherwise he can't exist. And here all the lies fall away. And that's why they know much more about what's happening, those who are on the inside of the fence, than those who live on the outside.*

Although Uldis himself is no longer at the centre of his account, the locus of narrative is now attributed a central importance for human experience.

Uldis refers to the many synonyms in Russian for prison, but for him they are all gateways to fundamental truths about the system.

> *In the large* peresiylkas,[5] *a synonym would be a selection prison. ... The selection prisons are real houses of chaos, real madhouses. There is terrible chaos and panic and terrible things happen. And people get sent out in all directions. People met there. In my opinion the biggest selection prison is in Moscow – the so-called Krasnaya Presnya.[6] It's a vast, enormous prison. Every day tens of echelons [special trains] would leave from there. And people from the whole of the Soviet Union met there. From the east, from the north, from the west. ... And as there was nothing to do there, for example, we couldn't read novels or watch television ... [laughing] there was absolutely nothing to do there. Many played cards, but most people tried to sharpen their minds. For example, I always raised this question of how many there were. ... And so we started counting. In the selection prison there are people from all the Gulags. ... And each prisoner knows how many zones there are in the Gulag: 20 or 30, sometimes even 40, in one Gulag. And they know, give or take a few, how many prisoners are in each zone. And in this way we started counting. And that's how we arrived at a figure. And according to our calculations – and they were fairly reliable – during the years before Khrushchev's amnesty there were 35 or 40 million. Moreover, they weren't pensioners or children but for the most part men in their prime. That was a dangerous force which had to be divided. And the Soviet administration knew how to break up prisoners. They set them apart by separating them into so-called castes, or groupings, I can't call them classes. There were thieves, reformed thieves, (so-called* sukas), bespredel'niks,[7] *anarchists. There were about five or six main groupings.*

My concern at this point was that Uldis was distancing himself from his past, that he was no longer speaking from experience and instead was theorizing. I interrupted his narrative by asking him to tell me more about himself and what precisely happened to him. His reaction was one of alarmed incomprehension:

> *Mmm. I completely fail to understand your question. I don't understand it precisely. How what happened? To do with what I'm telling you now?*

I explained that I wanted to hear not just about the system, but about his own experiences within that system. My attempt at being directive failed:

> *My experience is that I started getting interested in the history of the system, from the time that I was first imprisoned as an adolescent. I was interested in why one zone breaks down a fence and rushes into the other zone. And in every zone there are approximately 10,000 prisoners. They stab each other to death, and why is that so? Why with the help of the administration are there such groups wandering around the zone, groups of prisoners, with a historical personage, Pivovarov, at their head and his chief assistant, Grushchenko.[8] At that time they incited these groupings against each other. ... That's why the Gulag history is very interesting. Because the Soviet administration understood that if they don't divide all the imprisoned into hostile camps then the uprisings will repeat themselves. There were very many uprisings. There were uprisings in Norilsk,[9] where I too was injured in the leg.*

Although the passing reference to his leg injury clearly establishes Uldis's authority to speak about Norilsk, he does so as a political theorist or historian might do. That sense of authentic presence which gives life to his adolescent memories no longer informs these memories. This also applies to his memories of forced psychiatric treatment recounted in a generalized third person.

After that the medical period started. If a person can't be broken by physical means then he was broken with the help of doctors. Well, the person would disappear from the zone. He doesn't get tried. He isn't sent anywhere else. But new people come and ask after him. 'Yes, of course, he's gone to Kazan special hospital, he's gone to Blagoveshchensk, he's gone to Arzamas.'[10] There were so many. The nearest to us was in Kaliningrad. And in that way the reckoning started. And it was the same with us. For example, in 1984 some fool took it into his head to burn down a bridge, a wooden bridge, not far from Liepāja. And then a large commission arrived from Moscow headed by a general. I knew his surname but I've forgotten it now. And the general told everyone that the person who burnt down the bridge was sick. Because he'd burnt the bridge just at the time of the October celebrations. That he was going against Soviet power. But only a sick person could set themselves against Soviet power. If he is intelligent, if he is normal, he will not go against Soviet power. Because Soviet power cannot be undermined, it is invincible, and it would be the same as fighting a windmill. And if you take such a step you're not in possession of all your faculties. You have a pathology. That's why you have to be cured. He wasn't embarrassed to speak out, to propagandize among the locals in Liepāja. In this way we prepared ourselves in the zones: if by chance they should want to take revenge on us we would be sent to the special hospitals. Because we were considered psychopathic personalities.

Uldis recounts these happenings as an observer. However, when he moves on to talk about a diagnosis of insanity, pathology and cure he introduces the second person pronoun. As a rhetorical device it works to draw the listener into his predicament where he might otherwise set him apart. The *you* emphasizes the randomness of the labeling and the fact that it could befall anyone. His description of the psychiatric procedures continues in the second person:

Now for example, Riga's central prison, the second block, on the ground floor, the second or third cell had been transformed into an out-patients' department. And the outside specialists would go through there; in clinical jargon they were called pikminutka, in Latvian that would be translated as 'the little five minute'. You are suddenly called out from the cell, although you've been in the examination cell for about half a year. You're called out and the convoy takes you. You wonder where you are being taken. You're not being taken to the bathhouse, you're not taken for interrogation, and they take you into the second block where they've installed the clinic. Yes, our precious doctors are sitting there in white coats. 'Your surname?' The person gives his surname. 'On which article are you here?' Such and such an article. 'You can go.' And he has attached the 57th article.[11] He doesn't even know at the time. Well, of course, he knows from stories that he now has the 57th. But he is disappointed that nothing was asked, that he wasn't physically examined.

I was not altogether certain whether Uldis had himself undergone such experiences and asked whether that had happened to him. 'Yes, it also happened to me. With me it happened in 1976.'

It was, however, difficult to get an account of what had actually happened to Uldis. He claimed that he had not suffered through his experiences:

I was given special food. But other people were badly affected. It was a label. When you leave the prison again nobody takes you on for work; you can't get a driving license; very many rights are denied to you; you are always on the register; at any instant if you cause discomfort to a person, of course a person with power, you will be wiped away instantly, either to a psychiatric hospital or prison.

Uldis's personal experiences are hidden behind the generalities. His alarmed reaction to the suggestion that his account was not personal enough made me reluctant to press him, I did not find out in what way these restrictions had affected his own life. It is, however, interesting that Uldis has reverted to the pronoun *you*. The most difficult and painful of experiences can only be mentioned by putting me in the role of the subject.

Discussion

I have drawn upon Uldis's life because it illustrates so many of the difficulties of recalling and giving an account of events which combine to undermine the self. His narrative also illustrates the many rhetorical and literary strategies upon which people draw in order to circumvent these difficulties. State-perpetuated violence was not recognized; it was a non-event. Violent death and deportation could not be publicly acknowledged. Official attitudes towards people who had been killed, had disappeared, or had been deported were condemnatory, and this condemnation extended to their families. There was guilt by association; in Goffman's language, courtesy guilt (1963). However, because such guilt was well-nigh universal, ways of circumventing it had to be found. The introduction of lessons in writing autobiography for school children was one way of translating such guilt into ambiguous but socially acceptable language. However, although the official position accommodated personal histories in this way, it was at odds with personal feelings and knowledge; the open expression of grief and mourning was suppressed. Parents, by and large, tried to protect their children from knowledge of the labour camps because of the difficulties they might then experience in living in Soviet Latvia. The paradox is that although they have not been told the younger generation feel that Siberia has been rammed down their throats. The feeling and the terror have been communicated without their substance. This situation persisted for some fifty years throughout Soviet rule. Thus the narrative reconstruction of lives in Latvia is pitted not only against the intractability of the memories but also against many years of autobiographical self-censorship.

Steve Buckler has set out the reasons for the lacunae in Holocaust history (1996). Certain kinds of events resist incorporation into a full human narrative. They are beyond the familiar moral and temporal frameworks for human action. I agree with Craig Barclay (1996: 94) who argues that experiences of extreme victimization lack narrative elements essential to the construction of a coherent account of the personal past. Testimonies demonstrate the problems of translating unthinkable events into a coherent narrative. How can one bear witness to events which in the process of narration undermine the integrity of the narrator? The problems for victims of Soviet violence are no less. Informants express anxieties about their ability to find the right words and to make themselves understood. 'Will they be interested? Will they understand? That can only be understood by someone who has experienced it.' These were points I heard repeated again and again.

However, despite the voicing of such anxieties, narrators did manage to convey what they had been through. Sometimes it was by what they said, but as often it was by what they left out. Moreover, narrators employ various grammatical strategies to compensate for the 'meaning deficit' at the heart of their story. For example, there is a creative use of tense and narrative subject. Narratives are constructed around first, second and third person pronouns, sometimes singular and sometimes plural. Similarly, narrative action moves back and forth between the past and the present. Uldis conveys meaning not only by the content but also by the grammatical structure of his narrative. His shifting use of pronouns marks out the areas of his life which he is confident enough to remember as a singular *I*, areas where he has a supported, collective identity, and the areas which can be broached only by drawing the listener into the account. Changes in pronouns point to shifting sources of identity.

Uldis also conveys meaning by changing the tense of his narrative. His childhood and adolescent exploits are set in the past. However, when he comes to describe prison life he switches to the present tense. The use of the present is a signal that the narrative is now entering a witnessing mode and that what is recounted is of special significance for the narrative as a whole. Uldis is here witnessing fundamental truths about his experience of prison, even though the narrative lacks an identifiable witness as subject. The movement from past to present in certain portions of narrative links in with Dori Laub's contention that Holocaust memories are experienced, as it were for the first time, in the retelling (1992).

However, the semantic heart of this narrative is split between the heroic adventures of the adolescent and the historian who theorizes but does not recall the many labour camps and psychiatric hospitals in which he spent so many years of his life. The adolescent adventurer reverses the direction of the journey: instead of running away from Siberia, he runs towards it. In doing so he provides the older man with a story which offers him a habitable identity and one which can be shared. It is his first 'victory', and one which enables him to skim over the lacunae during the later periods of his life.

When pressed about his personal experience in labour camps, Uldis stated firmly that his experience was linked to his academic interest in the system. When asked about his psychiatric experience he compared the improved diet of the hospital with his earlier diet in prison. Having tried and failed to redirect his narrative I felt I had to respect his wishes.

So where is the subject of this narrative? To whom does it belong? Does it belong to the personal witness? To the collective subject? To the cultural hero *Sprīdītis*? To the system? To the generalized other? Or does it belong to you and me – to us as listeners and readers? Perhaps it is a story that is destined to remain homeless – perpetually searching for a subject.

I will end by letting the narrative speak for itself:

> *There are some good and honest doctors who abide by a professional code. Well, perhaps now it's easier for them to be honest. But in those years. ... For example, there was a diagnosis – twilight mind or twilight consciousness, but we can describe it as a twilight era. It was the era which was a twilight era. In the twilight era events took place which could be presented any way one wanted.*

Acknowledgements

I wish to thank Ruth Levitas whose article 'We' (1995) first alerted me to the importance of looking at pronouns, and Martin Dewhirst and Michael Erben for their reading of the paper. I am grateful to the ESRC for funding my fieldwork in Latvia.

Notes

1. Kārlis Ulmanis (1874–1942) was elected Prime Minister in 1918 following the declaration of independence. Following the coup of 1934, he also assumed in 1936 the role of President. After the Soviet occupation in 1940 Ulmanis was arrested and deported to the south of Russia where he died in prison in 1942.
2. Here Uldis is thinking of the adventure writers Jack London, James Fenimore Cooper and an Irish writer of romances and adventurous yarns, Thomas Mayne Reid (1818–83).
3. A *feldscher* is a medical assistant, normally with two to three years' medical training.

4. *Zemnīca* is Latvian for a dwelling dug into the ground, of a kind widespread throughout Siberia.
5. *Peresiylka* is Russian for a transit prison camp.
6. Krasnaya Presnya is the name of the prison and the poor district near Moscow in which it is located.
7. *Suka* is Russian for bitch and *bespredel'nik* for a thief. Uldis is using standard terms for describing the criminal hierarchy of the Gulag. For a fuller discussion see Rossi (1987).
8. Pivovarov and Grushchenko are prison leaders encountered by Uldis. I cannot find mention of them in any history book.
9. The uprisings in Norilsk took place in the summer of 1953. They spread to Karaganda and Vorkuta. The army was called in to control the prisoners and many hundreds were killed.
10. For a fuller discussion of the relationship between Soviet psychiatry and political repression see Bloch and Reddaway (1977).
11. Uldis is referring to clauses of the Soviet criminal code. Article 57 was invoked in cases of alleged mental illness. Clause 58 related to offences against Soviet power and was most frequently invoked to justify deportation and imprisonment.

12

THE EXPROPRIATED HARVEST: NARRATIVES OF DEPORTATION AND COLLECTIVIZATION IN NORTH-EAST LATVIA

Lord I knew that thou art an hard man, reaping where thou has not sown, and gathering where thou hast not strewed.

Matthew 25: 24

This chapter is based on extended visits to the parish of Drusti, in the province of Vidzeme in Latvia between 1992 and 1993. My introduction to Drusti was through a seventy-year-old country woman who replied to my newspaper advertisement inviting people to write to me about their health. Māra wrote at considerable length describing not only her medical history but also her life history and in so doing a slice of the social history of the parish. I first met her in the summer of 1992. Not only was she a willing and fluent talker, but she was keen to introduce me to friends and neighbours.[1] Since Latvian is my first language, all interviews were conducted in Latvian.

Drusti covers an area of some 120 square kilometres and during the period of Latvia's independence (1919–1939) it had a reputation for being a prosperous and progressive parish. A secondary school was built in 1930, and there was a resident doctor and a pharmacy. The population in 1935 was 1,521. In 1950 it was only about 1,200, and by 1993 it was down to 797. Because of its relative prosperity, Drusti suffered more from deportations, especially during the drive to collectivize in 1949. In March 1949, 180 people were deported, twenty of them children. As many inhabitants testified, there was considerable pressure to leave outlying farmsteads and move into the village centre where several typically Soviet-style blocks of flats were built. Farms were abandoned, particularly in outlying areas of the parish. In 1938 there had been a total of 274 farms. Forty-five of these were affected; thirty-eight of them now lie abandoned and many others are inhabited by people who are too old to work. With collectivization the landscape and architecture of the parish were changed.

There is a consistency between the remembered past in Drusti and the shape of twentieth-century historical events in Latvia. The independence period from 1919–39 is generally considered an economic success story in which the development of agriculture based on small farms flourished. The first Soviet invasion of 1940, although it affected country people less than townspeople, created widespread terror and alarm and is associated with the targeted arrest and killing of people in senior positions. It ended with the German occupation in July 1941 which lasted until the autumn of 1944. The second Soviet occupation lasted from 1941 to 1991. The years after the Second World War are referred to as the times of chaos. A resistance movement of forest partisans persisted for many years, creating the feeling that the war was not yet over. The sporadic arrests after the war took on a broader, systematic character in preparation for collectivization. Impossibly high agricultural taxes during 1947 and 1948 were followed by the arrest and deportation of one tenth of the farming population of all three Baltic countries – Latvia, Estonia and Lithuania. These events play a major role in the autobiographical accounts of Drustians.

I needed no persuasion to anchor my research in this particular locality. Just as the personal narratives I was hearing fused history and memory, fact and fiction, so too the landscape represented a fusion of art with reality. Drusti has a special enchantment. It embodies features singled out in literature and painting to represent the quintessentially Latvian landscape. This created for me an uncanny sense of familiarity. On my way to distant farmsteads I was confronted by views which appeared to be replicas of the landscape paintings of the Latvian impressionist painter Purvītis.[2] The countryside is gently undulating, with forests providing a dark frame for cultivated farmland. The parish is renowned for its seven lakes but has countless smaller ones, which, though they do not earn a place on maps, give unexpected delight. In summer the meadows are covered with a luxuriant growth of wild flowers. In winter the landscape has a bleached ethereal air. I was captivated.

Drustians have varied memories of the past, whether of the independence period, the war or the post-war period. It is hardly surprising that the memories of those deported differ from those who watched and were left behind and from those who organized the deportations. Similarly, memories of peasants forced into collectivization are different from those few who benefited from the changes. However, underlying these differences are certain themes and metaphors which unify both the narrative and to a certain extent the community, and enable people to carry on living with their neighbours. Thus, notwithstanding sharply differing experiences of Soviet rule and varying degrees of willingness to accommodate themselves to it, Drustians have carried on living alongside each other.

It has been argued by Jerome Bruner and Carol Feldman (1996) that autobiographical events are determined not by the nature of the lived past but by the needs of the story.[3] My own position is that both are important: lived events circumscribe what can be told, but the story determines whether and how they are told. However, as soon as the selective principle behind autobiographical events is acknowledged, this introduces the question of how such selection is made. The answers seem to lie in the autobiographer's relationship to his or her social group and to the wider society. Bruner develops his argument by claiming that shared values shape individual accounts and thus constitute them as members of a particular group. Conversely, group identity is constituted by the life accounts of individuals.

> Any group that wants to constitute itself as a lasting or important one has to develop shared stories that not only define the group's identity, but also provide a means whereby individual members can guide their own discovery of meaning in their own lives. If people are to go beyond what merely happened to what it meant to them, they need to share stylised genres of story, poetry, oratory and history to mark their shared meanings off from the quotidien banalities of everyday life and talk (ibid.: 1996: 295).

Autobiography is a popular genre in Latvia and narratives are structured around certain shared metaphorical themes in the way that Bruner and Feldman suggest. Moreover, the publication of life stories, particularly those of survivors' stories since 1990, relates to the independence movement and the need to establish a national identity (see, e.g., Līce 1990). However, they are not simply about oratory, and such an interpretation would not be recognized by the narrators themselves.

The fascination of all narratives of the personal past lies in their dual nature. They both reach out to past worlds and in the course of their telling construct new worlds of meaning. Latvian narratives use the image of the harvest to meditate on the theme of power and powerlessness. However, despite their metaphorical style, accounts were given as testimonies to past violence and destruction. The conviction of the teller and the spirit of the tale do not guarantee truth, yet these memories speak of events which have left a mark not only on the hearts and minds of the people but also on the very landscape and its shrinking population. Although people describe real events, collective and mythical perspectives are introduced which transform them into a new kind of reality.

The harvest metaphor suggests a number of connotations which are the subject of many Drustian narratives. Perhaps not surprisingly for a farming community, narrators recalled actual harvests, citing precise quantities and dates. However, harvests gleaned and harvests spoiled also appeared as metaphors to convey experiences of agency and victimhood; of power and oppression. The harvest is the physical culmination of the farmers' agricultural year, but it also provides a wealth of symbols and meanings. The harvest forms part of a network of meanings which includes temporal sequencing, causality, agency, justice and fairness. Thus the good harvest evokes the idea of predictability, order and balance; work has results, bears fruit and is rewarded. The spoiled harvest, by contrast, reverses the natural course of events; it introduces the idea of work and effort being in vain, of not reaping one's just rewards, of unfairness – in short, of being a victim.

Latvian poetry represents the Soviet invasion as a bitter or spoilt harvest. For example, the poem 'The Terrible Summer' by Edvarts Virza, which he wrote in 1940, refers to the bitterness of the honey harvest. It is part of an earlier tradition which promotes Latvian as the language of ploughing and sowing, as in these lines by Rainis, the national poet (1864–1920):[4]

We draw strength from the earth
Rich rye seed flows through us all
We are a people for ploughing, not war.
 We suck strength from the lap of the earth.
(translation VS)

These literary formulations have fused with the natural preoccupations of a farming people in such a way as to frame the memories of the Soviet occupation. Many narratives of the personal past recall the Soviet invasion in terms of a harvest filched from the peoples' grasp. For example, Ilga remembers talking to her mother about the meaning of communism.

> *And I know that mother and I went into the garden to weed and I asked her. 'What is the Soviet Union actually?' I asked that for the first time – I must have been eighteen and I asked her what it meant, although I already knew how they lived. And she replied like this: 'We're weeding potatoes now, but I ... don't know who will harvest them.'*

The role of informers too is linked to harvesting. Here is Rasma describing one such neighbour:

> *And then one spring we were planting potatoes and as he walked past he said, 'Carry on planting, but I'll be harvesting in the autumn.' And do you know it was quite ironic, we were harvesting the potatoes in the autumn and he was buried in the churchyard ... buried in the churchyard. And who did it? People from the forest who were hiding at the time. They knew about his ravings and what he was doing to innocent people. During that time none of the people who lived in the forest dared to come to us.*

However, behind the metaphorical meanings of the harvest lie very real preoccupations. The nadir of the *kolkhoz* (collective farm) movement was

accelerated by the bad weather of the summer of 1952 as Milda, a former
Communist Party secretary, describes:

> *Well, at the beginning during the early years when each kolkhoz was still*
> *separate, particularly Gaisma, then we had our own directors, you understand,*
> *and then people actually worked and conditions were quite normal for about*
> *three years, that was until about 1952. Then in 1952 we had the so-called wet*
> *year when the rain started falling on 13 August and rain met snow. The corn had*
> *grown but it couldn't be harvested. That was 1952. It was the wet year. Potatoes*
> *were good, corn had grown well because we still had fertilized soil. But it*
> *couldn't be harvested. And we mowed and mowed, and it started to snow and*
> *then that had an effect on the next year.*

The memory of that year serves for many as a symbol of spoilt land and
crops; above all 1952 marks the watershed between harvests which drew
upon the labour of earlier years and the depletion of those earlier
investments.

Collectivization

For most of the inhabitants of Drusti, collectivization is associated with
arbitrariness, unreasonableness and injustice. These feelings and ideas are
embodied in memories of harvests neglected, wantonly spoilt or
appropriated. The subversion of a natural order, of cause and effect,
underlies many accounts of collectivization. Neglected, unfertilised earth
cannot yield a harvest. The image which many narrators evoked was that
of animals too weak to stand in the spring and having to be carried out to
pasture. An inversion of seasons revokes the accustomed temporal order.
And most importantly, the balance between action and intended result,
between labour and its fruits, is destroyed.

Here is Māra, my first informant, describing collectivization:

> *Yes, everything was taken away. We didn't have a lot of land, just ten hectares,*
> *and that husband of mine had got it in mind never to join the kolkhoz. And the*
> *bigger farmers didn't sow wheat, that autumn they didn't sow anything, because*
> *they understood that in future they wouldn't be able to pay the taxes or hand in*
> *the levies. But we planted a large area of beautiful wheat and we had clover and*
> *then we had to give it all away and we had to give all the animals away, we had*
> *to give away the horse, we had two horses. We gave them away. And then in*
> *Khrushchev's time then it was hard. Then they wanted to destroy the private*
> *farms. They took the land away gradually and left half a hectare. But finally it*
> *went to the state farm, to the sovhoz. Khrushchev had a plan to make everyone*
> *work ... We were left with even less than half a hectare and they even measured*
> *round the house. Our house was on a little hill, planted around, well, like a*
> *Latvian farmhouse, we were just left with the fenced-in yard. Then we dug up*
> *the fruit bushes with a spade so that we could plant potatoes. We couldn't mow*
> *the hay until the sovhoz had mown their hay. We could only do it in September,*
> *but by that time it was already cold outside and the rains had started. It was very*

difficult with the hay. Then we were only allowed one cow and one pig. That was towards the end of Khrushchev's time. I don't even remember the year. Towards the end of Khrushchev's time – we were six people, the two of us, my mother and the three children – six people. One pig was taken away, we didn't hand it over straight away. And the land was taken away and the cow … I think we had about 0.15 hectares. Now they write in the papers that in that time of destruction they wanted to destroy cows altogether, just to make people work in the collective farms. Because my husband was the only worker, I had three children and my mother was old, we couldn't manage with one person's wages. We needed … well, more. But where would we get more? We didn't get anything. We didn't get anything, but I just know that we had to give one pig away and we kept one and the one that was given away was given for very little money. We sold a big pig and in the autumn Khrushchev was no more and suddenly we were allowed to have as many as we wanted. We were allowed to keep more pigs, but it turned out that for the big pig's money we could only buy little piglets. And then I remember the market and my husband saying 'we have to buy two piglets, we have to buy two piglets.' But I said, 'We'll rear them and have to give them away again. 'We can't manage with one, and so we bought two. And then things changed again and we could keep more.[5]

Joining the kolkhoz for Māra was also associated with forced forestry work:

When we joined the kolkhoz, then we had to go right up to the Estonian border to do forest work, I don't even know how many kilometres it came to. And then we would go there and stay there for a longer time. Some two weeks or so. We had to take food with us and then we would find somewhere to live. There was chopping and carrying and the whole winter would go like that. The timber was for the government. It was prepared for building material or something like that.[6] *There were timber levies, whether one wanted it or not, that's how it was. Whatever they wanted they imposed, and that's how it was with the land, with the horses. If you won't do it we'll take the horse away and give it to someone else. One was forced to do things. And in the years after the war, there were the huge levies; meat was levied from the big farmers. We had a small plot of land, just ten hectares, the levies weren't so big, but those who had more land couldn't grow that much and when they'd finished the threshing the* slaucitāji *(expropriators) would arrive, one is supposed to say the* priekšnieki *(directors), they arrived with their horses and took everything, cleaned everything out, everything that had been harvested.*

Such narratives are the closest that we as listeners and readers can get to the past experience of these Drustians. These accounts tell us what it is like to be at the receiving end of brute force and arbitrarily changing rules and the way in which this leads to a loss of the sense of oneself as an independent agent. Alasdair Macintyre's (1992: 213) reminder that we are not only the principal agents but also the principal authors of our lives points towards some important interconnections. The force of Māra's account derives not only from her testimony to past suffering, but also from her ability to convey the impact on herself and her family.

I feel I am being strangled. I cannot stand all the irregularities. There are no rules.

Latvian peasant women, like some social theorists, are preoccupied with problems of anomie and weep over the lack of meaning in their lives. Skaidrīte remembers the consequences of collectivization for her father. Skaidrīte was born the sixth and youngest child in a forester's family. In 1928 with the help of a loan from a relative her father bought a farm and some sixty hectares of land in Drusti. At the time of the Soviet invasion the loan had still not been paid off. Throughout her account Skaidrīte emphasizes the arbitrary and senseless nature of Soviet rules.

> *In the country we felt it less, but when the levies started we did feel it. Such-and-such an amount has to be handed over and just so. Not at first, but later the sorting started: those who had less land had less to pay, but the old farmers, they started calling them* budži *(rich peasants), and they imposed taxes on them that couldn't be paid. In the first year they imposed 18,000 roubles on us. That was the tax. Then we had to hand over tons of grain, potatoes; little was left for ourselves. But with the money it was like this: in the first year they said that they would impose the kulak tax and if you couldn't pay, then who knows what they would do with you. So we struggled. The first year we sold butter. I would take suitcases to Riga that you couldn't lift and a little suitcase full of money back home. They were cervonci, worthless money.[7] Then we sold a cow so that we could manage to pay the 18,000 after all. We paid it. The next year they imposed 30,000, and it was clear that we could not pay that. That was 1948.[8] We waited to see what would happen next. We wondered whether we would be deported or what. But we tried to hand in the grain, the potatoes. Very little was left in the granary. And then one autumn day, it was October or November, father was called to Cēsis. There was no transport. He had to take the horse; after the war all the railway lines were destroyed. Father went off, some people from the parish wanted a lift, and he didn't return. Neither the horse, nor father. We made enquiries in Cesis and the parish. Apparently he'd been arrested for not paying his taxes. The horse had been taken too. The horse was tied up in the yard and taken with the cart and all ... disappeared.*

Skaidrīte's father was put in Cēsis prison for two weeks before the trial. This is her account of the trial:

> *He'd just turned eighty, bent and white-haired. Two military policemen were guarding him. Murderers aren't led the way he was – being an old man. And then he was led into the court room. People had been called in, half of Cesis, to hear the kulak (rich peasant) being tried. The terrible enemy of the state. There was a man called Freiberg who said that he hadn't paid the money, that he was an enemy of the state, that he hadn't paid one rouble in taxes, what could one do with a person like that. Yes, grain had been handed in but the money had not been paid. What should the punishment be? The court deliberated. Well, they return and say one year's imprisonment with confiscation of all possessions to compensate for the thirty thousand roubles. The last word, the guilty man was allowed the last word. My father, all grey and bent, stood there and said, 'All the taxes that I could pay I have paid, but such a tax I could no longer pay, because the previous year I paid eighteen thousand. Well, what can I say. I ask the court*

to be merciful'. All the courtroom, all the people who had gone there, they were all crying, because it was a terrible sight, such an old man. I can't forget that.

Deportations

However, it was actual deportations of family, friends and neighbours which propelled people in Drusti and throughout Latvia into the *kolkhozi*. The deportations were swift and unanticipated. On the night of 25 March 1949, 50,000 men, women and children were deported from Latvia.[9] They constituted one tenth of all farming people. Since land had already been confiscated, the definition of a *kulak* was used retrospectively. In practice, of course, there was a large element of arbitrariness in the compilation of lists for deportation, and local envy and animosities were sometimes exploited. The deportations had the desired effect of speeding collectivization. According to Misiunas and Taagepera the proportion of collectivized farms rose from eleven to fifty per cent in a month (12 March to 9 April 1949). By the end of 1951 more than 98 per cent of all Latvian farms were collectivized (Misiunas and Taagepera 1993: 103). Deportation hit Drusti particularly hard, with some 16 per cent of farms destroyed as a consequence. Thus deportations destroyed individual lives, farms and the landscape. Massive disused agricultural buildings disfigure the land. However, deportation has also come to be central to Latvian national identity and 25 March is now a national day of commemoration. Albertīna's first teaching job was in Drusti in the immediate post-war period; this is her account of March 1949.

> *Well, it happened unannounced, suddenly. We went to school and saw that horses and carts had driven into the school courtyard with people and boxes and little bundles. We were surprised to see them all there. Then the militia arrived in the school and asked for the children. The parents had already been taken and put in the carts ... I don't know where they were taken. Then the militia asked for the children to be handed over. We teachers said we had no right to hand the children over and that we can't do that. Then some parents came to fetch them, others were taken anyway without our permission. Others fled ... those children. One little girl and her brother had taken refuge in my flat. I didn't know that they'd hidden there. And when everyone had gone away I went into my flat and the poor dears who'd been meant for deportation come towards me.[10] Everyone was alarmed. Alarmed. Both teachers and children. We couldn't concentrate on the lessons any more. And you could say that there were no more lessons. That day there was no more teaching.*

The theme of victimhood is reinforced by the knowledge that those doing the transporting were themselves roped-in for the task.

> *Those were just the farmers themselves with their carts. There were many who had been taken for* skūtis *(corvée). They were taken to the parish hall and then to Cēsis. No news came to the school of where they were taken or where they*

were. Nothing. We didn't know about the parents or the children. We didn't know where they were.

Jānis Arājs, a retired schoolteacher now living in Drusti, was working in a school in north Vidzeme at the time:

> *As everywhere, there was a deportation plan. A certain number of people. No one knew why. I and the headmaster of the school, also a young man, were called out to the parish hall and both of us were locked in a room. I don't know why. We were simply locked up and that was it. We didn't know what was happening outside. All night people were brought in and interrogated. In the morning I hear someone the other side of the door saying in Russian 'Now we can let those bandits out. We have enough'. And it seemed to me that we were being held in reserve and if they'd been short we would have been taken. But thank God they weren't short and we were set free. But the children ... Better not ask all that. When a lamb is taken away from the flock for slaughter, even then the farmer feels pain. It is terrible, it is a terrible situation which words can't describe.*

Inta was a schoolgirl in her fifth year at school when the deportations occurred.

> *I do remember. They drove into the school and called out the surnames for the children to come out. They were collected together and driven off. There were the Puķīsī, Asari ... I don't remember the names terribly well, but I do remember the feeling of alarm, because we didn't understand where they were going to be put and where they were being called. We didn't know they were being taken to Siberia.*

To dwell on the narrative strategies used to remember deportation is not to deny its reality or the terrible impact it had on people's lives. It is simply to recognize that narrators are authors as well as agents or victims. Accounts of the deportation of children convey the community's sense of victimization.

Fifty years of Soviet rule would not have been possible without some degree of complicity amongst a significant minority of the population. However, many of those who appeared to support the Soviet authorities share the same polarized world view of the system versus the victim. For example, Milda, who was involved in rounding up the deportees on the night of 24 March 1949, also presents herself as a powerless and unknowing victim.

> *Yes, on 24 March shortly before work was finished, about five o'clock, at that time we had to work until six, we got written instructions that on 24 March at ten o'clock in the evening we have to come to the parish executive committee in very warm clothes. Well. Of course we were very alarmed and confused and didn't know what was happening or who was to do what or what had to be done. Well ten o'clock arrived and we went to the council in the parish house. Well, then, we look, we didn't know how many were there, how many had been given instructions, what is going to happen. All the executive committee members were there, the librarians and club workers were there and a few more*

still. With all the people doing skūtis *perhaps there were more than twenty. And then there were the* istribiteli *[Russian, literally 'destroyers'].*

I wanted to know what the destroyers were actually supposed to destroy.

Well, what were they supposed to destroy? Istribiteli ... *it was a kind of translation from the Russian language, it's a term ... well they had weapons, like today's home guard have weapons, and ... and ... and ... they had a weapon. So we arrived, one person arrives after another, then we see and ask one another 'Do you know anything? Do you know anything? Do you know anything? What's going to happen? What's going to happen? What's going to happen?' Well, nobody knew anything. Nobody knew anything. Well, then we asked the* partorg *(party secretary) what we were supposed to do, the people were made to do* skūtis *anyway. She said 'Wait at two o'clock, on 25 March at two o'clock, they will arrive from Cēsis and tell you what has to be done. Wait.' And then we waited. And really at two o'clock armed uniformed men drove up and said ... that ... a transfer of people to another place of residence would take place. Nobody mentioned Siberia or said where they were being taken ... another place of residence. It is Stalin's order ... signed ... it was read out from some piece of paper. Well, we really didn't have any idea about Siberia. A transfer, a transfer of people, well what were we supposed to do? Well, we were instructed that we have to find ... they had read out that people could take possessions with them, only not animals, as many possessions as they want and we were told that we were to list the possessions and that we had to find a farmer to look after the animals until further notice. That was the plan. And the soliders knew straightaway where each was to go, and those three stood there and then the chairman of the executive committee and the partorg allocated each one of us as possession-inventorizers and animal-caretaker searchers to each of the three soldiers and we didn't know where we had to go. The soldiers told the* skūtnieks *who was driving the horse where they had to go.*

Independence Remembered

Memories of life in the 'Latvian period' and of life under Soviet rule mutually sharpen and bring into focus the themes of agency and its loss, of control and its absence, of direction and meaninglessness. Memories of pre-war youth and childhood are essential to conveying the full meaning of irregularity, unpredictability and victimhood under Soviet rule. The sense of having no control over one's life during the Soviet period contrasts sharply with earlier memories. Hard work and sufficiency form a thematic backbone to many recollections of childhood and Jēkabs's terse comment on his childhood can stand for many others.

We were farm workers. We lived and we worked. I went herding cattle; there was no time to wander around.

Rasma's memories of childhood also emphasize self-sufficiency.

We weren't rich, but it sufficed, we had enough to eat. There was a lot of work. My parents worked very hard. They kept cows, sometimes five, sometimes six. Then they would take the cart and go and see where they could arrange to mow some hay. That's how they managed. We had enough, but we weren't rich.

Jānis's narrative spells out the links between work and self-sufficiency:

My parents were servants. We didn't live particularly grandly, but we had enough. In the country it was usual to get work with a farmer. My father was a man of parts: he could put his hand not only to farm work but he could also do roofs. He knew how to thatch, which was rare in those days. He was also a bricklayer. Thanks to his skills we didn't experience want. My mother was a housewife. She made sure we had gloves and socks. I had a brother – we were two children in the family. We were both sent to primary and to secondary school.

Even those who do not have good memories, such as Austra, recall the independence period in an idiom quite different from the Soviet one:

My memories are very bad, because when mother and father married they had nothing. They rented land, for labour, they went as farm labourers to farmsteads. All those farms ... we were seven children in the family. A big family. I was the fifth. Because those were hard days. Sometimes there were bad harvests when we couldn't pay. We had to give ... when we were graudnieki *[sharecroppers] we had to pay back in corn. A fixed amount to the farmer. If it was a good harvest then fine, if it was bad then things were hard. That's how we left. It must have been 1919 when we quit altogether. The bad harvests started. I can't quite remember, but everything drowned. We had such land that everything drowned and we simply couldn't pay the farmer. We couldn't pay him and so the family split up. We were already growing up. We were of an age for my brother to volunteer for military service so that somehow or other he could get a living. One went to Riga ... two went to Riga. We were split up. And one brother went to Russia. That was in 1918 ... 1919.*

Despite her impoverished childhood Ausma goes on to emphasize the importance of work:

We were all kept busy. My father was very orderly and industrious. And he had accustomed us all to the land so that we could survive, because otherwise we wouldn't have survived if we hadn't all worked. And that's why to this day I love the land. And working the land is ingrained in me. And from there we came to Līzuma Near Līzuma, that's a bit further. How many kilometres I'm not sure. There is a farmstead there, Zosupītes, we took the house there on rent. That's where the year of the bad harvest was. There was very poor soil there, you couldn't grow anything but the meadows were grand. In my childhood it was this way: my brothers mowed and my father mowed and I had to mow alongside them. When I couldn't manage anymore they would help me, but I had to start mowing very young.

She contrasts the hard life of her childhood with later forms of oppression involving terror:

I didn't like the barons because my father had been told what the times of the barons were like. He didn't have any terrible tales to tell – they must have been earlier. [Ausma is referring to accounts of physical punishment and brutality.] *But there was oppression. There was forced labour. One had to go. There was no terror in my time, but one had to work hard, terribly hard. We didn't have land, you couldn't buy land. We went picking wild berries, mushrooms, we went to market to Gulbene and we went on foot carrying everything, and mother had made butter, cheese and cottage cheese, so that we could buy clothes.*

Austra, like all the other narrators, confirmed that the family had enough to eat.

Things were not at all bad with food because father worked hard and we kept animals. We had eight cows, sheep, calves. So although we had a large family we were fed. But we didn't have much in the way of clothes. If we went to some occasion we would try to spare our shoes by carrying them underarm.

Māra too remembers her childhood in terms of hard work.

I was born in the pagasts [an administrative district].[11] My parents hadn't yet built their house. We lived in the neighbour's house and the land was just nearby and they owned nothing except those rooms. The state gave a loan and we only had to pay one fifth of the cost of the building materials. The state helped; we were the jaunsaimnieki *[new farmers].[12]*

However, when Melānija remembers her childhood home her memories are happy.

When I dream I often dream of that house. Then when I wake up in the morning, I feel happy and have a sense of lightness. It seems so pleasant, although during the day I don't think that at all. But generally, I had a hard time to do with that herding. The work was hard. I had to get up early in the morning, the grass was wet, there was dew and my feet were constantly wet. Sometimes there was thunder and a storm. I was frightened. Then sometimes if there was a storm my mother would come.

Discussion

Drustian narrators attempt to recapture the past as they have lived it. In doing so they single out events such as collectivization and deportation. They do not do so because such events serve the ends of their story – indeed, some terrible events make very poor stories – but because these events demand explanation; they need to be fitted into a coherent story. In this respect Latvian memories differ from those of the French villagers described by Zonabend (1984: 196) in whose memories the war figured hardly at all. So which kinds of harvest are important for Drustian narratives? Are they the ones which fill bellies or those which offer an image of orderly life, of life as it should be lived? My answer is that both are important, but that the grain or potato harvest must be given precedence. However important to human understanding, the metaphorical harvest is dependent upon the 'real' harvest from which it draws emotional sustenance. This is not to suggest that the two can now be prised apart. Once metaphor becomes established it may transform its parent source. However, the power of harvest symbolism derives from the plain fact of human dependence on food.

The narrative 'I' moves between these two harvests. As agent or victim it is more interested in the grain harvest, as author it draws upon the metaphorical harvest. Both personal and literary narratives are dependent in some fundamental sense upon the real harvest and the real world. However, this is not to deny intertextuality. Literary and historical texts influence narrative and this is particularly true in Latvia where literature and the writing of history from a Latvian perspective have played a central role in the shaping of Latvian national identity. In trying to make sense of a victimized past, events are transposed to a world of meaning which draws upon text and metaphor. Indeed, whatever might be of use in creating meaning and coherence is roped in.

One characteristic way of doing this is by using the vocabulary of serfdom which offers a concise way of conveying the experience of powerlessness. The vocabulary used to describe the first phases of deportation and collectivization is borrowed from an earlier period of history. The provision of obligatory transport for deporting neighbours and the taxes imposed on farmers after the war were referred to by the words *skūtis* and *nodevas*, both terms belonging to the organization of serfdom. *Nodevas* referred to the agricultural produce which the manorial lord was entitled to exact; *skūtis* is the term for labour which the manorial lord was entitled to exact from peasants in return for their use of land. *Skūtnieki* refers to the peasants themselves when they give this labour. Neighbours drafted in to transport the deportees on the first leg of their journey are also described as *skūtnieki*. Most people had little choice over whether to co-operate with this process or not, but the language in which these events is described removes deportation from the realm of actions which might attract praise or blame to one of inevitable historical structures.

Memories of the post-war period evoke resonances of accounts of earlier history, perhaps those read in school textbooks. For example, here is an extract from Māra's first letter to me:

> The hay could only be mown when the feed for the kolkhoz was ensured, that was in late autumn. If someone had mown some hay from rough pasture around the bushes earlier, that was taken away to the communal barn. It was no use saying my family is big, my children are small.

And here she is describing the same problems when I met her in her farmhouse:

> The government wanted to restrict people so that they wouldn't rely on their own work, but work for free for the kolkhoz. One's own small piece of land, one's own hay could only be mown by stealth, so to speak – one had to mow

secretly. One couldn't mow hay in good weather, one had to do it for the kolkhoz *first, and for oneself only late in the autumn. The fodder was so bad that it was difficult to keep cows, only one could be kept and even that one was thin. Once I had mown the hay in good weather, then they came and took the hay away.*

The tone and focus of her concerns has resonances with that of a voice some two centuries old. Garlieb Merkel (1769–1860) was the son of a German pastor living in the province of Vidzeme not far from Drusti. His writing, influenced by Rousseau and the French revolution, was the first to address the social condition of the Latvian peasantry:

At haymaking, at harvest, at every big task the peasant farm had to supply three, four or five people or however many the manor demanded, so that all those capable of working were collected together early in the morning. Meanwhile the peasant's farm was motionless; one field was not sown, his hay was rotting, his seed was sprouting. But what did that matter? The manor had taken advantage of the good weather and was not worried about any more losses (Merkelis, 1999: 56, translation V.S.).

Whether the similarities between Māra's letter and Merkel's writing derive from recurring experiences or from textual influence and borrowing is impossible to establish with certainty. Both literature and personal narrative draw upon experience, but texts break free from the circumstances of their creation and take on lives of their own, making appearances in the remembered personal past of many Latvian narrators. Thus it is likely that Māra's recollections of her relationship with the *kolkhoz* authorities are shaped both by her actual experiences and by her childhood lessons in history. Similarly, memories of the Ulmanis period[13] reflect both experience and the requirements of narrative structure. Farmers were encouraged to buy their own land with the help of government loans. The result was, indeed, an agricultural success story, but at the cost of extreme hard work. However, the full development of the harvest metaphor demands a contrast between spoiled harvests and successful harvests, and it is this contrast which is achieved by the recollection of hard work and its fruits.

In their particularity and in their simultaneous search for a wider reference, these testimonies show how narrators in remembering the personal past have two sets of allegiances: to former experience and to the current need for explanation and meaning. The final shape of narratives, their combination of testimony and metaphor, is an expression of these dual allegiances.

Acknowledgements

I wish to thank Martin Dewhirst, Māra Kalniņš and Ian Hamnett for their critical reading of this paper and the ESRC for making the whole thing possible.

Notes

1. My sample snowballed to thirty-four. All interviews were recorded and later transcribed. In some cases, as with Māra, no questions were needed – I was merely a willing listener. In other cases I fed in the occasional question. Recordings varied between one and four hours.
2. Vilhelms Purvītis (1872–1945) was born in Zaube in Vidzeme.
3. In their article 'Group Narrative as a cultural context of autobiography' (1996: 293) Jerome Bruner and Carol Fleischer Feldman examine the way in which three drama groups develop distinctive genres of recalling the past.
4. Jānis Pliekšāns, pen-name Rainis (1864–1920), was a member of the Social Democratic party from 1891. He was active in the struggle for independence and his prolific literary output included poems and plays.
5. According to the 1935 agricultural statutes of Soviet Russia, applied to Latvia under Soviet occupation, each household could have one cow, two young calves, one sow with piglet (or two piglets without the sow), ten sheep and goats and twenty beehives. In Khrushchev's time the rules were tightened. From 1971 onwards permission had to be sought from the *kolkhoz*.
6. Obligatory forest work was widespread between 1945 and 1949, 1946 and 1947 being particularly bad years. The rules were issued by the Council of People's Commissariat for timber felling, transmitted to the Latvian government and then to local executives. These local officials decided on requirements from particular individuals. Country people were forced to sign contracts promising to deliver stipulated amounts of timber. Availability of transport was not taken into account.
7. When cervonci were first issued by the Soviet Socialist Republic in 1922, one cervonec was equivalent to ten golden roubles; later, people started calling a twenty-five rouble bill a cervonec. Their post-war worthlessness was a reflection of post-war inflation.
8. In 1947 taxes were 40per cent of estimated revenue; in 1948 they rose to 75per cent.
9. Deportation and mortality statistics are a contentious issue. In 1953 Jānis Kalnberzins (1893–1986), first secretary of the Latvian Communist Party, reported that 119,000 people were deported, but no further information was made available. Recent Soviet data gave a figure of 64500 deportations before 1950. However, exiled historians cite considerably higher figures. Edgars Andersons gives an estimate of between 108,000 and 216,000 (Latvju Enciklopēdija 1962–82: 318 Amērikas Latviešu Apvienība); Arveds Švābe of 540,000 (Latvian Encyclopaedia, 1950: 480 Tris Zvaigznes, Stockholm). According to the data of the Baltic Council there were between 180,000 and 200,000 deportations before 1953. Of those deported in 1949, 5,073 died during deportation.
10. Different tenses are used by narrators. Particularly dramatic, violent or painful events are recounted in the present.
11. *Pagasti* are administrative districts. From the seventeenth century they reflected the manorial division of land. With the emancipation of serfs during the nineteenth century *pagasti* created a forum for peasant voices. A notable change was the substitution in 1811 of *zemnieku valoda* or peasant language for keeping records of agricultural duties and taxes in the *vaka* books. At the time of the Soviet occupation in 1944 there were 516 *pagasti*. In 1950 these were replaced by 56 *rajoni* but in daily life *pagasti* continued to figure. See Arveds Švābe, 1930.
12. Māra's parents benefited from the land reforms of the 1920s. Land was requisitioned from the German barons and distributed to landless peasants. New farmers were helped in developing their farms by low-interest government loans. The legislation transformed Latvia into a nation of smallholders. Farms could not exceed fifty hectares.
13. Kārlis Ulmanis (1874–1942) was the first elected Prime Minister of Independent Latvia and his name is synonymous with the period of independence.

13

NARRATIVES OF LANDSCAPE IN LATVIAN HISTORY AND MEMORY

Our native hearth
Is burning in the sky
In order to come home
We do not open the door
But the cover of a book.

We cannot learn from a snail
Because home is not a refuge for us
But we will be a refuge for the homeland.
                                        Māra Zālīte

Background to Research

My fieldwork was carried out over a period of ten months between 1992 and 1993 and three months in 1999 and involved listening to over a hundred life histories. My proposed study was of neurasthenia, the most commonly used diagnosis in the former Soviet Union which relates to such symptoms as tiredness, anxiety and irritability – conditions most of us are familiar with at some time or another under another name. As so often happens in anthropological projects – particularly those dealing with illness – I found the fieldwork expanding, in my case moving inexorably back in time to events some forty or fifty years old. I heard stories of imprisonment, expropriation, deportation and return. However, these stories were not only concerned about the unfolding of events in time, they also interrupted the narrative sequence in order to describe the places of their early experience and thus to recreate landscapes of memory for themselves and their listener. There is a short book by Poulet (1963), which argues that

Proust's work is concerned not with time but with place and, in particular, with places lost. Latvian narratives too are concerned not only with the reconstruction of past times but also with the imaginative recreation of place. Description is as important as narration in Latvian autobiographical accounts in that it ties freewheeling accounts of movement and loss to recognizable and shared landscapes.

Roskill describes the interdependence of the visual and linguistic in the context of landscape painting and argues that there are certain conventions of transposability from visual images to linguistic descriptions.

> Space and time enter inevitably into the way that landscape is perceived. Things are taken as set apart from one another, in a fashion that entails both distribution and extension. But because of the parts played by imagination and recall here, in piecing together how the key features in question take up their places and what sort of ordering they imply, it is not at all clear that what happens spatially and temporally within an outdoor scene can be identified and responded to, independently of acquiring a language in which to do this (1997: 11).

The pastoral focus of Latvian painting and literature enabled this transposition from narrative eye to I to take place.

My point of departure for this chapter is a kind of paradox, which I would like you to consider. It concerns the way in which my Latvian narrators so often interrupt, or put on hold if you like, their narration of a rapid sequence of violent events in order to describe a seductive pastoral landscape and to take pleasure, albeit fleetingly, in the feelings thus evoked. For example, Jānis, interleaves his account of his train journey under arrest to a prison camp outside Moscow with a reference to the countryside: 'And then we were loaded into the wagons and we started the journey to the east. And I remember it was about 2nd or 3rd June and we passed through Lithuania and it was high summer and beautiful and I so much wanted to throw myself out of the wagon doors and run into the forest'. Pastoral form and feeling is intertwined throughout Jānis's and many other Latvian narratives. It suggests that pastoral is not incompatible with extreme experience but rather can help sustain the experience and its narrative representation. I find a parallel in a recent book on pastoral, which begins in an unlikely way by considering an episode from Primo Levi's *If this is a man* (1987). Levi and a fellow prisoner have found temporary respite from the regimented labour of Auschwitz: 'Levi's and Jean's sense of physical and conversational ease at noontime replicates, under painfully unlikely circumstances, a situation conventionally found in pastoral poems' (Alpers 1997: 5). Alpers uses this example to dismiss the case against pastoral on the grounds of its inability to 'envisage deprivation of this extent and severity' and to argue that the pastoral mode can indeed encompass the extremes of human experience (ibid.: 7).

I want to show that the pastoral mode of narrative is not merely compatible with the representation of extreme experience but that it creates the very possibility of such representation. There is, of course, a long and venerable tradition of mapping temporal sequences onto spatial theatres of memory (Yates 1966). These places are 'like all memory places, ... both a private site and a public location, a "commonplace" in a social even a national imaginary' (Mitchell 1994: 207). These public memory sites highlight the select nature of memory and what can and cannot be remembered. Narrators may feel unable to recall certain sites/sights and return instead to other more familiar and comforting landscapes. 'But describing the experience, recounting the experiential density of visual details, especially those trivial details that do nothing to advance the narrative, but "spread the narrative in space ... this way of telling is too dangerous. It threatens to ... take the narrator "back in memory" to a place he cannot endure' (ibid.: 201–2). Instead, Latvian narrators interrupt their story to revisit a pastoral landscape where childhood memories are grafted onto a culturally shaped emblem of national identity. In doing so my Latvian narrators are following a tradition which connects pastoral writing with war. Indeed, Virgil, who is seen as one of the originators of Western pastoral poetry, wrote against a background of civil war and one of the protagonists in the *Eclogues* – Moeris – was dispossessed of his land. The ninth eclogue includes the lines:

> Oh Lycidas, we've lived to reach this – that a stranger
> (Something we never feared) should seize our little farm
> And say: 'This property is mine; old tenants, out!' (Virgil 1980: 97)

Latvian folk songs also attest to the interconnectedness of pastoral and soldiering themes. Most are sad such as the following:

> I have to go
> I cannot stay
> There is no one to harvest
> The rye and oats I sowed
>
> I have to go
> I cannot stay
> My horse stays behind
> Nurtured but not yet ridden.
>
> Whoever harvests my rye and oats
> Let him take my horse
> Let him take my horse
> And let him take my bride.

Some are angry and bitter:

> Take the plough yourself master
> To the big field
> Why did you hand over to the king
> So many young ploughmen?

For the narrator a pastoral landscape answers both to a psychological need and to a figural and rhetorical device which promotes the involvement and commitment of the listener in the story. The psychological need is for a still point in a story which careers unpredictably forward with no subject in control. The need for persuasive literary figures which promote involvement on the other hand derive from the compulsive need to testify: to make public the personal. Latvian narratives of violence and dislocation have as their constant reference point a pastoral past and this iconic past draws upon sedimented layers of meaning. As Empson has written, pastoral accounts succeed in 'putting the complex into the simple' (1935: 23). Golden age stories, which are a recurring feature of Latvian life stories, inhabit a pastoral landscape. The golden age story holds together individual and community history: individual experience is mapped onto a pre-existing narrative template. In short the pastoral theme in personal narratives represent an achievement of social connectedness.

Landscape in Historical Narrative

In freezing narrative action, story-tellers enter pastoral landscapes of memory. These are drawn not only from memory but also from a shared language and history and its associated images and stories. The personal story can only be told if it borrows a collective idiom.

Until the Soviet occupation and the attendant reconstruction of society Latvia was a predominantly agrarian society. At the end of the nineteenth century 70 per cent of the population of what is now Latvia were country dwellers. At the outbreak of the First World War that figure had fallen to 60 per cent. But shortly after independence the figures for 1920 are 76 per cent (Skujenieks 1938: 43). Present day figures reflect the Soviet introduction of heavy industry and the migration of workers from other parts of the Soviet Union to Latvian cities. The distribution between country and city has been reversed with some 70 per cent of the population living in towns. However, throughout history the Latvian countryside has been periodically emptied. History books recount how, following the invasion of Livonia by the armies of Ivan the Terrible; one could not hear a cock crow from Riga to Tallinn. The First World War saw a mass exodus of three-quarters of the population of Kurland. And there is, of course, the more recent Soviet experience with its large-scale deportations of people and attack on the physical face of the landscape in the name of amelioration programmes which has resulted in the emptying of the landscape and a reversal to a wilderness of untended bushes and undergrowth.

Indeed, it could be argued that Latvian identity was forged in the countryside. Serfdom, which tied Latvians to the land and yet denied them land of their own, created a passionate longing for land. The nationalist movement of the 1850s and 60s created a literature, which was pre-dominantly pastoral. It also gave pride of place to the folk songs, collected by Barons in the 1890s, which represented human life as rooted in nature and came to be seen as representing the quintessential Latvian spirit. The high literacy rates suggest how influential these publications were in shaping values and feelings. It is no accident that the epicentre of the 1905 revolution moved very quickly from the towns to the countryside and was able to draw upon centuries of suppressed bitterness. Kārlis Ulmanis, the first president of Latvia after the declaration of independence on 18th November 1918, was head of the Farmer's Party. One of the major govern-ment reforms during the period of independence was the redistribution of land to the landless thus creating Latvia as a country of small farmers. With the first Soviet occupation in June 1940 it is the countryside which is seen as bearing the brunt of the onslaught and as being the site of resistance. Land of relatively modest sized farms of 30 hectares and above was confiscated as were farm dwellings. During this first year of occupation some 35,000 people were also arrested and killed with a view to systematically eliminating the intelligentsia, the business class and, indeed, anyone in a position of power or influence. The Soviets had known how to strike at the heart of national identity with their two-pronged attack on land and people. As a result the German invasion of the following summer encountered a demoralized and terrified population many of whom saw the Germans as liberators. Confiscated land was restored, but those relatively few country folk who had collaborated with the Soviet occupiers were in turn expropriated. It is probably the restoration of land and property which helps to explain why the German invasion is described not as an occupation but as a period of time. With the advance of Soviet military forces in the autumn of 1944 there was a resurgence of fear for life and livelihood. Many thousands of Latvians sought refuge in the forests. Plakans (1995: 155) estimates that in the post-war period these numbered between 10,000 and 15,000. Misiunas and Taagepera (1993: 83) quote a figure of 40,000. The forests were thought to hold the only hope of national regeneration. As Schama writes in another context: 'By retreating to the realm of the bison, the depths of the primeval forest, those later survivors of national disaster in the nineteenth and twentieth centuries would find asylum, succour, the promise of re-emergence' (1995: 42) The importance of collective farming to the Soviet enterprise entailed a major onslaught on both people and landscape. Latvian farmers were used to living in independent farmsteads and had no wish to join collective farms. Draconian measures had to be implemented to persuade them to do so. Taxes imposed on farmers in 1947 and 1948 gave an indication of what was to come. For farmers classified as *kulaks* (rich peasants) a tax of 40 per cent of estimated income was imposed in 1947 and 75 per cent in 1948. In practice incomes were overestimated and farmers were unable to pay the taxes. Despite this softening approach only 8 per cent of farmers had joined the *kolkhozi* (collective farms) at the beginning of 1949. On 25 March 1949 one tenth of the rural population, some 50,000 men women and children, were deported to Siberia in an attempt to persuade the rest to join the collective farms. Many were deposited in the region of Tomsk. Since land had already been confiscated the definition of a kulak was used retrospectively. In practice there was a large element of arbitrariness in the compilation of the lists for deportation and local envy and animosities were sometimes exploited. Those who survived deportation and exile often had no homes to return to and their return to the homeland could also be painful. The deportations had the desired effect of speeding up collectivization. Misiunas and Taagepera (1993: 103) quote a figure for collectivized farms of 11 per cent on 12 March and 50 per cent on 9 April. By the end of 1951 more than 98 per cent of all Latvian farms had been collectivized. They imposed a different face upon the landscape: whereas farm dwellings had been scattered over the landscape the Soviet system of collectivized farming required workers to live in artificially created villages consisting of medium rise blocks of flats. People living in outlying farmsteads were forced to move to the centres of administrative regions thus reversing centuries old patterns of scattered rather than village settlement. Figures 13.1 and 13.2 show how such farmsteads look today.

Amelioration was the blanket term used to cover all such acts of aggression carried out against farmers and their land in connection with collectivization. The term was used to describe the draining of marshy land as well as the destruction of farmsteads, wells and roads leading to remote

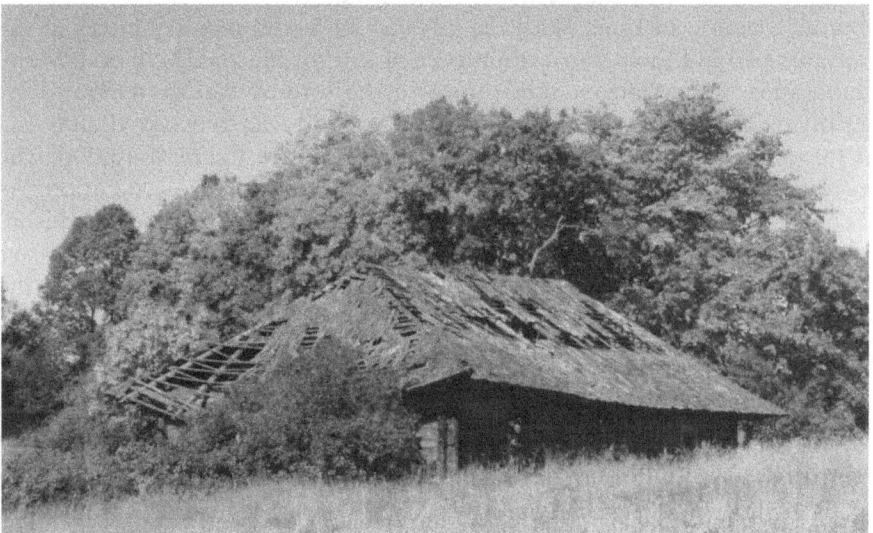

Figure 13.1: Abandoned Farmstead, Drusti

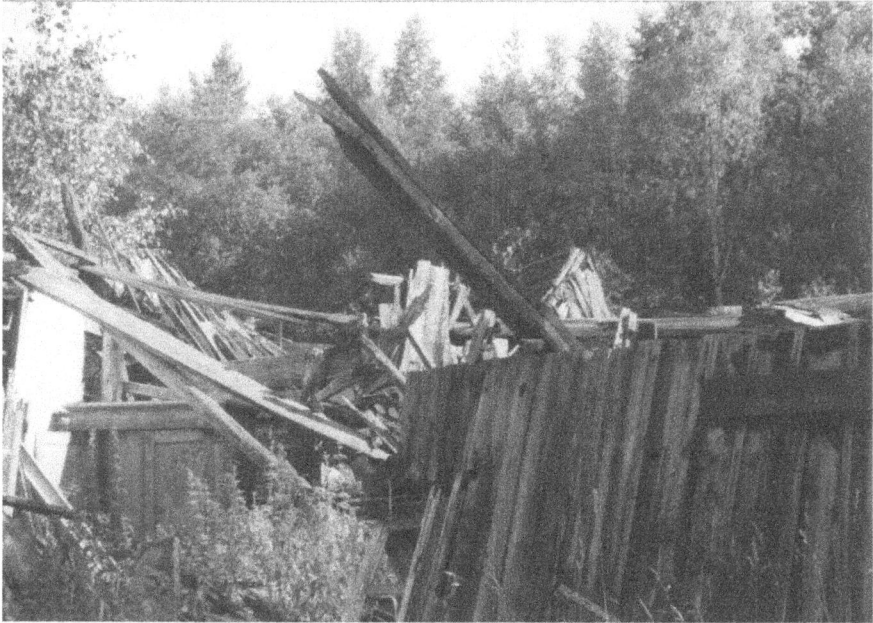

Figure 13.2: Abandoned Farmstead, Drusti

farmsteads. Indeed, some marginal zones near the sea became prohibited areas as Figure 13.3 shows. Not surprisingly the use of the term amelioration by Latvian country people was strongly ironic. In driving farmers out of their remote farmsteads Soviet authorities were not only ensuring ease of surveillance and control but also striking at the central symbol of Latvian identity: the small, single farmstead situated on a slight incline and fringed with forests.

The Promotion of Latvian Art

However, the rural character of Latvian identity was shaped not only by historical events but also by a self-conscious direction of the education system and of artistic enterprise. School children during the independence period were obliged to spend three weeks a year working on farms. The ethnographic museum, which was set up outside Riga in 1925 and covered several hundred hectares, turned traditional country life into an art form. Painting had lagged behind literature in Latvia. Indeed, the art historian Siliņš gives a new meaning to still life in the Baltic context he describes *Livländisches Stilleben* as 'a period of sleepy stillness in social, literary and art matters' (1979: 275). But all this changed during the independence period under Ulmanis who was particularly concerned with the

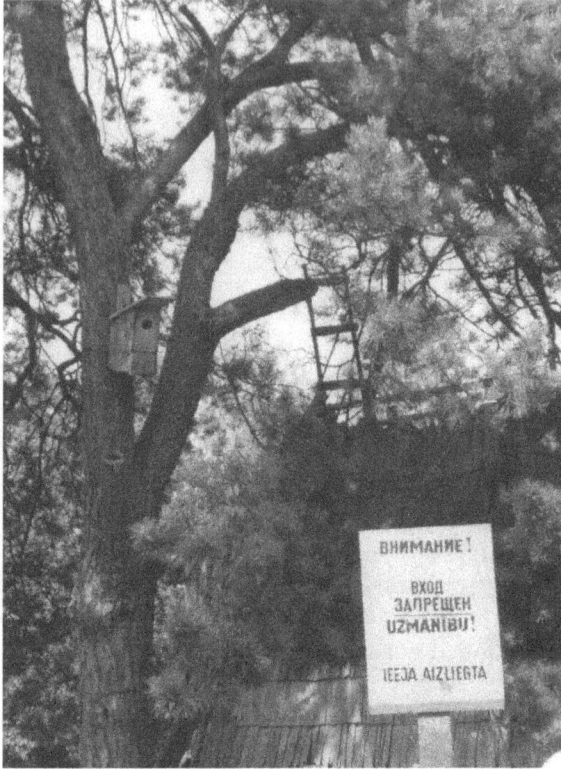

Figure 13.3: Forbidden Coastal Zone

popularization of literary and visual arts on the grounds that it would promote national self-confidence. Exactly two years after the declaration of independence on 18 November 1918 the Cultural Foundation was significantly established on the day of independence to promote and give financial support to the arts. Its self-avowed rationale was closely linked to the development of national identity. 'The Latvian nation has suffered so much that it wants to speak at long last ... Our nation is like a jug that has just been taken from the kiln and wants to ring out. In its roots it has remained healthy, but it wishes to be still more unified and to create its art and its spiritual life' (Kultūras Fonds 1928: 3–4). Indeed, throughout the 1920s and 30s the Cultural Foundation was active in the support of the arts. Considerable sums of money were given in prizes; for example Purvītis received 500 lats in 1921 on his birthday. In the 20s the average sum given for study abroad was 1,500 lats. Publishing, including art books, was heavily subsidized. Art museums were founded in the provinces in Cēsis and Talsis. Several exhibitions were mounted in the provinces throughout the 30s. In 1939 a travelling exhibition was organized which stopped in some fifty places throughout the provinces. The work of artists was subsidized by generous government purchases of paintings.

Between 1935 and 1938 the Cultural Foundation purchased paintings from two exhibitions to the value of 25,000 lats (Siliņš 1990: 18). The association of Latvian artists formed in 1929 argued for 'art with a Latvian content and form' (ibid.: 409) In practice, this involved a certain ambivalence because both government and artists recognized the need for foreign travel and study but it certainly served to promote landscape painting. One of the goals of this painting was the promotion of attachment to landscape and the perception of its beauty. Indeed, a synonym for beautiful is the Latvian word *gleznains* which is translated literally as painting-like – a good example of life imitating art or landscape perceived as art. Ulmanis himself contributed to an exhibition catalogue with the words: 'We must take care to honour works of art and also to honour artists and to see to it that they can work in peace' (ibid.: 18).

The result of this cultural policy was to broaden the category of those observing the landscape so as to include not only the recently emerged intelligentsia and urban middle classes but also those who lived in the countryside and worked the land. Of course, another way in which this was done was through calendars. Painter (1996), in his fascinating study of owners of reproductions of Constable's cornfield, explored the diverse and autobiographically specific ways in which artistic images enter ordinary people's lives. But such images also create profound commonalties in ways of seeing. Raymond Williams has suggested that what is significant is not the landscape in itself but the sensibility of the observer: 'The self-conscious observer ... this is the figure we need to seek: not a kind of nature but a kind of man' (1993: 121). Latvian art and literature, I am suggesting, combined to transform small farmers into these kinds of self-conscious observers and to elevate the farmstead as a root metaphor of Latvian culture. As Bishop has claimed in relation to Constable's paintings, so too Latvian painting was 'not just concerned with evoking memory but also with organizing memory landscapes' (1995: 54).

To summarize: actual historical events, the meanings ascribed to those events and artistic representations of landscape have all contributed to the specifically Latvian experience of landscape and place. The rural landscape has been the site of deprivation, violence and suffering. However, it has also been the source of hope for a better future. Artistic and literary representations have reaffirmed that hope by emphasizing the enduring qualities of landscape, which dwarf historical and biographical changes. Perhaps the best known Latvian painter is Purvītis who painted the landscape of Vidzeme in spring, summer, autumn and winter.[1] Purvītis's landscapes of the changing seasons are shown in Figures 13.4, 13.5, 13.6 and 13.7. As in the serial paintings of Monet who studied the same subject under different conditions, repetition serves to essentialize the landscape.

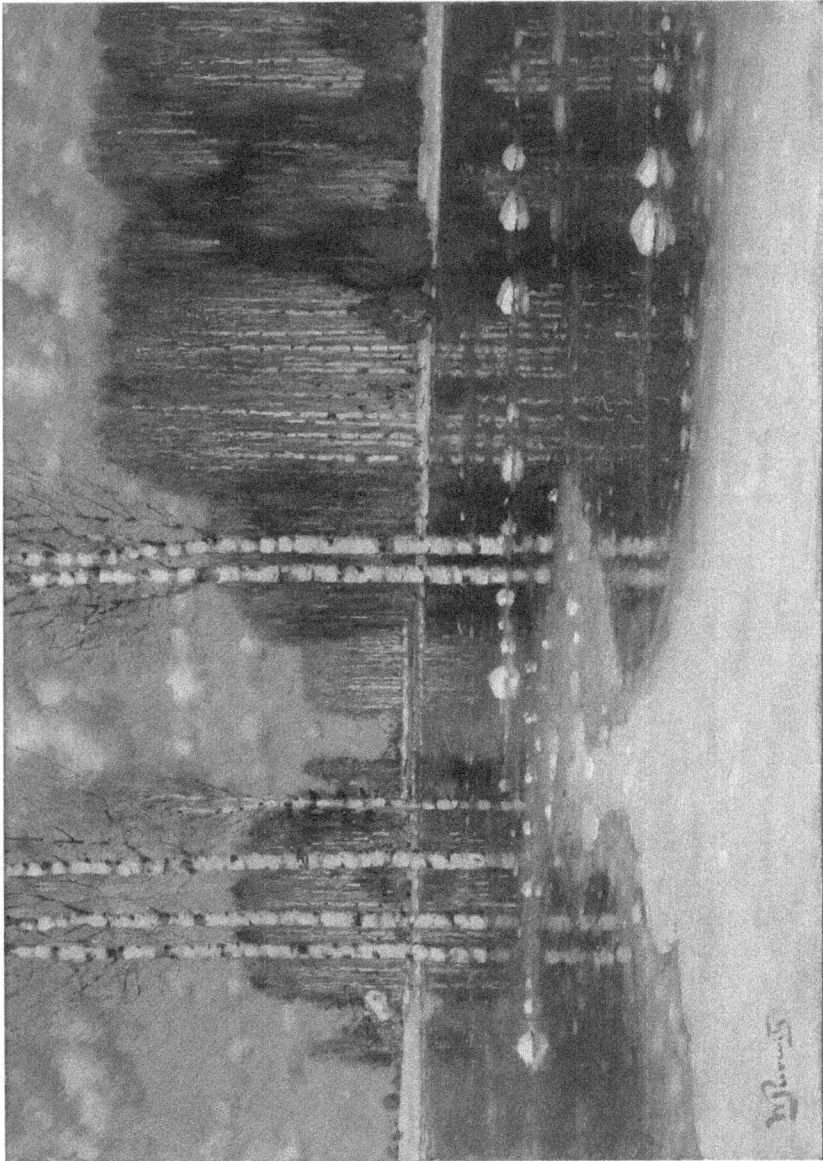

Figure 13.4: Landscape painting by Vilhelms Purvitis, Early Spring
Reproduced with permission of the Latvian National Museum of Art in Riga

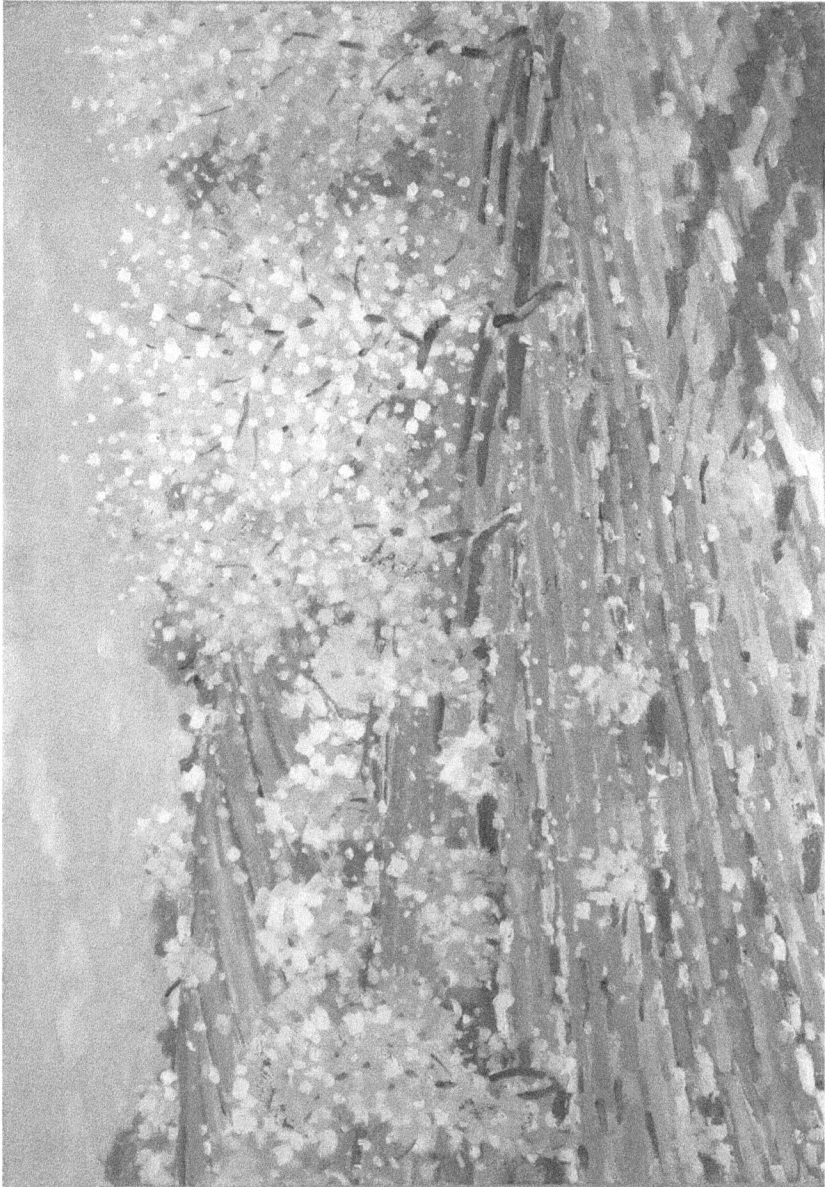

Figure 13.5: Landscape painting by Vilhelms Purvītis, Spring
Reproduced with permission of the Latvian National Museum of Art in Riga

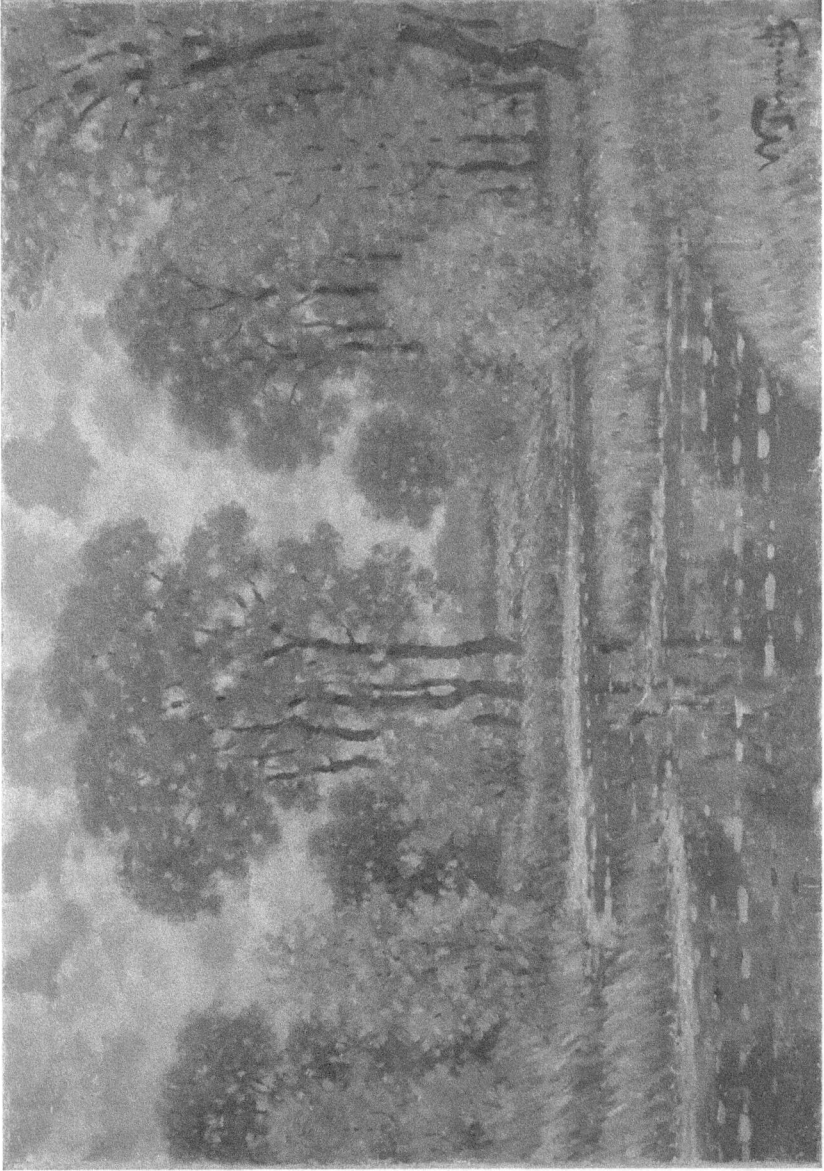

Figure 13.6: Landscape painting by Vilhelms Purvītis, Summer
Reproduced with permission of the Latvian National Museum of Art in Riga

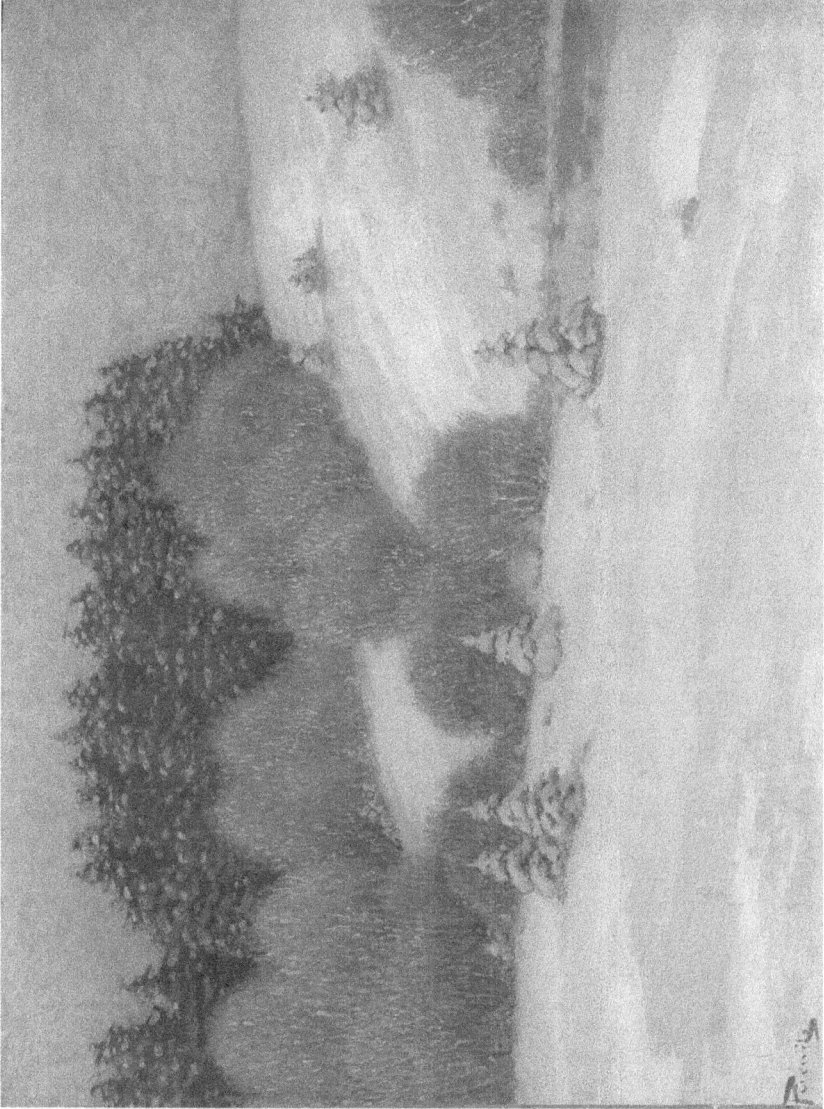

Figure 13.7: Landscape painting by Vilhelms Purvītis, Winter
Reproduced with permission of the Latvian National Museum of Art in Riga

Tucker writes: 'These paintings chart the passage of the sun across the stacks with such specificity that they collectively form a kind of chronometer' (1990: 84). Tucker argues compellingly that Monet's retreat from the city to the country was linked to the need to provide an untroubled image of national identity during a period of history when France was particularly under threat. So too Purvītis's depopulated images of the Latvian countryside served to consolidate and unify the identity of Latvia as an emerging nation.

Narrative Extracts

Most narrators take time to locate their childhood in an idyllic pastoral setting, which emphasizes solidity and permanence. Lidija insisted on recalling her childhood before she moved on to describe her many later bereavements:

> *We weren't particularly poor. My mother with a grand gesture had bought a cow. It was a brown Latvian cow. I don't quite remember but she must have been about seven years old. She was a well-built cow. She was called Laura. Nearly every household had a cow, but they were smaller, ours was built like a ship. My mother looked after her well and it was interesting that there was a shepherd's path. First came the house and then to the right of the house there was a beautiful alley of lime trees and beyond that there were more lime trees. So the landscape was very beautiful. And then there was the yard and the cellar and beyond that the shepherd's path again. And then in the mornings all the inhabitants would let their cows out onto the path. But the cows wouldn't go anywhere, they waited for Laura to appear. And then when Laura appeared, then they all fell into line with Laura at the head. Laura was the leader. It was interesting that when they returned home: Laura came first with her head in the air, she had beautiful large white horns. And she gave very good milk, quite a lot, but most important it was sweet as cream.*

The elements of this narrative – namely, trees, alleys and cream – suggest permanence, order and plenty, all things which were painfully lacking in Lidija's later life.

Trees are particularly important symbols of permanence and figure in many accounts of childhood. Orchards play an important role in Anna's recollection but are coupled with more sinister events:

> *I was born in the farmhouse that my great grandfather built more than a hundred years ago. There were large lime and apple orchards around. And my childhood came to an end there on 25 March 1949, in the morning half-light, in the dawn. On waking I saw soldiers in the room with daggers. My grandmother dressed me and then I remember that father took me in his arms and carried me out into the courtyard ... I was six. It was my seventh year. My seventh birthday took place in Siberia in the region of Tomsk.*

Childhood is associated with age and permanence in Uldis's account:

My roots the clan of Vērsis comes from the direction of Kurzeme. We come from the region of Kuldiga. For example, in Kuldiga there is a bridge built of bricks. It's one of the oldest in Europe. That was built in its time by my great grandfather – Indriķis Vērsis.

Memories of forest partisans conjure up a magical world far removed from the experience of fear, famine and cold that was the everyday reality for many. Emma spent seven years hiding in the forest with her husband. However, the very real fears of being captured are assuaged by the protective powers of the forest and its animals.

It was a terrible time, continual fear of ambush. To the animals in the forest we were one of them. Like us the stags slept during the day, but during the night they would go to a clearing or a meadow to eat. They would go past us, but when there were chekists (members of the cheka) about they would bark re, re, re. The whole forest resounded and we knew we were being surrounded. Then we had to stay put. That's how God protected us. There was a spring and I went to fetch water from there. There is a wolf sitting at the side of the path looking at me. As I go past I say quietly to him: 'Go home, little wolf, go home.' And he laid his ears back and didn't touch me. And so the animals helped us.

Perhaps the most important role of landscape is in the memories of exiles. For the inmates of prison camps conversation about the landscape of home was a gift reserved for special occasions such as birthdays and name days. Men remembered landscapes but found it more difficult to talk about them and share them with fellow prisoners. Miervaldis, imprisoned in Mordovia, in the 1950s has this to say:

We never spoke of those times when we lived well. Because we spoke about today, about what we would do because we each had our duties. Later when I was transferred to the mine, to the coal mine – then, of course, we only spoke about what had to be done and whether the plan was filled. Well, we might tell some jokes or pull each others legs. But specific memories about how things had been – that was very difficult, very painful. Of course, I thought my own thoughts. Very often I walked Riga's streets, along the boulevard beneath the lime trees. There were dreams that perhaps one day we would succeed in returning. That was the hope and you see one could only survive with that hope. The alternative was death.

Without landscapes of hope prisoners simply gave up the will to live.

Women were more ready to share pastoral memory as a means of supporting each other. This is Ilze speaking:

A close person was very important there, terribly important. To celebrate a nameday, a birthday, we spoke about our childhood. Maybe one didn't talk about one's case. But one's childhood, one's youth – one definitely described that. Because we had nothing else from the outside world. It was the only thing left – a close and sincere relationship. It was the only good thing left. Support from each other.

Such narrative extracts support Elie Wiesel's wonderful insight: 'God's punishment contains its own reward, namely, the ability to long for a paradise lost' (1996: 28).

Recollections of the return to the homeland from exile or imprisonment in Siberia are also part of a pastoral vision. The return from Siberia was associated with restrictions on where one could live, with practical problems of accommodation, access to medical treatment and schooling as well as with ostracism from cowed neighbours and relatives terrified of possible repercussions from, and their association with, the returnees. All of these problems have a place in the narrative accounts. However, they do not intrude upon the lyrical accounts of homecomings to landscapes where time has stood still. This is Andrejs's account of his return to his parents' summer house after imprisonment in Karelia.

> *I got out in Koknese station, I look, the station is bombarded, the culture building is bombarded. And quietly I go along the roads of Koknese, along by the old park. And then I entered it and saw those old alleys of trees, the old pond and then I felt that the old branches were like outstretched hands. That was exactly how I was welcomed.*

Figure 13.8 shows the landscape around Koknese with the frozen River Daugava.

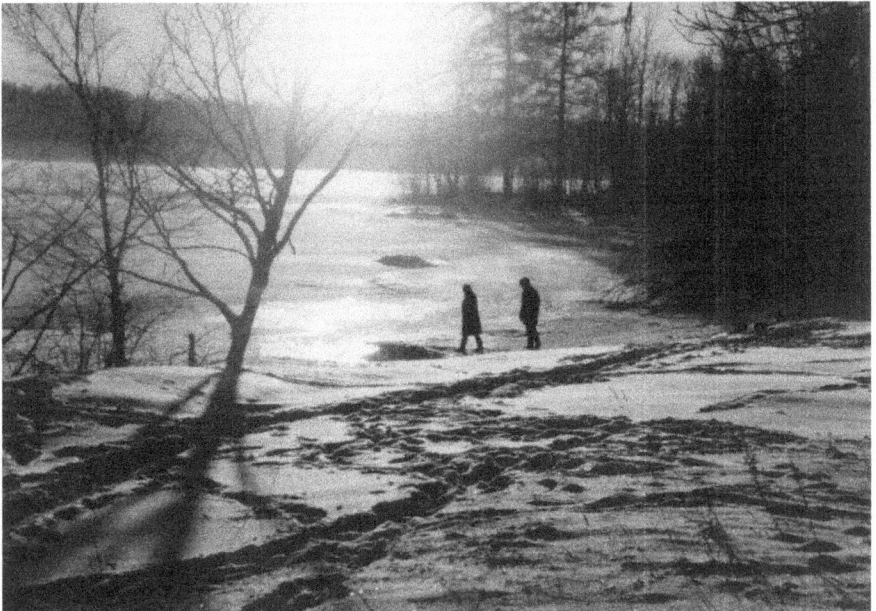

Figure 13.8: Koknese and the Frozen River Daugava

Discussion

Western literary traditions of pastoral writing incorporate a number of themes. The central thrust of pastoral is a longing for a lost innocence and happiness. Images of childhood and youth are central to this emotional constellation (Skultans 1998a; 1998b). Things natural and simple are valued above art and artifice and the country above the city. The pastoral tradition has influenced both literary and artistic conventions and feelings and attitudes of ordinary Latvians (see Alpers 1997: 13). Much of Latvian literature and art from the second half of the nineteenth century is pastoral in content and feeling and it has played a significant part in shaping Latvian notions of identity and attitudes to nature. Thus I want to argue that although the form of pastoral transcends geographical and social difference, yet its flesh has fed upon the specificities of local history and culture. The emotional power of pastoral, its seductiveness if you like, derives from its contrast with a difficult present. 'Nostalgia posits two different times, a problematical present and a past which is the object of yearning' (Bishop 1995: 57).

The intimate and cared for landscapes represented in literature and art draw their emotional power from these other darker landscapes which they overlay but which have a place in shared memory. Thus the images of pastoral landscape serve both the needs of the shared national story and the autobiography of the storyteller. Pastoral landscapes provide a balance for earlier landscapes of devastation both in historical and individual narratives. They serve to ground the life stories of those whose experiences have taken them to bleak and empty landscapes. In either case the symbols and images of pastoral evoke desire and longing which make detachment impossible (ibid.: 61). No wonder then that landscape has been described as 'the parachute cords of identity' (Schama 1995: 74).

Folk songs or *dainas* are replete with references to landscape and both are potent symbols of Latvian national identity. Oral folk poetry and song offer a distillation of shared experience drawn from many centuries when official records bore no relationship to the actual history of a subjugated peasant people. The collection of these songs played an important part in the national awakening and the formation of a shared national identity. They were at the centre of the song festivals which from 1872 onwards attracted tens of thousands of participants from different parts of Latvia. The words and tunes of these songs are familiar to all Latvians from home and from school. Indeed, it has been suggested that one such song, 'Pūt Vējiņ' or 'Blow Wind', is the true national anthem of Latvians. These songs construct a vision in which the natural, human and supernatural worlds are intertwined. Oak and lime trees symbolize men and women. The apple tree is frequently associated with orphanhood, a state which itself has come to symbolically represent the Latvian nation.

Landscape integrates a number of dualisms: it provides a common ground for symbolic and natural worlds, it draws together past and present, the individual and community, and personal biography and a common history. Meinig puts this so well when he writes: 'Any landscape is composed not only of what lies before our eyes but what lies within our heads' (1979: 33) The Soviets were well aware of the central importance of landscape for identity and took pains to destroy the sites of mythical stories and to transform the landscape of isolated farmsteads. What they failed to reach was the internalized symbolic landscape which provides an anchor for so many life stories.

The Latvian experience of landscape must keep in balance and negotiate between these dualisms of the physical and symbolic. While acknowledging the importance of metaphor I do not agree with Schama's claim: 'Landscapes are culture before they are nature; constructs of the imagination projected onto wood and water and rock. ... But ... once a certain idea of landscape, a myth, a vision, establishes itself in an actual place, it has a peculiar way of muddling categories, of making metaphors more real than their referents; of becoming, in fact, part of the scenery' (1995: 61). Landscapes are nature first and are constantly revisited to provide new metaphors. My position then is pegged out by Ricoeur's programmatic work on narrative. 'Language is not a world of its own. It is not even a world. But because we are in the world, because we are affected by situations, and because we orient ourselves comprehensively in those situations, we have something to say, we have experience to bring to language' (1976: 20–21). So too it is because we have lived in particular landscapes that we have the wherewithal to construct metaphorical landscapes which in turn colour our experience of landscape and place. Our reading of the landscape will inevitably be influenced by both the physical experience of landscape, by our particular autobiographies and the symbolic frames we have come to share in looking and talking about landscape.

According to Jackson 'Landscape represents the last and most grandiose attempt to create an earthly order in harmony with a cosmic order' (1979: 154). Images of Latvian landscape enable us to understand local conceptions of that order. These images are distillations of what is given in nature, of historical and autobiographical experience and of shared values and aspirations. In short we find: 'a translation of philosophy into tangible features' (Meinig 1979: 42) As the Latvian American geographer Bunkše (1990) demonstrates, Latvian conceptions of *glītums* or pleasantness embody, when applied to landscape, qualities valued for their contribution to Latvian ethnic identity: tenderness, industry, concern for nature.

Landscapes are storehouses of experience; they are the quintessential place. 'Its collective meanings are extractable and readable by later inhabitants. This symbolic housing of meaning and memory gives place temporal depth' (Platt 1996: 112). What we know about the past influences how we see the present.

On the other hand, landscapes are not just symbolic playgrounds. They are impregnated with the memory of historical events. In this connection the geographer Tuan quotes a conversation between the physicists Bohr and Heisenberg: 'Isn't it strange how this castle changes as soon as one imagines that Hamlet lived here? ... Suddenly the walls and the ramparts speak a different language' (1977: 4) To give a personal example, forests spoke to me in a different voice since I knew they had provided my grandfather a temporary hiding place from the KGB. So too the Latvian perception of forest and farm landscapes is changed by knowledge of what took place there.

My argument then is that accounts of a violent past involve both narrative sequence and intensely experienced descriptive passages and that we must look particularly to the descriptive passages for shared meanings. But as Mitchell reminds us 'Description threatens the function of the system by stopping to look too closely and too long at its parts' (1994: 194). If we tarry too long we can become locked in the past and bring narrative progression to a halt. Mitchell refers to ekphrastic hope as the pleasure and consolation we derive in rendering one medium in terms of another in giving a verbal description of visual objects and ekphrastic fear as the anxiety lest we are too successful in doing this and lose the original altogether. So Latvian descriptions of pastoral embody a contradiction: they hold out hope and yet they contain a fear lest the landscape will speak of the brutalities it has witnessed.

Note

1. For a historically situated discussion of Latvian art, see Mansbach (1997: 141–78).

14

ARGUING WITH THE KGB ARCHIVES: ARCHIVAL AND NARRATIVE MEMORY IN POST-SOVIET LATVIA

The history of the Baltic states since the Second World War, their violent Soviet annexation, the extent of political dissent and the more recent ambiguities in government attitudes towards the Soviet past all serve to underline the importance of an anthropology which recognizes the creative and dissenting power of the self. This chapter will argue that the possibility of political dissent, both as expressed in action and in narrative, as well as our understanding of it, hinge upon the restitution of an enlarged and to some extent autonomous self. The opening of the KGB archives in Riga, the accessibility of hitherto closed files and their critical reading by my informants call for a re-evaluation of the moral status of voice and self within anthropology.

The interpretation of my field material draws upon the argument that the neglect of the self has been closely linked to the neglect of 'empirical studies of moralities' (Howell 1997: 8). In the drive to theorize the otherness of customs, traditions and values, questions of individual moral dilemma, choice and commitment have been neglected. Anthropologists have tended to see their informants as vehicles of social values rather than as moral agents in their own right. Conceptualizations of the relationship between individual and society must have enough depth to be able to encompass situations of political dissent, where the source of moral judgment lies not within society but within the individual. The Latvian situation offers examples of experience *in extremis* but also represents crucial potentialities of all human identity and experience.

Anthony Cohen has argued extensively against the neglect of the self by anthropologists: 'Anthropologists did not attribute any importance to the problem of what these structures actually meant to those who populated them. In this kind of theoretical scheme, people, individuals, were important only as structures in themselves, or as related to structure in some identifiable way' (1994: 14). By contrast, Cohen argues that individuals construct their relationship to society on their own terms. 'Self-consciousness ... provides a means through which individuals construct the terms of their membership, establish the meanings of selfhood and society to them, and rehearse their rights to their selves' (ibid.: 79). The self is not socially constructed but holds in balance and takes up a moral position towards the various social identities available to it. The self judges the identities available to it, discarding some and investing others with moral significance. Cohen refers to the Mbuti, for whom the integrity of society depends upon the integrity of the self (ibid.: 33), but clearly this understanding of the relationship between self and society has wider application. My Latvian informants insisted upon their own integrity in the face of an unjust and dishonest society.

The self is closely linked to the idea of agency. My own view builds upon Taylor (1985) and Frankfurt (1988) and sees the essence of agency as lying in wanting to be particular kinds of people even when this leads to disagreement and social exclusion. Taylor argues that there are two senses of agency: according to the first sense, agency concerns the ability to put a lifeplan into action; it concerns strategic power. But according to a second sense agency concerns meaning and value. 'Agents are beings for whom things matter, who are subjects of significance' (1985: 104). This second sense is by far the more important in that it identifies what it is to be human. Latvian narratives suggest that things matter most precisely where the execution of life plans is most restricted. In contesting the reliability of the KGB files, narrators assert the importance of their lived experience and reclaim their identity as agents. This view of agency runs counter to that of Giddens who proposes a different model: 'Agency refers not to the intentions people have in doing things but to their capability of doing those things in the first place' (1984: 9). Commenting on this, Cohen observes that individuals 'seem doomed to be perpetrators rather than architects of action' (1994: 21).

My interest in the anthropology of self has been aroused through the narrated life stories I collected between 1993 and 1994 (see Chapters 7, 8, 10 and 11 this volume, and Skultans 1997, 1998a). My initial interest was in neurasthenia, a nineteenth-century diagnosis, which had exceeded its medical shelf life in the West. As Wessely argues it 'disappeared because it [has] ceased to be useful to the doctor' (1994b: 195). Neurasthenia was, however, welcomed by the countries of the Soviet Union and communist China, where it was given an extended lease of life and a new identity. No longer characterized exclusively by exhaustion, it came instead to be associated with heightened anxiety and sensitivity. If, as Kirmayer suggests, neurasthenia is, indeed, 'a commentary on the vicissitudes of modern life' (1994: 100), then it can also serve to distinguish between those vicissitudes in different societies. While in Western society neurasthenia came to be seen as a consequence of the speed and relentless routines of life, the lay interpretation of neurasthenia in Soviet society linked neurasthenia with the unpredictability and lack of control over one's life course; in short, the powerlessness of the individual against the state. So while my original aim had been to explore medical and lay understandings of neurasthenia, my informants took charge of the project and redirected my attention to what they thought was important, namely, life testimonies.

These stories seemed both to belong to people in a special way and at the same time to have a place within a broader historical narrative. They compel the listener or reader to enter the world they describe. My passionate involvement with these stories has been attributed to my Latvian origins. I was born in Riga, left as a refugee aged six months but was brought up speaking and reading Latvian. I am a 'halfie', to borrow Abu-Lughod's (1991:140) apt description of a woman belonging to two cultures. This hybrid status encourages the recognition of others as equals rather than simply as exemplars of their culture. Because certain cultural assumptions are shared and familiar, attention is focused on difference rather than similarity. I do not, however, see identification as simply about shared cultural origins. Rather, my long-standing respect for the particularity of stories derives from the recognition that in an important sense these texts embody the selves of others (Skultans 1974). My informants' sense of themselves depended upon these retrospective quarrels with the files. Rorty, following Nietzsche, claims that to accept another's version of oneself and one's life is to fail as a human being (1989: 28). Contesting KGB accounts, no matter how formulaic and repetitive they may be, is important. Authoring one's own life and thereby laying out what one cares about, what should matter in human life, acquires great urgency in this context. It represents the only kind of power we have in life. Rorty puts it thus: 'The final victory of poetry in its ancient quarrel with philosophy – the final victory of metaphors of self-creation over metaphors of discovery – would consist in our becoming reconciled to the thought that this is the only sort of power over the world which we can hope to have' (ibid.: 40). This may be true for all of us but it is particularly true for those deprived of liberty in is most basic sense.

Language and the State Archives

The opening of the state archives in 1997 gave me the opportunity of matching oral testimonials with the archival records. However, while the original reference of these stories was to relatively undocumented episodes in the history of Soviet Latvia, their telling and retelling drew attention to language itself and the contrasting uses to which it was put. Through the strange hermeneutic exercise of scanning their old files, radically different uses of language emerged juxtaposed in the act of reading and questioning the text. The fundamental difference between the language of the archive and my informants' language lies, I suggest, in their purpose and allegiance. The allegiance of the language recorded in the archive is to social structures and institutions; that of my informants is to preserving a sense of moral and personal integrity. The language of the archive is characterized by its formality and concern with consistency. On the other hand, the language of my informants is concerned with the relationship between words and experience and the right that that experience gives them to make moral judgements. In the meeting between texts written some fifty years ago and their present-day readers new and unanticipated meanings emerge. The encounter with the files highlights the difference between institutional and personal uses of language. It also makes room for the personal creativity which, Rapport argues, has been submerged and 'drowned out by the rigours of social structure' (1997: 41). Moral outrage is reignited through the encounters with the KGB files.

In Bakhtin's important sense, the KGB files are monologues, since they involve 'a denial of the equal rights of consciousness vis-à-vis truth' (1984: 285). The Czech linguist Mukarovsky characterizes monologue and dialogue in terms of activity and passivity (1977: 96). In monologue, only one participant is active. This certainly applies to the written records of the KGB interrogations where the interrogator exercises total control over both the questions and the answers. In dialogue, on the other hand, the two parties to the conversation take turns in being active and passive. Each allows their utterance to be penetrated by the other. Many of my informants had been subjected to some hundred or more hours of monologue. But the desire to prise the monologue open and transform it into a dialogue had not disappeared. Perhaps the constant stream of people intently perusing their files in the state archive are there because, after all, 'To be means to communicate ... To be means to be for another, and through the other for oneself' (Bakhtin 1984: 287). Without acknowledgement from another the sense of self becomes precarious – hence the unremitting need to reopen the dialogue.

Velody has written of the 'privileged topology or siting' of archival documents (1998: 2). Often archives are housed in important buildings in city centres. By contrast, Latvia's state archive was found in an unprepossessing building in a dilapidated inner suburb of Riga called – appropriately enough – the Moscow suburb.[1] Unlike the Stasi archives which employ more than three thousand staff, the Riga state archive employs only a handful of individuals. This marginal location reflects the uncertain status of these records. Certainly there are resonances with Echevarria's discussion of the etymology of the term 'archive' and its connection with the arcane: 'So archive suggests not only that something is kept, but that which is secret, encrypted, enclosed' (1990: 32). And later he writes: 'Archives keep the secrets of the state' (ibid.: 33). The ambivalent status of the archive, as both containing and creating knowledge, is also remarked upon by Borneman (1997: 76).

Spurred on by curiosity and the importance of reported dialogue and represented speech in the life stories of my narrators, I spent some twelve weeks during the summer of 1999 reading the files of my earlier informants whose life stories I had recorded in 1993 and later invited them to join me in re-reading their files. Altogether we worked on the files of some twenty informants. The files were handwritten in blue or black ink, and sometimes in pencil, by several hands. Some ran to ten or more volumes, each some 200 pages long. Any person who had been arrested, imprisoned or deported would have a file. The daily newspaper *Diena* estimates that the secret police held files on some 80,000 Latvian citizens (Upleja and Titavs 1998).

The files are meticulously written and logically sequenced. The interrogation protocols give us the answers of the accused as faithful echoes of the questions. The form and vocabulary provided by the question shapes the answers given. For example, Emma Priedīte is asked: 'When did you join the bandits' group and which group was it?' Her answer comes back like an echo: ' I joined the bandits' group in March 1948'. But in our joint perusal of the file Emma adds: 'They write just the way they want. You could confess or not confess, they wrote just what they wanted.' The precision and rigidity squeeze out meaning. Anita Siliņa's file has the question: 'Tell me about your father's and mother's *kulak* (rich peasant) descent'. Her reply follows the shape of the question: 'My father and mother were descended from *kulaks*.' And later there is the question: 'How many workers did your *kulak* farmstead exploit?' Again, the reply is simply an inversion of the question. 'Our *kulak* farmstead exploited three seasonal workers.' Anita's later response sums up her scorn for such versions of the interrogation process: 'And look at all these declarations and interrogations of former neighbours – you can see from the text that they're all written to a standard pattern, invariably the same questions. In my view they're meaningless'. The coherence of these files is over-determined and self-validating and if evidence is needed against the coherence theory of truth then it can surely be found here.

Havel's play *The Memorandum* (1980) demonstrates the absurdity of precisely this kind of official, over-determined self-referential language that bears no relationship to experience. All my informants challenged and contradicted the files in numerous ways. For example, Emma is alleged to have supplied the group of bandits with food and brandy. Her reaction on reading this is: 'That's sheer madness! Where would I get any food? I didn't even have anything to eat myself'. She was also accused of writing anti-Soviet leaflets on a typewriter. Her response to this is: 'Rubbish! No one in our group had a typewriter while I was there. We didn't have a typewriter'. She summarizes her feelings by saying: 'They wrote just what they wanted. They made it all up'. And on seeing me writing she exclaims: 'Good God! You're not going to write all that nonsense down, are you'. Lienīte has this to say about her interrogation by the KGB: 'But then I understood that I couldn't trust anyone or believe a single word. If they say there is no tape-recorder then one is certainly being taped. In my father's time there certainly weren't any such tapes. Millions of people were interrogated but I don't think they were taped. Interrogations were written down. They wrote to incriminate them, to be able to sentence them. The most important thing was to find new names, new surnames. They asked people to mention names simply so that the register would grow.'

Although many pages are taken up with the interrogations, the files contain no dialogue. They are monologic. It is this complete absence of dialogue that makes them so extremely oppressive and ultimately I felt corrupted by them. These files are about the politics of quotation: how much of the original meaning is preserved when it is re-sited among the words of others. For example, Ieva recollects talking about her time as a girl-guide during the interrogation. 'Yes, guides. I said I was a member because they had the photographs. He asks what sort of an organization it is. I said it was a youth organization, an international organization, I said it was founded by the Englishman Baden-Powell, wasn't it? And it encouraged kindness towards old people and a respectful attitude towards nature. We went on excursions, and also of course a kind of patriotism but that doesn't appear anywhere.' The archive translates her words into a language that suits its own purposes: 'At the time I was living in bourgeois Latvia and I was a member of two bourgeois nationalist youth organizations'. The file refers to the girl-guide groups as 'cells', thereby attributing them with revolutionary intent. In another context, Mishler describes the way in which doctors maintain control and continuity of discourse by relocating the patients' talk to a different semantic world: 'The symptom is thus transformed by being relocated to a different province of meaning' (1984: 123). Just as the KGB interrogators extract statements and reposition them within their own orders of meaning, so too do the informants extract ironic meaning from the files by repositioning and playing with the words of the KGB officers. Ieva asks me: 'Well, I ask you, would an imprisoned person add bourgeois nationalist at the end of every sentence? Not on your life!' She takes issue with the use of the term cell. 'Well, forgive me, but I would never let such a word as cell pass my lips.' There is almost a physical repugnance against taking the words of the KGB formulaic texts into one's mouth. Reading the file on her father, Lienīte Sestule says of a fellow partisan: 'Here he is called a bandit, but my tongue doesn't want to pronounce the word bandit'. Referring later to her father's statements she says: 'Here they're referred to as bandits, but I doubt whether father called them bandits, he would have called them forest brothers.'

The recorded interrogations of Miervaldis Ozoliņš deal with his possession and circulation of volumes of 'bourgeois literature'. Among the books in his possession was a book of Rilke's poetry. Miervaldis recalls the following interchange in which the interrogator's unfamiliarity with literature transforms the name of the metaphysical poet into *rīkle*, the Latvian word for throat: 'And I remember that at one reading we read and discussed the poems of the German poet Rainer Maria Rilke. And the interrogator said, "Who is this German poet Rikle?"' The interrogator's mistake is recalled and the error in syntagmatic sequencing is put to metaphorical use: it provides such an apt image of the way in which the ideals of Miervaldis and his literary friends were transformed into fodder for the *cheka* (state secret police) and swallowed up. This entire narrative episode makes fun of the *cheka*'s misguided pursuit of verbal metonymic. In making fun of the interrogator's ignorance Miervaldis is following a revolutionary tradition. In Arendt's words: 'The greatest enemy of authority, therefore, is contempt, and the surest way to undermine it is laughter' (1970: 45).

The Russian historian Kozlov, writing about the handling of denunciations in Soviet Russia, emphasizes the almost ritualistic role of language: 'The NKVD[2] authorities used a special bureaucratic lexicon when submitting documents for investigation, as if to "program" into the investigating office a certain attitude towards the facts' (1996: 890). This lexicon was all about binding the writer and reader together. He describes the denunciations as 'trying to activate in the consciousness of the reader a whole system of symbols that reflected the basic ideological and political preferences of the government ... The use of applicable ideological codes was supposed to set up a special almost intimate relationship between the informer or denouncer and the regime and to indicate that the author was deserving of special trust' (ibid.: 883).

The KGB files in Riga exemplify this; they are constructed around a restricted and highly repetitive lexicon. But while the denouncers referred to by Kozlov were writing for the KGB officers, it is not at all clear for whom the files in Riga were written. Clearly not the accused narrators, who were not allowed access to them, nor of course for me or any other researcher. Fitzpatrick (1996: 866) has written that denunciation was one of the few ways in which agency could be exercised in authoritarian societies. But although agency was clearly restricted in Soviet Latvia, denunciation does not appear to have been common. Certainly, I found no letters of denunciation in the files I looked at, even though the interrogators repeatedly invited verbal denunciations. For example, Aija Jundze's father was asked many times who attended his church services and in whose houses his prayer meetings were held, but he refused to offer any information.

The Interrogation Protocol

The files record the times of the interrogations and the names of the interrogators who took turns to question. On average interrogations lasted some five or six hours. Each interrogation protocol is signed by the accused as being a true version of events. But signatures were often extracted under duress and the accused were often asked to put their signature to writing they could not understand. Elza Glaudāne recalls being interrogated through an interpreter. 'There was an interpreter and usually the interpreter sat by my side. And he just wrote and wrote. And then I asked him what he was writing at such length and he said, "The Russian language is very rich. There's not so much to say in Latvian." And then I just had to sign, to give my signature'. Emma Priedīte also spoke of the meaninglessness of the signature: 'It's all nonsense. A lot of nonsense that they write there – they give the answers they need. Some of the questions haven't even been asked. And the replies certainly weren't like that. They just want a particular reply and in the end they say sign.' Looking at her father's file, Lienīte doubts whether her father actually signed his name: 'Maybe it is my father's signature, this is my father's signature, but this isn't, this definitely isn't my father's signature.'

Although the written versions of these interrogations run to a hundred or so pages, they are extremely abbreviated versions of the oral exchanges. Since the starting and finishing times of interrogations are given, I could work out that one handwritten page represents about an hour of interrogation. However, although the interrogators are named, the actual authors of the files, the scribes if you like, are not identified. If there is no author there is no one to argue with. So these are strange documents with no authors and no addressee specified. Sessions vary in length, a short session lasting some two to three hours and the longest recorded fourteen hours. Looking at her father's transcript of six hours of interrogation Aija Jundze had this to say: 'But it's a wonder that they wrote that [the time] down. Usually they didn't write it down. [Aija is wrong in this instance.] Look, here's another session ending at 12.30 a.m. I think they wrote the time down because the interrogators were paid extra for overtime.' Later she adds: 'It seems as though that man enjoyed writing.' However, by and large the transcripts tended to underestimate the length of the interrogations. For example, Elza's interrogations appeared to last about two hours according to her files but this is what she has to say: 'I was called out repeatedly. I was a whole year in the cellars of the *cheka*, a whole year, and they were always calling me for interrogation. It wasn't just for a few hours. They called me every day for hours on end.'

Whatever the precise length of the interrogation, the subjective experience was of never-ending questioning, as Elza Glaudāne recounts: 'Particularly at the beginning, it wasn't a question of every few days. We were called out every day.' Antonija describes the effects of this continual interrogation: 'We couldn't get any sleep. We were completely crazy, as if sleepwalking. In my case it was like this: I didn't listen to what he said because I didn't understand Russian. The interpreter would still be reading out the protocol and I was ready to sign my name. I was just glad to be able to get away.' And yet the written text is presented as a verbatim record of what took place with a series of questions and answers. Each session concludes with the statement 'The interrogation protocol has been read out to me and what I have said has been correctly recorded' and nearly always bears the signature of the accused, one interrogator and, in cases where the accused could not speak Russian, of a KGB interpreter. We do not have any grounds to assume that all KGB employees involved in the interrogation signed the protocol.

The interrogation protocol provides a lens whereby all events and experiences are reduced to a narrow lexical and semantic band. The vocabulary – consisting of a small set of terms such as 'nationalistic', 'chauvinistic', 'bourgeois', 'reactionary', 'anti-Soviet', 'ideologically harmful', 'oriented towards the west', 'hostile towards Soviet power' and 'anti-Soviet activity' – find infinite applications. Indeed, it is the absurdity of the supposedly coherent that calls for a retrospective dismantling. As political rhetoric increases, so the factual content or the power to connect with the world, decreases, as Bloch (1975) has argued. Small wonder that the need to challenge the files continues to be so important. Certainly, the files bear no relation to the way informants recollect their experience.

The need for dialogue does not disappear, however, which is how I am drawn in. My narrators prefaced their responses with questions such as 'well I ask you' (*nu es tev prasu*) or 'you tell me' (*nu saki man*):

> *Well you tell me: at that time would I have said that I lived in bourgeois Latvia, that I was a member of two bourgeois nationalist youth organizations? That's been added on, the bourgeois nationalist, so that we could be blamed don't you see? To make it seem that I'd said it myself.*

The divergence between social and political categorizations of the person and the individual's own view of what has happened and what should have happened is acutely evident in Anita Siliņa's encounter with her mother Emīlija's file. Anita is simultaneously reading and translating from her mother's file:

> *On 1st March 1949 there is a statement made by Senior Lieutenant Skripov: he has examined the case of the kulak family, of Emīlija Berķe, daughter of Janis and has found that they correspond – how shall I put this – the Latvian Soviet*

ministry has found ... Well, this family corresponds. Let's say that this family falls within the category that has to be driven outside Latvian territory.

However, Anita's mother was a servant and her parents landless, and she remained convinced that she had been wrongly categorized. Anita reads out her mother's letter asking that she be repatriated:

On 25th March 1949, I, Emīlija Berke, daughter of Jānis born Emīlija Rage on 28th April 1914 in the Valka region, in the parish of Ēvele of a working-class family was arrested together with my little girl, Anita, born 8th January 1945 , and deported to Siberia. I do not understand and neither was it explained to me why I was deported, because my parents, my father and mother, worked all their lives as servants, and I too started to work for kulaks from the age of ten. Only after the consolidation of Soviet power was I granted 15 hectares of land in the parish of Ēvele which I cultivated until the time of my deportation. I have never been a member of any political or military organizations, neither during the German occupation nor the Latvian period, and I have never worked against the Soviet state. My brother Jūlijs, son of Jānis, who worked in the dairy in Ēvele, was called to fight in the great patriotic war, and died for the fatherland in 1945. Taking the above-mentioned into account I contend that I was wrongly deported and I am turning to you as minister of home affairs in Latvia to plead for your protection so that my daughter and I be taken off the register and be allowed to return to Latvia.

Anita's reflections on her mother's and her own early experiences challenge official categorizations. She muses on whether the fact of having been born out of wedlock has any bearing on the turn of events:

I think there were very many people like my mother and I who were unjustly and pointlessly treated. Because looking at these chapters I too do not understand why my mother and I were deported, because she was a servant. And if she gave birth to a daughter outside wedlock should that be punished? I don't understand – a woman has given birth and not given up her baby. After all, she brought me up. So I really don't know whether that is the greatest sin. My mother didn't deny that she was a servant and my mother told me that I was born outside marriage. I didn't learn anything new from the files, I didn't make any discoveries, absolutely not. The only thing I learnt was that these people who wrote all this are totally indifferent to who one is or isn't and that they were totally clueless about all the family ties.

All my narrators complained of the extreme indifference of interrogators to individuality and feeling. Perhaps this added to the heightened emotional tone of the encounters with the files both for the narrators and for myself. These stories demand identification and active participation and make distancing difficult. My narrators' accounts raise questions about Ricoeur's theory of distanciation as central to narrative discourse, each taking the narrative further away from the experience (1976). The meaning of what is said about an event leaves the event behind. The meaning of the text surpasses the intended meaning of the speaker. The text breaks free of its social and historical context. And finally the text ceases to be concerned with reference (see Thompson 1984: 179). Judged alongside Ricoeur's characterization of narrative, these extracts demonstrate their allegiance to a very different genre of testimonial discourse and one that precludes distanciation.

Let me give an illustration. This is an extract of an interview with Mudra, a sixty-year-old woman. She is in fact the daughter of one of my earlier narrators, Malvīna, who died in January 1999. Malvīna was accused of giving shelter and food to her brothers who were forest partisans. She was sentenced to five years' prison camp, leaving behind three young children including Mudra, then aged six. Here we are slowly reading her mother's file together:

> *400 kilograms of rye*
> *400 kilograms of barley*
> *350 kilograms of oats*
> *90 kilograms of summer wheat*
> *500 kilograms of potatoes*
> *'A lot,' I say.*
> *'A lot,' she agrees.*
> *'A lot, plenty,' I repeat.*
> *She replies, 'Well, there was everything. The house was full. But when father returned [from prison camp in Siberia] there was nothing. The house was empty.'*

The rest of this narrative is accompanied by tears and sobbing. Mudra goes on to describe the famine they experienced as children. The only thing they ate for months were the boiled ears of corn. But what upset her most was the fear that she might need to defecate at school and the possibility that other children might see what she had eaten.

But what meaning does this transcribed KGB text retain if it is indeed distanciated in the several ways Ricoeur suggests? Severed from our subsequent dialogue and the events of expropriation and family rupture which in turn resulted in motherless children and famine, the text is reduced to a meaningless inventory. The participants in the dialogue – Mudra and myself – seek to share the experience. Mudra chose to tell me about her shame at school and I chose to select that part of the dialogue for this chapter. The text only makes sense as one individual's experience of a particular episode of Soviet history. Historically decontextualized it becomes meaningless. And the ostensive reference of this text, namely the KGB file and its reading, contribute to a more complete understanding of this dialogue. Throughout these readings of the files there is a contestation of archival truth and a polarity between the authority of the state and individual experience which belies Hann's claim that:

> The assumption of an overriding antagonism between state and society is futile. If these terms can serve at all, their task must be to investigate their complex and continuous interactions. This certainly should not be restricted to the mapping of political opposition to authoritarian regimes. Radical opposition to socialism

was restricted to small, politically conscious fragments of populations, and it should also be remembered that many of those who struggled to change communist systems did so from space they managed to create within the state including its large education and research establishments (1996: 9).

This characterization of the restricted nature of political opposition certainly does not apply to Latvia, and few of my informants could be described as belonging to an intellectual elite.

From Personal Misfortune to Social Injustice

A major focus of anthropological interest in Eastern Europe has been on the way in which post-Soviet societies reckon with the past. Much of this work has been concerned with macro social and political structures. Borneman (1997), for example, has examined the important role of accountability, retribution and restitution for the establishment of civil society. He describes the way in which the Stasi archives are used to transform individual narratives of misfortune into public narratives of injustice. The archives are consulted to confirm transgressions against the individual. Borneman writes: 'Without reliable corroborative evidence ... the experience of the victim remains merely a misfortune and not an injustice' (ibid.: 72). The implication is that, whereas individuals experience suffering, the moral evaluation of this suffering comes from society. My purpose in this chapter has been to concentrate on the claims to moral authority of individual voices in a context where legal processes for establishing accountability are unevenly developed. The process of finding objective corroborative evidence of unjust imprisonment and exile is fraught with difficulty in Latvia, just as it is in former East Germany, as Borneman recognizes: 'If the GDR was an Unrechtstaat (an illegal state), as many claim, a criminal band unconcerned with truth or justice, then its own data banks and archives are of questionable reliability' (ibid.: 72). Accountability must, Borneman argues, rest upon the rule of law and Borneman draws heavily upon the writing of Lon Fuller (1969) – principally the idea of the 'inner morality of law' – to make his case. Havel makes the same point when he asks 'whether an appeal to legality makes any sense at all when the laws – and particularly the general laws concerning human rights – are no more than a façade, an aspect of the world of appearances, a mere game behind which lies total manipulation' (1986: 93–4). My intent in this chapter is not to deny the contribution of the law in recognizing injustice, demanding retribution and bringing about accountability. However, my focus is on personal narratives as the place where ideas of moral right and wrong are developed and nurtured. In the absence of archival reliability it is even more important for anthropology to recognize the individual as a locus of moral judgement and authority.

Latvia, like the other two Baltic states, has instigated extensive procedures of retributive justice. With the declaration of independence in 1991, a legal commission was set up to deal with the issue of *reabilitācija* or the identification of miscarriages of justice. Anyone who considered that they had been unjustly imprisoned or deported during the Soviet rule could apply to be rehabilitated. Altogether some 40,000 people have been rehabilitated since 1991. Rehabilitation involves the public admission that the person has been wrongly punished. All those deported or imprisoned in March 1949 as part of the drive to collectivize farming have been rehabilitated as a matter of course. Others arrested during 1940, the first year of Soviet occupation, whose alleged crimes related to their position in society – i.e. bourgeois, capitalist, plutocrat – have also been rehabilitated. Soldiers conscripted into the fifteenth and nineteenth Latvian divisions of the German army have been rehabilitated. Those suspected of being involved in the killing of the Jews have not been rehabilitated. Of those requesting rehabilitation 95 per cent have been granted it. Apart from the important fact of restoring personal dignity, rehabilitation carries with it a not insignificant package of material benefits that include: the restoration of appropriated property; the issue of two government certificates per year of deportation or imprisonment which can be used in lieu of cash to acquire property or land; cheaper or free transport; reduced prices for medicine; and an earlier retirement age of fifty-five.

However, while the government has been active in the legal restitution of individuals, very few of the perpetrators of these crimes have been brought to justice. Only three KGB agents have been tried. One reason for this is that during the break-up of the Soviet Union a large number of the most important and incriminating files were taken to Moscow, thus removing evidence and making the prosecution of KGB agents difficult. However, another reason is the extensive earlier involvement of government ministers with the KGB. Although the extent of KGB activity in Latvia did not reach the scope of Stasi activity in East Germany, where Childs (1998: 94) suggests that there was one full-time operative per 165 inhabitants, it was nevertheless considerable. The daily newspaper *Diena* suggests that there were some 4,800 security agents active in 1991, yielding a comparable figure of one agent per 520 inhabitants. Few workplaces were without a KGB agent. Politically sensitive institutions such as universities were put under special surveillance (Zālīte 2000). In the context of fifty years of Soviet rule it is difficult to place people in discrete, mutually exclusive categories of those for and against the political system. Havel puts it thus: 'for everyone in his or her own way is both a victim and a supporter of the system' (1987: 53). He also remarks that 'society is not sharply polarised on the level of actual political power, but as we have seen, the fundamental lines of conflict run right through each person' (ibid.: 91).

So while it is true that Latvia, along with the other two Baltic states, has 'engaged in substantial retributive justice' (Borneman 1997: 10), retributive justice has been somewhat one-sided in its exclusive focus on the victim and not the perpetrator of the crime. While the government has sought to make extensive reparation to the victims of violence, the perpetrators of these crimes have not been brought to justice. According to Borneman's definition of democratic states, one of the elements is in place but two are missing. Borneman's argument is that accountability is central to democracy. This accountability involves not only reparation for victims, but the punishment of wrong-doers and the re-evaluation of unjust laws and government policies. Without these processes of accountability, Borneman predicts repeated cycles of violence (ibid.: 144–45). According to these criteria, Latvia is an imperfect democracy, since the triangle of crime, victim and criminal is missing two of its corners. These missing links, I would argue, heighten the imperative need felt by former victims for a continuing dialogue with the past and a personal voice which speaks of things as they really were.

A paradoxical outcome of these legal anomalies is that dissidents have been rehabilitated although the government position is that they were imprisoned under a just law (Titavs 1998). We have victims without crimes or perpetrators of those crimes. Torpey describes a similar conundrum in East Germany: 'The discussion turned on the division between the proponents of the legal positivist view, which privileges the principle *nulla poena, nullum crimen sine lege* (no punishment, no crime without a law) enshrined in article 103 of the Federal Republic's Basic Law, and those who argue for the natural law notion that prosecution could proceed on the basis of a "higher law"' (1998: 197). In *Beyond Justice*, Heller writes of criminal law: 'The sense of justice demands that the legal system of the absolute tyrant should be disobeyed. Morality and legality are not in contradiction here (as sometimes happens when the legal system is unjust but not evil), for in the criminal legal system there is no law, only the semblance of law' (1987: 179). The legal commission set up to deal with these issues has drawn a distinction between those inhabitants who were exiled and imprisoned without trial in the post-war years and later arrests and imprisonments that were carried out under the rubric of the criminal law. In practice, however, the distinction is an academic one since only a tiny handful of state security officials have been tried.

The Testimonial Pact

The contradictions that surround attitudes to rehabilitation and retribution in Latvia have implications for my informants' continuing conversations with the past. The absence of a consistent government policy to past injustices fuels the need to revive and reframe the verbal exchanges with their interrogators. I have already written of the subversion of my original research plans by my informants (Skultans 1998a). It is, of course, not at all unusual for the focus of anthropological research to change during the course of fieldwork, but in this case there was a real sense in which my informants took charge. There was an implicit expectation that I would endeavour to disseminate these testimonial narratives as widely as possible. Informants insisted that their narratives should not be made anonymous. Their unhesitating acceptance of me derived, I think, from an assumption that we belonged to a community whose members might have diverse histories yet shared a common destiny.

Closer attention to the nature of testimony illuminates the inevitability of fieldwork developments. Latvian narratives share the essential characteristics of testimony, which is defined as:

> an authentic narrative, told by a witness who is moved to narrate by the urgency of a situation (e.g. war, oppression, revolution, etc.). Emphasizing popular oral discourse, the witness portrays his or her own experience as an agent (rather than a representative) of a collective memory and identity. Truth is summoned in the cause of denouncing a present situation of exploitation and oppression or in exorcising and setting aright official history (Yudice 1996: 44).

Furthermore, testimonial is grounded in experience and concerned above all with referential truth: 'perhaps more than any other genre in the past, [it] has foregrounded the issue of what is real and has been defined ... as a trace of the real' (Gugelberger 1996: 5).

Because testimony by its very nature makes claims to truth through experience, it demands an active involvement on the part of the listener/interviewer, it depends on the interviewer identifying with the speaker's community and sharing their moral position.

> Unlike the private and even lonely moment of autobiographical writing, testimonies are public events. [They address] a flesh-and-blood person, the interviewer who asks questions and avidly records answers. The narrative, therefore, sometimes shifts into the second person. The interlocutor and by extension each reader is addressed by the narrator's appeal to 'you' ... When the narrator talks about herself to you, she implies both the existing relationship to other representative selves in the community and the potential relationships that extend her community through the text. She calls us in, interpellates us as readers who identify with the narrator's project and, by extension with the political community to which she belongs ... Rather the testimonial produces complicity. Precisely because the reader cannot identify with the writer enough to imagine taking her place, the map of possible identifications through the text spreads out laterally. Once the subject of testimonial is understood as the community made up of a variety of roles, the reader is called in to fill one of them (Sommer 1996: 152).

I was drawn into the testimonial narratives in precisely this way. Rather than an intense and intimate identification with the narrator of an autobiography, I was drawn into a moral landscape where, as the testimony unfolded, my identifications moved between the speaker and her mother, father and others who peopled these narratives. I use the term moral landscape advisedly because the entire story serves to establish a moral point. A single event, such as an arrest, has a ripple effect that affects a whole life. And the course of one person's life is linked to many others and repeated many times over. Sommer uses the word complicity, which, of course, suggests the illicit. Certainly, life histories were told in opposition to earlier official versions of Soviet history at a time when it had become possible to give one's own account. And yet these testimonies of suffering were not encouraged. A 1999 article in *Diena* was entitled 'The West Does Not Want To See Our Tears', and argued that dwelling on the sufferings of the past would make acceptance within the European Union more difficult. A new kind of forward-looking identity which focused on economic progress and consumer sophistication was called for. However, Borneman warns against ignoring 'the trope of suffering' if stable democracy is to be achieved; personal suffering must be transformed into social injustice. It is against this background that my relationship with my informants has to be viewed. I was linked to them not so much in complicity but through an implicit authorial pact in which the narrators entrusted me to co-author and disseminate their testimonials. Their preoccupation with things as they really were, with the contestation of official history, were concerns which, as the recipient of their testimonials, I was expected to share. The opening of the state archives simply provided an opportunity for expanding the earlier testimonies.

Voice and the Poetics of the Self

Experience, self and personal voice are central to the testimonial use of language, but have no place in other dominant theories of language. Austin's *How to do Things with Words* (1962) provided a landmark in the shift away from the representational functions of language to its persuasive and performative functions. His discussions of the illocutionary function of language, its power to bring about a certain state of affairs, has directed attention to the institutional frameworks and power structures that underpin language and make illocutionary acts possible. This shift in the focus of attention has been registered by the introduction of a new term, discourse, that recognizes the interpenetration of linguistic and power structures. Discourse promotes an indexical view of linguistic power: namely, the recognition that official languages by definition have greater authority and, therefore, greater powers to denote. Havel puts this well:

'The principle involved here is that the centre of power is identical with the centre of truth' (1986: 36). It is argued that linguistic competence and power do not simply relate to a command of language but a command over one's audience. This linguistic authority relates to institutional position. Thus language always uses borrowed authority: 'authority comes to language from outside' (Bourdieu 1991: 109).

Whilst there is an obvious sense in which these Latvian narratives are framed by the collapse of communism and could not have been voiced during the Soviet period, their meaning is not exhausted by the frame. The collapse of the Soviet Union may be a necessary, but not a sufficient, condition of their production. The delegated view of linguistic power fails to recognize individuals as moral selves on a par with the anthropologist. The indexical view of language recognizes the social persona but not the individual who stands back from society and reflects upon it. Indeed, we could argue that the tighter the institutional control and bureaucratization of language, the less meaningful it becomes.

Ieva's file refers to her diary which contained anti-Soviet writing and poetry. This is how she responds to her file entry: 'Well, I did have one such poem that I wrote in 1941. They found the diary somewhere or other and had torn the page out. I still remember the poem.'

And I [VS] persuade her to recite it:

In these dark days happiness is snatched from me
And words of joy fall silent on my lips
And searing pain which dwelt afar
Crushes my soul with searing envy.

Words speak to us even when the speaker is powerless: Ieva is old and impoverished. Recall also sixty-year-old Mudra: the rhetorical power of Mudra's narrative derives not from her status but from the juxtaposition of mountains of corn with a child's shame at producing faeces containing undigested corn and which speak of a famine diet.

Let me give another example of what I call narrative power. This is Mudra taking up her mother's story and describing how she perceived her mother after her long years in Siberia: 'Even though she was dear to me she was ... it seemed to me she'd somehow become coarse ... I don't know how to put it in words [crying]. She'd become harsh in a way ... she wasn't soft any more. We'd waited for her as little children, she used to take us on her lap and cuddle us and hold us close to her [crying]. Her hands were loving and firm, her hands were tender. But then later she was completely ... well bony ... her body was like a man's. The first time when I caught sight of her when she came to my school and they said, 'That's your mother'. From her face and her appearance I couldn't recognize her, I was almost afraid. She came to embrace me, but in my memory the whole time were her tender caresses, but she was hard now and it felt as though a man was embracing you. That's how it was. What can one do? That's life.'

Again narrative power lies in the skill that juxtaposes a child's memory of infinite tenderness with the fear of a skeletal embrace. The power of language is here linked to its intimate relationship with experience. It does not take its shape from a succession of frames but rather from a life that has been lived. The Italian philosopher Cavarero makes a similar point: 'Indeed ... while a story results from every life, no life can result from a story' (2000: 144). These narratives draw upon deep sedimentations of feeling: sadness and anger related to years imprisoned, youth lost, health damaged and lives irreparably fractured. These feelings could not be articulated under Soviet rule but neither did they spring into being with the collapse of the Soviet Union. What Rapport (1997: 40) refers to as 'the drive to individuality' is expressed through a poetics in which the particularities of experience combine with an idiosyncratic use of language to give us a powerful sense of a unique self.

Throughout these dialogues with the archive there is an appeal to experience and to truth which raises the vexed question of reference. We know that we can no longer make easy assumptions about the relationship between events and their descriptions. The world does not have 'a preferred description of itself' (Rorty 1991: 21). Silverstein refers to this idea as 'referential cleanliness': the idea that certain standard ways of speaking are able to get closer to reality than others (1998: 292). When a particular language or dialect is given higher status and prioritized, 'language acquires a "thinginess" such that the properties language takes on are continuous with other objects in the culture' (ibid.: 290). Certainly, the authors aspired to that kind of ontological status for the KGB files. They make special claims to defining reality and override the experience of others, shaping it to their will.

However, these files have not only imposed unwanted linguistic structures, they have damaged peoples' lives and deprived them of freedom. Thus the reading of the files provides an important opportunity for reasserting moral agency. Informants use personal experience to construct narratives that make a moral point. They speak of relationships torn apart, children unnurtured and talents undeveloped. The persuasiveness, feeling and poetry of these narratives are opposed to the rigid coherence of the language of the archive and seek to undermine the language of Soviet power. Rorty invites us to see language as a kind of 'evolution, constantly killing off old forms' (1991: 18) and this is what we see here. The old forms in question here are the political rhetoric of the state archives. Bloch's analysis of political oratory (1975: 12–13) linked formalization, with its multiple restrictions on verbal expression, to coercive power. However, formalization can only be achieved by emphasizing the metonymic pole of language and eliminating the metaphoric. Precisely for this reason metaphor plays such an important role in challenging formal political language. Bloch writes: 'It is really a type of communication where rebellion is impossible and only revolution could be feasible' (ibid.: 20). Bloch uses the metaphor of the tunnel to convey the restricting experience of being a party to formal oratory (ibid.: 24). However, although he is right about the impossibility of rebellion his discussion does not take account of the possibility of linguistic challenge and deconstruction opened up by retrospection. Precisely because political rhetoric becomes increasingly self-referring and any genuinely referential function disappears, my informants were concerned to re-instate reference. In so doing, they are also asserting their selfhood. There are parallels with Burridge's insights from new religious movements. He writes: 'the individual, using similar modes but transcending the given categories, rerationalizing and arguing antithetically, provides a moral critique and ideally seeks a closer fit with the goodness in the truth of things as he or she perceives them' (1979: 7).

Because what was written in the files determined the course of my narrators' lives, my informants felt the need to contest the claims even now. As Emma Priedīte said:

> *You know, I don't like it. I feel angry that they can say that you're supposed to have said something when you haven't said it at all. I'd never have thought that they could say that I'd said these things and made out that I'm guilty. I don't know. I just want to say, they can write anything, that they can write nonsense. I wouldn't want lies to be written about me. Untruths. There's no truth in what they write in those files.*

Perhaps because they had been unable to speak their minds at the time, speaking out now was still important: Elza Glaudāne sums it up thus:

> *Now it's easy to talk but at that time we were afraid. We didn't know what lay ahead of us, you understand. If I were arrested now I would be more clever. But you see, at that time we were afraid, we didn't know whether we would be shot or not. You see, we didn't know anything.*

No narrative can claim privileged access to the world's 'preferred description of itself'; the 'view from nowhere' is a mirage. And yet the authority to speak is rooted in experience. Alfrēdis Geidāns had a stroke in 1992 which impaired his memory for facts: names and dates elude him, but the memory of pain and torture is still vivid and brings tears to his eyes. He can no longer contest the KGB archive. In answer to my questions he pointed to his own personal archive: 'We must look in that pile,' he repeated, but the stroke has deprived him of the ability to access and interpret his own archive. Irvine has written: 'Not everyone who uses the term gold has to identify gold, but someone must be able to use the term gold in an authoritative way' (1989: 257). Which is why, just as there have to be goldsmiths who can distinguish between gold and plate, so we must listen to those who speak with the authority of experience.

Acknowledgements

My fieldwork during the summer of 1999 was made possible by a grant from the British Academy, for which I am grateful. I would like to thank Ēvalds and Terēsa Landra for their help in translating the files from Russian into Latvian. An earlier version of this chapter was given at the Auditing Selves conference in Manchester, November 1999, and later versions to the departments of Anthropology at Cambridge and Sociology at Aberdeen. I am particularly grateful for the comments of anonymous reviewers on earlier versions of this chapter.

Notes

1. Since my work there the Archive has been moved further away from the city centre to the new suburb of Imanta.
2. The earlier acronym NKVD (Narodny Komisariat Vnutrennikh Del) translates as the commissariat for the people's internal affairs. It was replaced by the acronym KGB (Komitet Gosudarstvenij Bezopasnosti) or the State Security Committee. However, the term favoured in popular usage for the secret police is that by which it was first known, namely, the Cheka.

15

VARIETIES OF DECEPTION AND DISTRUST: MORAL DILEMMAS IN THE ETHNOGRAPHY OF PSYCHIATRY

> He felt as though he had been sucked into a machine that was dismembering him into impersonal, general components before the question of his guilt or innocence came up at all.
>
> Musil (1997: 168)

Ethnographic encounters with patients and their psychiatrists bring ethical dilemmas into painful focus. The title of my chapter was deliberately chosen to reflect what I see as a central ethical problem in psychiatric practice. Deception and distrust characterize the relationship between Latvians and wider society and these qualities have inevitably come to shape the relationship between patients and their psychiatrists. What Frank describes as 'the subversive voice' (2001: 360) of suffering is a protest against the ideological voice of psychiatry.

The very rapid economic liberalization of the Baltic states and its problematic relationship with an unrealistic philosophy of limitless individual opportunity has made deception harder to pin down but has intensified distrust and isolated the subversive voice. The process of economic liberalization has scooped up psychiatric theory and practice. Earlier somatic diagnoses have been replaced by psychological diagnoses. Psychiatry, medicine and the social sciences have all been implicated in the process of fragmenting and reconstructing individual experience to fit in with what Smith calls their own specialist 'textually mediated forms of ruling' (1993: 212). However, in most cases such processes are ongoing and patients and respondents have become habituated and embedded within these discursive projects. Approval of medical or sociological texts is to be understood not as authentic approval but as capitulation to relations of ruling (Frank 2001: 356). Following Bourdieu (2002), I would describe some psychiatric interchanges as misrecognition and relate such misrecognition to contradictions between the philosophy and implementation of liberalism in Latvia and the consequences of such contradictions for individuals. Ironically, however, this knowledge has only been made possible at a cost of fudging issues to do with negotiated consent and transparency. In post-Soviet Latvia we can witness Western psychiatry in the process of trying to articulate its discursive project and to establish relations of ruling. As a result of the uncertain hegemony of a changing psychiatric discourse the discordant voice of patients' suffering is more apparent.

Latvia along with the two other Baltic states played a key role in accelerating the dismantling of the Soviet Union (Lieven 1993). These countries were keen to end their very real experience of Soviet oppression. At the same time their new democratic leaders were ready to embark upon an immediate and radical programme of economic reform. 'Latvia through numerous governments has not strayed from this liberal economic path. Its firm acceptance of the market and concomitant rejection of state interventionism has placed Latvia among the top tier of the reforming countries in the eyes of international financial organisations' (Pabriks and Purs 2001: 95). However, for many Balts these economic changes, involving as they did the end of socialist support structures such as free health care, brought about considerable personal hardship and insecurity. Political and economic liberalization affected every aspect of society including medicine and psychiatry for which charges were introduced in 1995.

My thematic interests arise without exception from my need to acknowledge the experience of individuals and to put on record my encounter with them. That is not to say that I wish to exclude theory altogether. But the task of anthropology as of philosophy 'is to say whatever can be said that is as general as the field permits' (Toulmin 1988: 348). My field, in this case, focused on the dialogue between patients and their psychiatrists: an exchange between narratives of despair and a discourse of diagnoses and medication. Patient narratives included a polyphony of voices that spoke of cramped accommodation, unemployment and poverty as well as of shame and self-blame. Through listening to these consultations I became interested in three areas. Firstly, in identifying the key features of change from a Soviet and socialist society to a liberal capitalist one that impinge upon lay conceptions of the self and narratives of distress. Secondly, in understanding how these shifts in culture have permeated the theories and treatment strategies of mental health professionals. And, finally, in mapping the extent to which understandings of lay people and mental health professionals converge or diverge and how this contributes to personal suffering. All of these questions have an ethical dimension. Radical economic and political changes have brought with them a shift in the locus of deception, which has resulted in guilt and shame for many. Under Soviet occupation the mismatch between official versions of history and actual experience could not be openly acknowledged but was keenly felt and easy to identify. The collapse of Soviet power has brought with it a policy of economic liberalism, which rests upon a conception of individual power that fits badly with the reality of everyday life. However, the philosophy of agency has powerfully penetrated individual psyches so that its mismatch with available opportunities is harder to identify. Psychiatrists play an important role in this process in that the language they use has a huge potential for affirming or diminishing self worth and in shaping conceptions of the self. And thirdly, an increasing divergence between lay and professional understandings undermines the project of finding meaning in illness.

These three concerns confronted my fieldwork throughout its entirety. It seems to me that they raise ethical issues of a more fundamental nature than those traditionally associated with anthropological research. They challenge but also transcend issues to do with autonomy, informed consent and transparency, both in relation to psychiatrists and in relation to their patients. What kind of autonomy is being given to patients? Miller distinguishes four different meanings of autonomy: namely, as freedom of action, as authenticity, as effective deliberation, and moral reflection (1981: 22). My encounter with patients and psychiatrists suggests that there is a tension and contradiction between their conceptions of autonomy. Psychiatrists appear to be concerned with nurturing a sense of autonomy to do with recognizing and conforming to a particular kind of patient role. Patients' concern with autonomy is of a different order and relates to moral deliberation and authenticity. This in turn raises the question of whether transparency within the research relationship is of paramount importance or whether it can be overridden in favour of making a long-term contribution to the well being of psychiatric patients. How can one negotiate the differences in ethical position of a Soviet grown psychiatry and British anthropology? To what extent do institutional constraints and official ethical guidelines influence the actual practice of psychiatrists? What are the ethical implications of listening to the misery of others with a view to translating such misery into an anthropological text? Frank writes of balancing on the edge between symbolic violence and silence (2001: 361). And finally, in what ways has the westernization of psychiatry altered the practice of psychiatry in Latvia and changed relations between doctors and their patients? The answers to these questions lie not in ethical theory but in ethnographic contextualization. We must look to areas that the early moral philosophers chose to ignore. Toulmin writes: 'In four sets of topics and spheres of thought, they were especially *un*interested: the "oral", the "particular", the "local", and the "timely"' (1988: 338). Toulmin argues that if ethics is to have meaning it must embed itself in ethnographic and clinical context. Others have argued that without ethnography ethics cannot survive: 'Theoretical systematization supposedly transubstantiates the water of moral experience into the wine of moral knowledge. Although the ritual may continue to play a role in the cathedral of academia, it remains peripheral to the outside world. There moral experience retains its primacy, and it is appreciating the primacy of experience and in providing ways of understanding and guiding that experience that ethnography can be useful' (Hoffmaster 1992: 1424).

Ethical questions are easier to formulate than to answer. My answers indicate the beginnings of an argument and the tentative mapping out of a moral domain. Autonomy, like freedom, has multiple meanings but essentially they relate to two dimensions. They are the freedom to act and the freedom to take up a moral position and to be a particular kind of person. Taylor (1985) and Frankfurt (1988) both argue that freedom in the latter sense is more important. 'Agents are beings for whom things matter, who are subjects of significance' (Taylor 1985: 104). Thus what matters to the patient must be recognized within the psychiatric consultation. Issues of transparency raise the question: transparency for whom? Rendering the research transparent to the psychiatrist might have made research impossible and thus ultimately have silenced the voice of the patient. And finally with regard to translating the misery of others into an anthropological text, my view is that by and large psychiatry carries greater risks of symbolic violence and misrecognition than does a humanistic anthropology. In part this is no doubt due to the greater institutional and financial backing of psychiatry. puts this well: 'The symbolic violence that any ideological discourse implies, in so far as it is based on misrecognition, is only operative inasmuch as it is able to make its addressees treat it the way it demands to be treated, namely with all due respect, observing the proper formalities required by its formal properties. Ideological production is all the more successful when it is able to put in the wrong anyone who attempts to reduce it to its objective truth' (2002: 153).

Although the three Baltic states are cited as an economic success story, as I have indicated, this has been at considerable human cost for large numbers of people. The problem for many middle-aged people is that they have learnt to live life, to play the game, according to one set of rules and that midway through their lives those rules have undergone a radical change. Playing by the rules no longer brings them the rewards they were promised. The result is a huge feeling of loss and wasted lives. Furthermore, the locus of responsibility for an individual's well-being has shifted from collective imaginings such as the state, history and destiny to the individual agent. Nuckolls has made an interesting attempt to relate histrionic and anti-social personality disorders to Weber's ideal types configured around moralism and materialism (1992: 37). These twin pillars of the capitalist self exert an influence beyond specific psychiatric diagnoses and combine to constrain individuals in a particularly painful grip, making them feel acutely responsible and ashamed of a lack of material success. The dramatic changes in conceptions of the self and responsibility remind us forcefully that the self has a history (Gergen and Gergen 1986; Bruner 1986, 1990; Rose 1997).

A unifying characteristic of both the Soviet and the post-Soviet era is an absence of trust in the workings of society. Numerous studies have shown that physical and psychological well-being are directly related to the levels of inequality in a society, rather than absolute poverty (Wilkinson 1996). And social inequality is in turn related to the levels of connectedness and trust between people (Putnam 2000; House, Landis and Anderson 1988; Berkman 1995; Seeman 1996). However, the absence of trust has had different mental health manifestations in the Soviet and the post-Soviet era.

Fieldwork Background

My own work has been carried out in Latvia since the summer of 1990. It has involved talking with people who described themselves as psychologically damaged and who may or may not have sought medical help for their condition (see Chapters 7, 8, 10 and 11 this volume, and Skultans 1997, 1998a). It involved talking to doctors and psychiatrists and, more recently, it has involved sitting in on psychiatric consultations as a semi-participant observer (Skultans 2007). Throughout my periods of fieldwork and in the transcription and interpretation of interviews I have been uneasily aware of the ways in which my work has fallen short of the formal guidelines suggested for ethical anthropological practice. But had I followed the guidelines in a strict sense my fieldwork could not have been carried out.

My chapter is based upon twelve months of fieldwork carried out in Latvia between 1991 and 1992, and seven months during 2001. During the first period of fieldwork I talked with more than a hundred people who considered their health, in particular their nervous health, to be damaged. In 2001 I spoke with psychiatrists and their patients. I was allowed to sit in on some 300 psychiatric consultations and to tape-record these consultations. Without a doubt, the location and focus of my research, particularly in 2001, brought the traditional ethical problems of transparency and informed consent to a particularly sharp edge. However, over and above these traditional concerns was an acute moral discomfiture that some psychiatrists were promoting an account of patients' distress that was totally at odds with the patients' views of what was wrong and why and, indeed, with my own perceptions.

Negotiating 'Consent' and Fudging Transparency

Negotiating consent to carry out an ethnography of psychiatric consultations reveals the unequal distribution of power between psychiatrists and their patients. The difficult part was gaining permission from psychiatrists to sit in on and record their consultations. Thereafter, the patient's consent appeared to be part and parcel of agreeing to the consultation as such. Patients were asked something along the lines of, 'You don't mind if the anthropologist from England listens to our conversation'. No patient refused permission for me to listen. Of the ten psychiatrists whom I approached two refused collaboration. The other eight showed an extraordinary degree of tolerance and generosity in overcoming distrust of my presence, fear of how I might judge their professional competence and the uses to which I might put the recordings. Their friendly generosity has placed me in a moral quandary. How can I square the hospitality and co-operation offered me by Latvian psychiatrists with my sometimes critical stance of their ideas and practice? The result is that I feel rather like a guest who eats a meal only to speak badly of the hosts cooking skills afterwards. I am not sure how to resolve this unease, save to say that ethical obligations form a hierarchical structure. Taken singly each has weight but taken together some override others.

Understanding other cultures on their own terms requires a certain suspension of judgement. And yet recent developments in epistemological theory have highlighted the naivety and unattainability of aspirations towards ethical neutrality. How to find a middle way between openness to cultural difference and ethical indifference is an ongoing problem in ethnographic research. The emphasis on transparency and openness in the research situation influenced largely by feminist practice has been shown to have major pitfalls of its own. Stacey has argued that it is precisely the closeness engendered by feminist ethnographic practice that is responsible for 'inauthenticity, dissimilitude, and potential, perhaps inevitable, betrayal' (1991: 113). Emotional connectedness and empathic understanding should not disguise the fact that the ethnographer and informant have different motivations in participating in the research. Glucksman describes this as 'the different and unequal relation to knowledge of the researched and researcher' (1994: 159). Renaming informants, respondents or participants does not empower them in any real sense. It may simply be a way of 'attempting to establish an egalitarianism in the research situation as a substitute for establishing it in the "real world"' (ibid.: 1994: 151). And as Smith argues obtaining approval for sociological texts is often not real approval but a form of capitulation (Smith cited in Frank, 2001: 356).

The American Anthropological Association has published a statement on ethical practice that contained the following injunction: 'In research, anthropologists' paramount responsibility is to those they study. When there is a conflict of interests these individuals must come first' (1986: 2). This statement poses special problems for the ethnographic study of psychiatric practice, which encompasses both psychiatrists and their patients. Whilst the statement recognizes the 'plurality of values, interests and demands' in the societies studied by anthropologists, the study of psychiatric consultations often encapsulates a conflict of interests that are particularly difficult to work with. Some of these misgivings may be resolved by the directive 'to contribute to an "adequate definition of reality" upon which public opinion and public policy may be based' (ibid.: 3). However, the equivalent British statement of the Association of Social Anthropologists is more cautious: 'The advancement of knowledge and the pursuit of information are not in themselves sufficient justifications for overriding the values and ignoring the interests of those studied' (ASA, 2007: 2).

Perhaps more than other areas of anthropological study cross-cultural psychiatry is faced with the problem of how to adjudicate between competing definitions of reality and normality. Some years ago Kleinman advocated a 'new cross-cultural psychiatry' (1977). His argument for the more radical approach of cross-cultural psychiatry rested on epistemological considerations to do with the social construction of knowledge. The imposition of Western psychiatric categories for understanding the behaviour of people in other societies was, he argued, a form of psychiatric imperialism. Each society has developed concepts for understanding disordered behaviour and to impose Western categories is to distort a reality that has already been filtered through local concepts. It involves imposing second-order categories on first-order categories and was, he argued, an illegitimate move.

These problems, which are a regular feature of ethnographic research, appear in a more acute form in the anthropological study of mental illness and its treatment. Disordered behaviour, which causes distress to the individual and those around them, rules out moral indifference. Unequal access to knowledge within a psychiatric consultation makes true equality difficult and inequality may in any case be further ensconced by institutional arrangements of inequality. A divergence between the individual's experience and psychiatric theories may feed a conflict of interests. Competition over the right to define reality acquires a new meaning in the triangulation that takes place between the anthropologist, the psychiatrist and her patients. And how does the demand for informed consent fit into the ethnographic study of psychiatric practice? What counts as informed consent in the context of a psychiatric consultation? Whose consent is required: the patient's, the psychiatrist's, or both? And given the conflict of interests and perspectives is it realistic to expect such consent?

The ASA ethical guidelines describe informed consent as expressing 'the belief in the need for truthful and respectful exchanges between social researchers and the people whom they study' (19—: 3). And moreover, it is not enough to be given consent once only. Consent 'may require renegotiation over time; it is an issue to which the anthropologist should return periodically' (19—: 3). In my case consent to listen and record consultations was obtained from psychiatrists through informal discussion who then asked for 'consent' from their patients at the beginning of the consultation. Typically, this took the form a cursory question such as: 'You don't mind if the professor from England sits in on the consultation, do you?' As I said earlier, permission was never withheld. Whether their agreement constituted informed consent is another matter. But certainly my presence in the consultations was not, I think, perceived as particularly unusual.

This ready agreement within the context of a psychiatric consultation is not only about informed consent. It concerns a clash of cultural and professional expectations. Medical consultations in Soviet Latvia lacked the privacy with which they are associated in the West. Access to consulting rooms is seldom restricted to a doctor and her patient. Besides the prescribing nurse who shares the consulting room, other staff and, indeed, patients frequently interrupt an ongoing consultation. Moreover, the ringing telephone regularly intrudes with other patients' problems as well as with the doctor's domestic troubles. Neither the boundaries of the patient's nor the doctor's problems are guarded as rigorously as they are in Western medical practice. Patients were, until recently, in charge of their own notes. In such contexts problems are publicly shared. However, the idea of informed consent only makes sense in the context of guarded boundaries and appropriated knowledge. To have pushed for more explicit consent would have been to challenge and possibly undermine the existing understandings and practices surrounding medical and psychiatric consultations in Latvia. Not only might my motives have become suspect but also those of the psychiatrist. The emphasis on returning to the issue of informed consent and renegotiating it suggests, in fact, that informants may wish to push the anthropologist's agenda out of their mind.

Changing Conceptions of Self under Communism and Capitalism

Weber first alerted us to 'the way in which "ideas" have, like switchmen, determined the tracks along which action has been pushed by the dynamic of interest' (1991: 280). But action is intrinsically connected to intention, which in turn brings in the idea of agency. But agency is itself a slippery term and means different things at different periods. Kemp has identified five types of agency: moral, embodied, volitional, behavioural and social, which may or may not co-exist (2004: 63). Under Soviet rule agency for many Latvians was confined to the moral sphere. It related to an individual's ability to take up a moral position despite an absence of behavioural and social agency. Paradoxically, under economic liberalism, which emphasizes the individual's power to change his or her life circumstances, there has been an erosion of moral agency. There has been an unquestioning internalization of a liberal philosophy of the self. However, in the absence of behavioural and social agency this uncritical acceptance of an ideologically enlarged conception of the self is a source of pain and discomfort to many. Thus the changes from a command to a market economy have been accompanied by equally painful intra-psychic changes. I would like to present images of social and psychological change by using excerpts from my conversations with psychiatrists and patients over a ten year span. My excerpts come from my fieldwork in 1992 and 2001. They illustrate the way in which both understandings of distress, the positioning of the individual *vis-à-vis* society, the divergence between lay and professional understandings of mental ill health and the sources of distrust and disconnectedness have changed.

In 1992 I had many conversations with Anna, a psychiatrist. Initially I was interested in her practice and her patients' problems. However, as we became friends the conversation shifted to her own life and the way in which she felt the events in her life had damaged her health. Her own shorthand term for her problems was summed up by the quasi medical term neurosis. She attributed the condition to herself and claimed that it had developed as a result of the particular course her life had taken and the historical and social conditions in which it was embedded. However, in making these claims and admissions Anna was making a connection with other Latvians.

For example, Anna says:

> *I don't for one moment consider that I am the only one who hasn't succeeded or something like that. I have always told myself that I am not the only one like that. The whole Latvian nation is like that. I think that every other family has all sorts of problems. You could call it destiny, or the situation or this communist epoch. I don't know how to put it more precisely: there is nowhere where this mystical epoch hasn't interfered and hasn't transformed life. My destiny isn't anything special. There are many more tragic destinies than mine.*

Anna's life history is almost a social history detailing as it does the problems of returning from Siberia and subsequent problems with accommodation.

> *People were very intimidated here. They didn't want to socialize freely. It was difficult to find anywhere to live, although houses were empty. They didn't let us in. We lived with relatives for three or four months, then we found a little old woman, she lived in a private house and she gave us a room.*

Anna also relates her neurosis as she terms it to her subsequent difficult living circumstances. I asked her whether she had sought help for her problems.

> *Well, I think I could be helped with the nerve illness. But I think that while the cause has not been liquidated, the cause of my neurosis, the cause of my stress, until I have peaceful home circumstances, at work I am tense, I have to listen to different people, different complaints, different characters, I have to be calm all the time, and when I go home I can't rest and again I have to hear... to be specific I have to hear various swear words addressed to me. Actually, I don't get any rest anywhere.*

But most of all I suffer from the fact that my children hear those rude Russian swear words. I'm not so concerned about myself, however unpleasant it may be, and the same goes for grandmother, but a child. Those children are growing up the same way as me – neurotic. A new generation of neurotics, because they're already afraid. A young child doesn't understand swear words. I remember that my youngest daughter was five years old. She comes in and calls me swear words. My daughter asks me what they mean. I have to tell her that those are bad words. It hurts me especially for the children, that a new generation will also suffer from accommodation neurosis.

The neurosis seems to have an existence that is almost independent of the individual. Accommodation neurosis suggests that the neurosis resides outside the individual. But at the same time Anna retains her ability and right to pass judgement on her difficult circumstances even though she lacks the ability to change her circumstances. Anna is typical of many doctors who in 1992 were ready to be open about their problems and see their source in the difficult circumstances through which they had lived and were living. Although psychiatrists during the Soviet era were perceived as agents of social control – some were indeed, involved in medicalizing political dissent – many others were ready to acknowledge the harsh impact of historical and social circumstances on individual well-being. The role of psychiatrists in promoting a misrecognition of the noxious influence of certain forms of social oppression has not been confined to the Soviet era.

Images of change in 2001 are drawn from thirty-five open-ended conversations I conducted in the polyclinic of a provincial town in north Vidzeme. This clinic had no psychotherapist or psychiatrist and for this reason the director of the clinic was happy for me to see patients who wanted to talk about their problems. I explained to the director that I was an anthropologist interested in social change and its affect on self-concepts and discourses of distress. A poster to that effect was put up in the clinic and a notice was published in the local chapter. However, it soon became clear that I was cast in the role of a psychotherapist. One patient opened the interview by saying that she had never consulted a psychotherapist but that she had seen psychotherapists in action in American soaps. All thirty-five of the patients who came to see me were women and all were struggling with extremely difficult financial and domestic circumstances. All the conversations were tape-recorded.

A unifying characteristic of all the accounts is that, whilst patients described their difficult circumstances and the impossibility of making ends, meet all adopted a judgemental and even a punitive attitude towards themselves and what they perceived as an inability to control their painful emotions and to cope. For example, Milda is a 46-year-old woman due to have an operation for a pituitary tumour. She blames herself for her lack of control:

The tears flow by themselves. Even if I don't want it the tears flow. It's some sort of weakness. It's bad. Probably someone else could control themselves but my tears just flow and flow. I don't know.

Nearly everyone used phrases to do with management, control, order and cultivation. The inability to manage one's finances is mirrored by an inability to manage one's self. As one 29-year-old woman said:

If there is order around me, then I myself feel ordered.

Aija is 47 years old and started the conversation as follows:

It all started because my husband has a job where he is supposed to be paid but isn't paid.

Aija herself cannot get a job because she has tiny stubs in place of teeth:

I can't get a job, for example, because I don't have teeth. A paradox so to speak. It's a kind of joke.

But it is a joke that makes her cry even as she talks about it. And she condemns herself for crying:

I cry over nothing. I always manage. I don't know how to find a solution. There's nothing to cry about.

Like many others she both manages in the sense of surviving and yet does not manage in any decent and meaningful way. The difficult financial situation creates a feeling of futility and purposelessness. A senior nurse at the polyclinic described it thus:

All my life I've saved, all my life. But I'm still short of money and short of money.

The financial difficulties are accentuated in cases of illness. Biruta is 46 years old and has an ailing 65-year-old mother and two boys who are studying and not yet financially independent. This is how she describes the problem:

Father had a bigger pension. At that time there were two pensions. And one pension could go on medicines. Then they could afford 20 lats and buy Cipramil, for example(an anti-depressant). But now there is just one pension. And during the winter my husband doesn't have a proper job and I still have to support my children and to pay the bills. I can't take my mother to the doctor and get all her prescriptions because mother's pension just won't cover them. She has heart, she has liver, she has kidneys, she has legs, she has back. Well you understand, when you have all the ailments, all the money goes on medicines. And now, for example, when she gets her pension she will have just 5 lats in her purse

The rhetorical detailing of ailments and precise sums of money serves to bring home the impossibility of making the sums add up in a satisfactory way. However, beyond the impossible sums and the paradox of not being able to get a job without teeth or teeth without a job lies the shame that such situations engender. The feelings of shame and self-blame are most acutely conveyed in the anxieties aroused by the ceremonial functions of school leaving. In Latvia, both during the Soviet era and continuing to the present, school leaving was associated with a number of public occasions demanding lavish expenditure on clothes for children and parents, and flowers and presents for teachers. Many women spoke of the nightmarish anticipation of these events. Of not knowing how to find the necessary money and yet being terrified of exposing the shame of their poverty to schoolmates, other parents and neighbours.

These extracts demonstrate important differences in the articulation of distress between 1992 and 2001. In 1992 abnormality was perceived as an attribute of social circumstances and their shaping of individual lives. People described their abnormal life (*šitā nenormālā dzīve*) as damaging nerves (*sadragā nervus*) in a very concrete way. It is the individual's life experiences rather than their personality, which is abnormal. The verb *sadragāt* is primarily used to convey the infliction of physical damage as in the case of using an insufficiently inflated car tyre or the scuffing of a shoe by a careless child. The term brings to mind a careless and brutal assault and its physical consequences. Here the explanations speak of the contingency of existence and suggest a fine understanding of the historical and social embedding of their lives. In 2001 the locus of responsibility for distress has shifted. Although life now presents an equally difficult, though different, set of circumstances, people do not judge their responses as inevitable and, therefore, in some sense appropriate. Instead, their distress is tied up with feelings of shame and self-blame. Whereas Anna in 1992 connected her feelings with those of others, Milda in 2001 distinguishes her responses from those of others: 'Probably someone else could control themselves'. These changes have taken place independently of the intervention of psychiatrists or psychotherapists, as my conversations in the polyclinic indicate. My own understanding of patients' distress pointed to contradictions between the new ideology of economic liberalism and the actual opportunities that were available to people. Indeed, I felt it was right to make my views known to patients if only to lessen the punitive burden of self-blame. In articulating my own position, at odds with that of the patients, I was, I suppose, trying to give them a lost sense of community and to relieve them of the burden of self-blame.

Changing Psychiatric Language

Psychiatry, as practised in Latvia, has until fairly recently been very much in the Soviet mould. This has meant that the psychiatrist's duty to the patient has been counterbalanced by what the Physicians' Oath of the Soviet Union (1971) calls 'the interests of society' and 'the principles of communist morality' (cited in Bloch and Chodoff, 1984: 114). Certainly, the social and political abuses of Soviet psychiatry have been widely publicized (Medvedev and Medvedev 1971; Bloch and Reddaway 1977; Lader 1977; Podrabinek 1980). These writings have largely dealt with the diagnosis of 'sluggish schizophrenia' and the ways in which it has been used to incarcerate and silence political dissidents. The misuse of psychiatry for political ends led to the expulsion of the Soviet Union from the World Psychiatric Association in 1983. They were readmitted in 1989.

For these reasons Soviet psychiatry, which has been held up as an extreme example of the potential abuse of psychiatry for political ends. Soviet psychiatry 'demonstrates, with grim clarity, how a system that appears to have only scientific origins and professional goals can, simply by virtue of its own nature as a systematic psychiatric technology, result in significant human harm' (Reich, 1984: 66). The development of Soviet psychiatry and, in particular, the diagnosis of 'sluggish schizophrenia' illustrates the dramatic ways in which psychiatric categories can come to influence the perception of behaviour and, therefore, the experience of patients. 'Those Soviet psychiatrists really saw the patients as schizophrenic; or, to put it another way, the system created a category, first on chapter and then, with training, in the minds of Soviet psychiatrists, which was eventually assumed to represent a real class of patients and which was inevitably filled by real persons' (ibid.: 71).

However, in the process of identifying the misuses of Soviet psychiatry, the everyday practice of psychiatry has been neglected and the ethical dilemmas encountered in all psychiatric practice have been glossed over. I would argue that it is precisely the ubiquity of certain psychiatric conditions such as neurasthenia that rendered them invisible. Conversations with Dr Alka, the principal doctor at the headquarters of the Riga emergency ambulance service, suggested that the majority of Latvians suffered from damaged nerves in some form or other. In people under thirty-five years of age this manifested itself as a dysthesia of the autonomic nervous system in Latvian *vegetativa distonija*. The Chambers dictionary defines dysthesia as 'a morbid habit of body, resulting in general discomfort or impatience'. Dr Alka listed chest pains, headaches, sudden changes in blood pressure as symptoms of *vegetativa distonija*. In patients over thirty-five the diagnosis was neurasthenia suggestive of a more entrenched condition that had moved beyond mere habit but was associated with similar symptoms. Dr Alka referred to the difficulty of distinguishing between functional and organic conditions:

> *Well, you see, we are afraid of overlooking organic illnesses. Because in principal almost every person has these neurasthenia problems. Those or some others, because all these social things leave a very heavy imprint on a person.*

Thus Latvian psychiatry embodied a paradox. On the one hand, it had assimilated a Pavlovian theory of character types, which accounted for a variety of weaknesses of the nervous system. Underpinning this categorization was a dualistic theory that divided people into social and egoistic types (see Chapter 7, this volume). But on the other hand, these diagnostic categories have a semantic complexity that included a critique of society. People, including doctors, described the dishonesty and disorder of society eroding their health in a very direct and brutal fashion.

Independence and westernization have brought with them many changes in psychiatric theory and practice not easy to describe under a single rubric. Two new helping professions have appeared, namely psychotherapists and psychologists. Experts from the Scandinavian countries, France, Germany and the United Kingdom travel regularly to Riga to give seminars and training courses. Considerable diversity has thus been introduced into psychotherapeutic practice. However, countering these centrifugal tendencies is the centripetal effect of the translation of the *International Classification of Diseases* into Latvian. Whereas earlier versions of the ICD were adapted to local

Circumstances, the *ICD 10* aims to be an exact translation. The large section 'Disorders of the Autonomic Nervous System' has disappeared. In their place have appeared psychoneurotic disorders such as depression, anxiety and acute panic disorder. The very active presence of two pharmaceutical companies, namely Solvay Pharma and Lundbeck, have also played a large part in shaping psychiatric treatment and theory. The monthly day-long conferences organized by pharmaceutical companies are well attended by provincial family doctors and psychiatrists. The diagnosis and discussion of disorders such as depression are linked to new possibilities of treatment. In some ways the sudden influx of a variety of drug treatments has become an iconic representation of the new market economy which in theory is open to all but in practice is beyond the reach of most.

In practice these diagnostic changes have led to changes that involve a fragmentation of feelings and their decontextualization. By and large psychiatrists are interested in the intensity and duration of feelings and their response to medication but not the circumstances that give rise to these feelings. This means that feelings are stripped of their narrative structure and come to be seen as quasi physical objects rather than socially embedded feelings. The novelist and philosopher Robert Musil captures this way of viewing human experience in his novel *The Man Without Qualities*:

> Who has not noticed how independent experiences have made themselves of
> humans? They have gone on the stage, into books, into the reports of scientific
> institutions and expeditions, into communities based on religious or other
> beliefs, which cultivate certain kinds of experience rather than others, as a kind
> of social experiment, and insofar as experiences are not merely found in work,

they are simply in the air ... There has arisen a world of qualities without a man to them, of experiences without anyone to experience them, and it almost looks as though, in the ideal case, people would no longer experience anything privately at all, and the comforting weight of personal responsibility would dissolve into a system of formulae for potential meanings (1997: 158).

Divergence in Conceptual Understandings and the Implications for Meaning Loss

The fit between clinical concepts of disease and lay concepts of illness is never perfect. Theories of disease involve generalization and aim to identify patients as instances of a particular disease. Illness focuses on the particularity, the non-repeatability and life-threatening quality of suffering. Illness is a prime example of the vulnerability and non-repeatability of human projects and the elusiveness of our aspirations for control (Nussbaum 2001: 42). However, there must be some degree of overlap for understanding and dialogue to take place. I would argue that during the era of Soviet psychiatry there was a divergence between professional and lay uses of language but that this served to disguise an underlying agreement in meaning and a fundamental solidarity between psychiatrist and patient. Doctors like Anna and Dr Alka were ready to admit that they themselves might suffer from neurasthenia. Although the psychological language of depression might prima facie suggest the possibility of convergence, in fact it has served to exacerbate differences between people by linking depression with vulnerable personalities. Dr Helga expresses this difference by saying: '*For the patient the doctor is more powerful. Because he is a more powerful personality and more unified. And that is more healthy for the patient. Because the process of re-constructing is quicker.*' The new psychiatric language, rather than promoting empathy and the recognition of suffering, has created hierarchical boundaries and a widening gap between local and extra local meanings.

Lack of consensus and dialogue compounds pain and creates confusion. The following excerpts from a consultation between Valerijs, a middle-aged man diagnosed as having depression, and the psychiatrist Dr Helga illustrate the way in which the diagnosis of depression serves to deny suffering and promotes non-communication. The patient's suffering has a narrative structure intimately linked to the chronological unfolding and contingencies of his work situation. The psychiatrist, however, introduces a medical discourse of 'insufficiency' that explicitly excludes the patient's concerns.

> *Patient: Fundamentally I had problems with work. Ours is a changeable situation. At the moment, for example ... It's very interesting that last year I came because of problems at work and as a result depression set in, nothing*

interests me and it's difficult to get involved in anything. And now after a year I have exactly the same situation, except that the firm where I worked ... Well, they just made me redundant without a reason. I asked them, 'What's the reason?' There's no reason. I've got no protection. At present the social security systems are insufficiently developed. A person is very vulnerable.

Interestingly, the patient uses the same term 'insufficiency' that the doctor later uses to describe his brain. There follows a conversational exchange in which there is a considerable amount of agreement and support for the patient partly because of my own interventions and sympathy for the patient's plight. The worthlessness of contracts and absence of employees safeguards is discussed. However, when the consultation moves on to address issues of health, the polyphonic and dialogic quality disappear and the psychiatrist begins to assert her clinical authority. Ironically it is I who move the conversation on to the subject of health.

V.S. And how is your health?
Patient: My health ... thank God. Well, it depends in what sense. I suppose in one sense it's good and in another sense it's so ... Well thanks to the medication, of course, it's good. I'd stopped. I told you I'd stopped taking the medicines. It must have been about a week. And then I felt straight away that dark thoughts started to crowd in upon me. I started to feel bad. I didn't think that would happen because I thought am I going to be dependent on medicines forever.

The patient's uncertainty and hesitation over what is wrong, why things are wrong and how to put them right emerge at this point. It is clear that there is a fundamental disagreement between the patient's and the psychiatrist's views of the problem. Valerijs is concerned about dependency and recovering a sense of his own agency whereas the psychiatrist seems to have in mind an explanatory model based on constitutional deficiency.

Doctor: That's not dependency Valerij. That's not dependency.
Patient: Yes, but I am dependent right now.
Doctor: No, it's not dependency but insufficiency. It's insufficiency. In the same way that, for example, you can have cardiac insufficiency, or lung insufficiency or liver insufficiency, so you can have insufficiency of the brain synapses. Or more accurately the mediators of the synapses.
Patient: But is it temporary?
Doctor: It is temporary. No, rather it can be compensated for. Temporary is perhaps not the correct description, it is compensatory.
Patient: Does that mean that I shall never be the same as I once was?

The directness of Valerij's question conveys both poetry and anguish and is in stark contrast to the psychiatrist's obfuscating and dilatory replies. She does not attempt to answer his question but instead pursues a pseudo-scientific theory.

Doctor: Why do you say that? If it is compensatory then you can compensate for the condition. It can be improved and maintained. But it needs long-term ... well

it needs a long-term foundation so to speak. Well just as for any insufficiency.
Because that's how it is in fact. And that's what we spoke about earlier – why
these disturbances recur. Because these are micro-organic disturbances. And as
we know – the organic does not get better by itself. It returns and it can only be
compensated for. That's why I compare it to weakness and insufficiency. It's to
do with the mediators of the synapses.
Patient: But if all the circumstances were very favourable, then perhaps one
could recover?
Doctor: Yes, but you need compensation.

In this sequence the psychiatrist defines the terms of the discussion. She
introduces the idea of 'the return of the organic', representing the patient as
its harbinger. The patient's anxious questions about dependency on
medication suggest that for him the psychiatrist's theories about compensation for insufficiency carry little weight. Certainly, the questions are not
addressed and issues of dependency are redefined as an organic defect.
Again the essence of the patient's emotive plea 'Does that mean I shall never
be as I once was?' is left unanswered. The question is about the patient's
sense of himself and the convoluted answer in terms of brain synapses does
not address the patient's anxieties. However, the patient does not give up
and tries to relate his problems to the social circumstances of his work,
thereby implying that recovery might just be possible. The interchange
between patient and psychiatrist illustrate the moral implications of
mind/body problems. As Toulmin argues: 'Far from being purely theoretical
questions about how we can distinguish psychological explanations from
physiological ones, the issues now become intensely practical ones, about
how we are to treat people at the crucial moments of their lives' (1988:
344). Toulmin is discussing medical technology and dying patients but his
point applies with equal force to patients consulting a psychiatrist.

Patient: Well, for example, what do favourable circumstances mean? Literally
one month ago favourable circumstances started to develop when I achieved a
more or less normal financial situation – well, according to today's standards
anyway. I sat down with my wife and we sorted our budget out. We knew we
could cover this and this and this. And that went on for a week and I was in a
very good mood and I was already starting to plan, I started to think about
tomorrow. And Monday I arrived at work and I had totally unexpected news –
I was told I had to look for other work. And immediately I stopped thinking
about tomorrow. So about tomorrow ... I just have today. I no longer have a
tomorrow. So to speak.
Doctor: Well, that's quite right.
Patient: In the stress situation I was in I felt ...
Doctor: Yes, quite right

The doctor's replies are perfunctory. Indeed, as the patient tries to elaborate
on his feelings she cuts him short. The patient then offers a symptom that
the doctor may be more ready to respond to.

Patient: My only complaint is that I'm terribly sleepy

At this point in the consultation the doctor at once becomes more alert and shows interest. However, when the patient voices the suspicion that his tiredness may be due to diabetes and that he should consult a different kind of specialist the psychiatrist bluntly contradicts him: 'That's not diabetes. That's hypochondria.' The psychiatrist then switches tack and seems to undermine her own previous model of disease.

> *Doctor: Well you see … You must understand that you shouldn't put demands on yourself. Otherwise you won't be able to start your internal motor. You can't buy strength in a shop. Unfortunately, even though many would like to. Surprisingly, many people want to.*

The patient's reply suggests that he has more insight into the implications of the doctor's approach than she does herself.

> *Patient: Well maybe if we develop in the capitalist direction, then we'll be able to buy strength.*

After discussing the combinations and strengths of the patient's various medications the doctor emphasizes the importance of rest for restoring his strength. Surprisingly in view of the fact that much of the discussion has been about purchasing medication to compensate for nervous insufficiency, she tells the patient that he cannot buy strength. Clearly the patient, although not the psychiatrist, is unaware of the negative connotations of the term hypochondria. When the patient makes a tentative suggestion that extends beyond the limits of the psychiatrist's professional competence, namely, that perhaps his problems fall within the area of another medical specialty such as endocrinology, the psychiatrist quickly abandons the organic model. Instead the pejorative term hypochondria is introduced which questions character and motives. Finally, the consultation is wrapped up by looking through the prescriptions. The psychiatrist effects closure by saying,

> *Doctor: If there is anything let me know. If anything is unclear? Yes?*

Much in the consultation has been left unclear and created bewilderment in the patient but clarity is confined to timing and dosage of medication.

Throughout the consultation the doctor skilfully directs the conversation away from the social polyphony of his life to something narrower and more tangible thereby asserting her clinical authority. Only when her authority is challenged does the organic model flounder. However, no real dialogue develops between this patient and the psychiatrist. The voices of the patient and psychiatrist extend in parallel without meeting. The patient's account encompasses both an interpretation of the social forces that give his suffering its particular shape and the existential anguish to which they give rise. He knows, for example, that, 'The market does not work in my favour'. As a consequence he describes his existential dilemma as having 'no tomorrow'.

So what do these voices from a psychiatrist's consulting room tell us about ethics? And how do they relate to my earlier discussion of self-understanding, psychiatric language and divergences of meaning? Latvian psychiatrists, like their colleagues elsewhere, have humanitarian and pragmatic goals, which are to do with reducing painful feelings and making life more tolerable for their patients. In order to put these goals into practice they focus on the efficacy of diagnoses and medications. However, my observation of consultations and the broader existential issues that these raise suggest that an exclusive focus on painful feelings and their alleviation is counter-productive and, indeed, increases suffering. The decontextualization and denarrativization of emotion are a powerful assault on the patient's search for meaning. They constitute a refusal to engage with the patient as a moral agent. By contrast, as an anthropologist my interests in the psychiatrist's habitual ways of dealing with patients and their responses was not primarily to do with efficacy but rather with the social forces that shape the understanding and practice of both. In having this broader social agenda I would like to think I was closer to acknowledging the suffering of the patient.

So where does this leave transparency within the research relationship? Transparency implies a certain congruence of perspective. But it may be that certain intellectual perspectives are, by their very nature, incongruent. Perhaps, therefore, anthropology is destined to remain opaque from the perspective of certain kinds of psychiatric practice. Notwithstanding the claims of hybrids such as Devereux (1978, 1980), medical anthropology is, after all, in the business of destabilizing, if not dissolving, psychiatric categories – the very tools of the psychiatrist's trade. The psychiatrist's pragmatic goals make them less aware of their own theoretical assumptions. The insistence on transparency, given the divergence of interests, might constitute an obstacle to getting on with the business of the consultation. Does this mean that anthropological fieldwork necessarily involves betrayal, and if so, how can it be justified? Was I listening to the misery of others with a view to gaining more publications and furthering my own career? Stacey reveals her ambivalent position over an informant's death providing her, as it does, with rich fieldwork opportunities (1991: 114). I suppose to be honest I would have to recognize that one's motives are always a varying mixture of the personal and the altruistic and that it is their combination that matters particularly as it affects the practice of ethnography at particular moments. If at the most painful culmination of a patient's story my concern is for my tape recorder rather than the patient then there is clearly something wrong with the combination. These are the dilemmas of witnessing that Behar attempts to identify. She writes:

> In the midst of a massacre, in the face of torture, in the eye of a hurricane, in the aftermath of an earthquake, or even, say, when horror looms apparently more gently, in memories that won't recede and so come pouring forth in the late-night quiet of a kitchen, as a storyteller opens her heart to a story listener, recounting hurts that cut deep and raw into the gullies of the self, do you, the observer, stay behind the lens of the camera, switch on the tape recorder, keep pen in hand? Are there limits – of respect, piety, pathos – that should not be crossed, even to leave a record (1996: 2)?

Her way of resolving such dilemmas is not to separate the ethnographic voice from the personal and emotional voice, but to write personally and vulnerably (ibid.: 17). How one puts this into practice is another matter, for there is no single model to follow. And yet I hope that an anthropological perspective, which includes the voices of both patients and psychiatrists and is both personal and critical, may make a longer term contribution to psychiatric practice and the well being of patients.

BIBLIOGRAPHY

AAA 1998. *Statement on Ethics Principles of Professional Responsibility.* www.aanet.org/committees/ethics/ethcode.htm (accessed 6th. June, 2007).

Abu-Lughod, L. 1991. 'Writing against Culture'. In Fox, R.J. ed. *Recapturing Anthropology: Working in the Present.* Santa Fe: School of American Research Press.

Acton, W. 1865. *The Functions and Disorders of the Reproductive Organs.* 4th.edn. London: John Churchill and Son.

Alexander, P. 1973. 'Normality'. *Philosophy* 48: 137–51.

Alpers, P. 1997. *What is Pastoral?* Chicago: University of Chicago Press.

Andersons Edgars 1962–82. *Latvju Enciklopēdija.* New York: Amērikas Latviešu Apvienība.

Anonymous. 1710. *Onania or the Heinous Sin of Self-Pollution and All its Frightful Consequences in Both Sexes.* London.

Anonymous. 1849. *Confessions of a Hypochondriac or the Adventures of a Hypochondriac in Search of Health.* London: Saunders and Otley.

Antze, P. and Lambek, M. 1998. *Tense Past Cultural Essays in Trauma and Memory.* London and New York: Routledge.

Ardener, E. 1975. 'Belief and the Problem of Women'. In Ardener, S. (ed). *Perceiving Women.* London: Dent.

Arendt, H. 1970. *On Violence.* London: Allen Lane.

Ariès, P. 1960. *Centuries of Childhood.* Harmondsworth: Penguin.

Armstrong, D. 1983. *The Political Anatomy of the Body: Medical Knowledge in Britain in the Twentieth Century.* Cambridge: Cambridge University Press.

ASA *Ethical Guidelines for Good Research Practice.* www.theasa.org/ethics/ethics_guidelines.htm (accessed 6th. June, 2007).

Aubrey, J. 1950. *Brief Lives.* Lawson, D. (ed). London: Secker and Warburg.

Austin, J.L. 1962. *How To Do Things With Words.* Oxford: Oxford University Press.

Babcock, B. 1980. 'Reflexivity: Definitions and Discriminations', *Semiotica* 30(1–2): 1–14

Bakhtin, M.M. 1984. *Problems of Dostoevsky's Poetics.* Translated by Emerson, C. Minneapolis: University of Minnesota Press.

Bakhtin, M.M. 1986. *Speech Genres and Other Late Essays*. Austin: University of Texas Press.

Bakhtin, M.M. 1992. *The Dialogic Imagination: Four Essays*. Translated by McGee, V.W. Austin: University of Texas Press.

Balint, M. 1964. *The Doctor, His Patient and the Illness*. London: Tavistock Publications.

Banks, J.A. 1954. *Prosperity and Parenthood*. London: Routledge and Kegan Paul.

Barbalet, J.M. 1992. 'A Macro Sociology of Emotion: Class Resentment', *Sociological Theory* 10(2): 150–63.

Barclay, C. 1996. 'Autobiographical Remembering: Narrative Constraints on Objectified Selves'. In Rubin, D. (ed). *Remembering our Pasts: Studies in Autobiographical Memory*. Cambridge: Cambridge University Press.

Barth, F. 2000. 'Boundaries and Connections'. In Cohen, A.P. (ed.) *Signifying Identities: Anthropological Perspectives on Boundaries and Contested Values*. London: Routledge.

Bauman, R. and Briggs, C. 1990. 'Poetics and Performance as Critical Perspectives on Language and Social Life'. *American Review of Anthropology* 19: 59–88.

Becker, E. 1963. 'Social Science and Psychiatry'. *Antioch Review* 23: 353–65.

Behar, R. 1996. *The Vulnerable Observer: Anthropology that Breaks Your Heart*. Boston: Beacon Press.

Bell, C. 1844 [1806]. *The Anatomy of Expression*. 3rd.edn. London: John Murray.

Bentham, J. 1970. *An Introduction to the Principles of Morals and Legislation*. Burns, J.H. and Hart, H.L.A. (eds). London: Athlone Press.

Berkman, L.F. 1995. 'The Role of Social Relations in Health Promotion', *Psychosomatic Medicine* 57: 245–54.

Bhaskar, R. 1993. *Reclaiming Reality a Critical Introduction to Contemporary Philosophy*. London and New York: Verso.

Bhattacharyya, D.P. 1986. *Pagalmi: Ethnopsychiatric Knowledge in Bengal*. Foreign and Comparative Studies/South Asia. Series II. Syracuse: Syracuse University.

Bhatti, R.S., Janakiramaiah, N. and Channabasunna, S.M. 1980. 'Family Psychiatric Ward Treatment in India', *Family Process* 35(1): 193–203.

Bishop, P. 1995. *An Archetypal Constable. National Identity and the Geography of Nostalgia*. London: Athlone.

Blackmore, R. 1725. *A Treatise of the Spleen and Vapours: Or Hypochondriacal and Hysterical Affections*. London: J. Pemberton.

Bloch, M. 1975. 'Introduction'. In Bloch, M. (ed.) *Political Language and Oratory in Traditional Societies*. London: Academic Press.

Bloch, S. and Reddaway, P. 1977. *Russia's Political Hospitals: The Abuse of Psychiatry in the Soviet Union*. London: Victor Gollancz.

Bloch, S. and Chodoff, P. (eds.) 1984. *Psychiatric Ethics*. Oxford, New York and Melbourne: Oxford University Press.

Borneman, J. 1997. *Settling Accounts: Violence, Justice and Accountability in Postsocialist Europe*. Princeton: University of Princeton Press.

Boswell, J. 1928. *The Hypochondriack*. (ed.) Bailey, M. Stanford: Stanford University Press.

Bourdieu, P. 1991. *Language and Symbolic Power*. Cambridge: Polity Press.

Bourdieu, P. 2002. *Outline of a Theory of Practice*. Cambridge: Cambridge University Press.

Bradley, F.H. 1888. 'On Pleasure, Pain, Desire and Volition', *Mind* X111: 1–36.

Bruner, J. 1986. *Actual Minds, Possible Worlds*. Cambridge, Mass. Harvard University Press.

Bruner, J. 1990. *Acts of Meaning*. Cambridge, Mass.: Harvard University Press.

Bruner, J. and Feldman, C. 1996. 'Group Narrative as a Cultural Context of Narrative'. In Rubin, D. (ed.) *Remembering Our Pasts: Studies in Autobiographical Memory*. Cambridge: Cambridge University Press.

Buckler, S. 1996. 'Historical Narrative, Identity and the Holocaust', *History of the Human Sciences* 9(4): 1–20.

Buduls, H. 1928. *Psihiatrija*. Riga: Valters and Rapa.

Bunkše, E.V. 1990. 'Landscape Symbolism in the Latvian Drive for Independence', *Geografiska Notiser* 4: 170–78.

Burgess, T. 1828. *The Physiology or Mechanism of Blushing*. London: John Churchill.

Burke, P. 1991. 'History of Events and the Revival of Narrative'. In Burke, P. (ed.) *New Perspectives on Historical Writing*. Oxford: Polity Press.

Burridge, K. 1979. *Someone, No One: An Essay on Individuality*. Princeton: Princeton University Press.

Burrows, G.M. 1828. *Commentaries on Insanity*. London: Underwood.

Burton, R. 1806 [1621]. *The Anatomy of Melancholy*. 11th.edn. London: J. and E. Hodson.

Bury, M. 1982. 'Chronic Illness as Biographical Disruption'. *Sociology of Health and Illness* 4: 167–82.

Calloway, P. 1992. *Soviet and Western Psychiatry*. Keighley: Moor Press.

Cavarero, A. 2000. *Relating Narratives: Storytelling and Selfhood*. London and New York: Routledge.

Cheyne, G. 1724. *An Essay of Health and Long Life*. London: Strahan and Leake.

Cheyne, G. 1734. *The English Malady or a Treatise on Nervous Diseases of all Kinds*. London: Strahan and Leake.

Childs, D. 1998. 'The Shadow of the Stasi'. In Smith, P.J. (ed). *After the Wall: Eastern Germany since 1989*. Colorado: Westview Press.

Claus, P.J. 1979. 'Spirit Possession and Spirit Mediumship from the Perspective of Tulu Oral Traditions', *Culture Medicine and Psychiatry* 3: 29–52.

Cohen, A.P. 1994. *Self Consciousness: An Alternative Anthropology of Identity*. London: Routledge.

Comfort, Alex 1968. *The Anxiety Makers: Some Curious Preoccupations of the Medical Profession*. London: Panther.

Connerton, P. 1989. *How Societies Remember*. Cambridge: Cambridge University Press.

Coveney, P. 1957. *The Image of Childhood*. Harmondsworth: Penguin.

Csordas, T.J. 1993. 'Somatic Modes of Attention', *Cultural Anthropology* 8(2): 135–56.

Curling, T.B. 1856. *A Practical Treatise on Diseases of the Testis*. London: John Churchill.

Damasio, A.R. 1994. *Descartes' Error: Emotion, Reason and the Human Brain*. New York: Grosset/Putnam.

Dandekar, H. 1986. *Men to Bombay Women at Home: Urban Influence on Sugao Village, Deccan Maharashtra, India 1942–1982*. Ann Arbor, Michigan: University of Michigan, Centre for South and South East Asian Studies.

Daniel, V.E. 1996. *Charred Lullabies: Chapters in an Anthropology of Violence*. Princeton: Princeton University Press.

Darwin, C. 1872. *The Expression of Emotion in Man and the Animals*. London: John Murray.

Das, V., Kleinman A., Lock, M., Ramphele M., and Reynolds P., 2001. *Remaking a World: Violence, Social Suffering and Recovery*. Berkeley: University of California Press.

Dawson, R. 1852 [1840]. *An Essay on Spermatorrhoea*. 6th. edn. London: Aylott Jones.

Descartes, R. 1988 [1649]. 'The Passions of the Soul'. In *Selected Philosophical Writings*. Translated by Cottingham, R. and Murdoch, D. Cambridge: Cambridge University Press.

Deutsch, H. 1944. *The Psychology of Women*. New York: Grune and Stratton.

Deutsch, H. 1965. 'The Psychiatric Component in Gynaecology'. In *Neuroses and Character Types*. London: Hogarth Press.

Devereux, G. 1956. 'Normal and Abnormal: The Key Problem of Psychiatric Anthropology'. In *Some Uses of Anthropology: Theoretical and Applied*. Washington D.C.: Anthropological Society of Washington.

Devereux, G. 1978. *Ethnopsychoanalysis: Psychoanalysis and Anthropology as Complementary Frames of Reference*. Berkeley: University of California Press.

Devereux, G. 1980. *Basic Problems of Ethnopsychiatry*. Chicago: University of Chicago Press.

Douglas, M. 1966. *Purity and Danger: An Analysis of Concepts of Pollution and Taboo*. London: Routledge and Kegan Paul.

Douglas, M. 1970. *Natural Symbols*. London: Barrie and Rockliff.

Doyle, J.C. 1952. 'Unnecessary hysterectomies', *Journal of the American Medical Association* 151: 360–65.

Durkheim, E. 1966. [1895]. *The Rules of Sociological Method*. New York: Free Press.

Durkheim, E. 1984 [1893]. *The Division of Labour in Society*. London: Macmillan.

Echevarria, G. 1990. *Myth and Archive: A Theory of Latin American Narrative*. Cambridge: Cambridge University Press.

Eglītis, I. 1989. *Psihiatrija*. Riga: Zvaigzne.

Ellis, W.C. 1838. *A Treatise on the Nature, Symptoms, Causes and Treatment of Insanity*. London: Samuel Holdsworth.

Empson, W. 1935. *Some Varieties of Pastoral*. London: Chatto and Windus.

Erikson, E.H.1975. *Life History and the Historical Moment*. New York: Norton.

Estroff, S. 1981. *Making it Crazy: An Ethnography of Psychiatric Clients in an American Community*. Berkeley: University of California Press.

Feldhaus, A. 1983. *The Religious System of the Mahanubhav Sect*. New Delhi: Manohar.

Felman, S. and Laub, D. 1992. *Testimony: Crises of Witnessing in Literature, Psychoanalysis and History*. London: Routledge.

Fenton, S. and Sadiq-Sangster A. 1996. 'Culture, Relativism and the Expression of Mental Distress: South Asian Women in Britain', *Sociology of Health and Illness* 18(1): 66–85.

Fernandez, J.W. 1995. 'Amazing Grace: Meaning Deficit, Displacement and New Consciousness in Expressive Interaction', in Cohen, A.P. and Rapport, N. (eds). *Questions of Consciousness*. ASA monograph 33. London and New York: Routledge.

Fernando, S. 1988. *Race, Culture and Psychiatry*. London: Croom Helm.

Field, M.G. 1967. 'Soviet Psychiatry and Social Structure, Culture and Ideology: a Preliminary Assessment', *American Journal of Psychotherapy* 21: 230–43.

Fitzpatrick, S. 1996. 'Signals from Below: Soviet Letters of Denunciation of the 1930s', *Journal of Modern History* 68(4): 831–66.

Fortes, M. 1959. *Oedipus and Job in West African Religion*. Cambridge: Cambridge University Press.

Foucault, M. 1971. *Madness and Civilization: A History of Insanity in the Age of Reason*. London: Tavistock Publications.

Foucault, M. 1973. *The Birth of the Clinic*. London: Tavistock.

Foucault, M. 2002. *The Archaeology of Knowledge*. Translated by Sheridan, A.M. London: Routledge.

Frank, A. 1995. *The Wounded Storyteller: Body, Illness and Ethics*. Chicago: University of Chicago Press.

Frank, A. 2001. 'Can we research suffering?' *Qualitative Health Research* 11(3): 353–62.

Frankfurt, H.G. 1988. *The Importance Of What We Care About: Philosophical Essays*. Cambridge: Cambridge University Press.

Freud, S. 1900. *The Interpretation of Dreams*. London: Hogarth Press.

Freud, S. 1930. *Civilization and its Discontents*. London: Hogarth Press.

Freud, S. 1931. *Female Sexuality: Collected Papers 5*. London: Hogarth Press.

Freud, S. 1960. *Totem and Taboo*. London: Routledge and Kegan Paul.

Freud, S. 1966 [1901]. *The Psychopathology of Everyday Life*. Translated by James Strachey. London: Ernest Benn.

Freud, S. 1973 [1933]. *New Introductory Lectures on Psychoanalysis*. Translated by James Strachey. Harmondsworth: Penguin.

Freud, S. 1985. *The Complete Letters of Sigmund Freud to Wilhelm Fliess, 1887–1904*. (Ed.) Masson, J.M. Cambridge, Mass.: Belknap/Harvard.

Fuller, L. 1969. *The Morality of Law*. New Haven: Yale University Press.

Gadamer, G. 1989. *Truth and Method*. 2nd. edn. London: Sheed and Ward.

Gaines, A.D. and Farmer, P. 1986. 'Visible Saints: Social Cynosures and Dysphoria in the Mediterranean Tradition', *Culture, Medicine and Psychiatry* 10(4): 295–330.

Gassmann, F., and de Neubourg, C. 2000. *Coping with Little Means in Latvia*. Social Policy Research Series. Riga: Ministry of Welfare of the Republic of Latvia and United Nations Development Programme.

Geertz, C. 1973. *The Interpretation of Cultures*. New York: Basic Books.

Geertz, C. 1988. *Works and Lives: The Anthropologist as Author*. Cambridge: Polity Press.

Geertz, C. 1993. 'Blurred Genres: The Refiguration of Social Thought'. In *Local Knowledge. Further Essays In Interpretive Anthropology*. New York: Basic Books.

Gellner, E. 1982. 'Relativism and Universals'. In Hollis, M. and Lukes, S. (eds). *Rationality and Relativism*. Oxford: Basil Blackwell.

Gerber, E.R. 1985. 'Rage and Obligation: Samoan Emotion in Conflict'. In White, G.M. and Kirkpatrick, J. (eds). *Person, Self and Experience: Exploring Pacific Ethnopsychologies*. Berkeley: University of California Press.

Gergen, K. 1994. *Realities and Relationships: Soundings in Social Construction*. Cambridge: Cambridge University Press.

Gergen, K.J. and Gergen, M.M. 1986. 'Narrative Form and the Construction of Psychological Science'. In Sarbin, T.R. (ed). *Narrative Psychology*. New York: Praeger.

Giddens, A. 1984. *The Constitution of Society: Outline of the Theory of Structuration*. Cambridge: Polity Press.

Gleason, P. 1983. 'Identifying Identity: A Semantic History', *Journal of American History* 69(4): 910–31.

Gluckman, M. 1962. In Gluckman, M. (ed). *Essays on the Ritual of Social Relations*. Manchester: Manchester University Press.

Glucksmann, M. 1994. 'The Work of Knowledge and the Knowledge of Women's Work'. In Maynard, M. and Purvis, J. (eds). *Researching Women's Lives from a Feminist Perspective*. London: Taylor and Francis.

Goffman, E. 1968. *Asylums: Essays on the Social Situation of Mental Patients and Other Inmates.* Harmondsworth: Penguin.

Goffman, E. 1963. *Stigma: Notes on the Management of Spoiled Identity.* Harmondsworth: Penguin.

Goldie, P. 2000. *The Emotions: A Philosophical Exploration.* Oxford: Oxford University Press.

Good, B.J. 1994. *Medicine, Rationality and Experience: An Anthropological Perspective.* Cambridge: Cambridge University Press.

Gugelberger, G. 1996. 'Introduction' In Gugelberger, G. (ed). *The Real Thing.* Durham, NC: Duke University Press.

Hacking, I. 1982. 'Language, Truth and Reason'. In Hollis, M. and Lukes, S. (eds). *Rationality and Relativism.* Oxford: Basil Blackwell.

Hacking, I. 1986. 'Making Up People'. In Heller, T.C., Morton, S., and Wellbery, D.E. (eds). *Reconstructing Individualism: Autonomy, Individuality and the Self in Western Thought.* Stanford: Stanford University Press.

Hacking, I. 1996. *Rewriting the Soul: Multiple Personality and the Sciences of Memory.* Princeton: Princeton University Press.

Hacking, I. 1998. *Mad Travellers: Reflections on the Reality of Transient Mental Illness.* London: Free Association Books.

Hacking, I. 1999. *The Social Construction of What.* Cambridge, Mass.: Harvard University Press.

Halbwachs, M. 1981 [1950]. *On Collective Memory.* New York: Harper Row.

Handler, R. 1994. 'Is "Identity" a Useful Concept?' In Gillis, J.R. (ed). *Commemorations: The Politics of National Identity.* Princeton: Princeton University Press.

Hann, C. 1996. 'Introduction: Political Society and Civil Anthropology'. In Hann, C. and Dunn, E. (eds.) *Civil Society: Anthropological Approaches.* New York: Routledge.

Hare, E.H. 1962. 'Masturbational Insanity: The History of an Idea', *Journal of Mental Science* 108: 1–25.

Harris, G. 1959. 'Possession "Hysteria" in a Kenya Tribe', *American Anthropology* 61: 1046–66.

Havel, V. 1980. *The Memorandum.* New York: Grove Press.

Havel, V. 1986. *Living in Truth.* London: Faber and Faber.

Healy, D. 1997. *The Anti-depressant Era.* Cambridge, Mass.: Harvard University Press.

Hegel, G.W.F. 1997. *Phenomenology of Spirit.* Translated by Miller, A.V. Chicago: University of Chicago Press.

Heller, A. 1987. *Beyond Justice.* Oxford: Basil Blackwell.

Hoffmaster, B. 1992. 'Can Ethnography Save Medical Ethics?' *Social Science and Medicine* 35(12): 1421–31.

Hollis, M. 1982. 'The Social Destruction of Reality'. In Hollis, M. and Lukes, S. (eds). *Rationality and Relativism.* Oxford: Basil Blackwell.

Homer. 1965. *The Odyssey of Homer.* Translated by Lattimore, R. New York: Harper and Row.

Horney, K. 1967. *Feminine Psychology.* London: Routledge and Kegan Paul.

House, J.S., Landis, K. and Umberson, D. 1988. 'Social Relationships and Health', *Science* 241: 540–5.

Howell, S. 1997. 'Introduction'. In Howell, S. (ed). *The Ethnography of Moralities.* London: Routledge.

Hume, D. 1932 [1734]. *Letters of David Hume.* Greig, J.Y.T. (ed). Oxford: Oxford University Press.

Humphrey, C. 1994. 'Remembering an "Enemy" the Bogd Khaan in Twentieth-Century Mongolia'. In Watson. R.S. (ed). *Memory, History, and Opposition under State Socialism*. Santa Fe: School of American Research Press.

Irvine, J. 1989. 'When Talk Isn't Cheap: Language and Political Economy'. *American Ethnologist* 16: 248–67.

Irvine, J.T. 1982. 'The Creation of Identity in Spirit Mediumship and Possession'. In Parkin, D. (ed). *Semantic Anthropology*. London: Academic Press.

Jackson J.B. 1979. 'The Order of a Landscape: Reason and Religion in Newtonian America'. In Meining, D.W. (ed). *The Interpretation of Ordinary Landscapes*. New York and Oxford: Oxford University Press.

Jadhav, S. 2000. 'The Cultural Construction of Western Depression'. In Skultans,V. and Cox, J. (eds). *Anthropological Approaches to Psychological Medicine: Crossing Bridges*. London: Jessica Kingsley.

Jakobson, R. 1971. 'Shifters, Verbal Categories and the Russian Verb'. In *Selected Writing of Roman Jakobson* volume 2: 130–47. The Hague: Mouton Press.

Jenkins, J.H. 1991. 'The State Construction of Affect: Political Ethos and Mental Health among Salvadoran Refugees', *Culture Medicine and Psychiatry* 15: 139–65.

Johnson, W.O. 1939. 'Emotional Disturbances with Pelvic Symptoms', *Southern Surgeon* 8: 373–83.

Jones, E. 1924. 'Psychoanalysis and Anthropology', *Journal of the Royal Anthropological Institute* 54: 47–66.

Jones, S.A. 1994. 'Old Ghosts and New Chains: Ethnicity and Memory in the Georgian Republic'. In Watson, R.S. (ed). *Memory, History and Opposition under State Socialism*. Santa Fe, NM: School of American Research Press.

Kafka Franz 1994 [1925]. *The Trial*. Harmondsworth: Penguin.

Kakar, S. 1982. *Shamans, Mystics and Doctors: A Psychological Inquiry into India and Its Healing Traditions*. Delhi: Oxford University Press.

Karvé, I. 1965. *Kinship Organisation in India*. 2nd. edn. Bombay: Asia Publishing House.

Kemp, M. 2004. *Agency and Discourse on Distress*. Unpublished PhD thesis, Department of Psychiatry, University of Bristol.

Kemper, T.D. 1984. 'Power, Status and Emotions: A Sociological Contribution to a Psychophysiological Domain'. In Scherer, K.R. and Ekman, P. (eds). *Approaches to Emotion*. Hillsdale, NJ: Lawrence Erlbaum.

Ķīlis, R. 1996. 'Social Memory as a Constituent of Collective Identity in Latvia: the Case of Deportations' Unpublished paper given at the European Institute, London School of Economics, 5 March.

Kirk, D. 1964. *Shared Fate*. Glencoe, Ill.: The Free Press.

Kirmayer, L. 1988. 'Mind and Body as Metaphors: Hidden Values as Metaphors'. In Lock, M. and Gordon, D. (eds). *Biomedicine Examined*. Dordrecht: Kluwer Academic Publishers.

Kirmayer, L. 1994. 'Editorial: A Symposium on Neurasthenia and Fatigue Syndromes', *Transcultural Psychiatric Research Review* 31: 99–100.

Kirmayer, L. 2003. 'Failures of Imagination: The Refugee's Narrative in Psychiatry', *Anthropology and Medicine* 10(2): 167–85.

Kleinman, A. 1977. 'Depression, Somatization and the "New Cross-Cultural Psychiatry"', *Social Science and Medicine* 11: 3–10.

Kleinman, A. 1982. 'Neurasthenia and Depression: a Study of Somatization and Culture in China', *Culture, Medicine and Psychiatry* 6: 117–90.

Kleinman, A. 1986. *The Social Origins of Distress and Disease: Depression, Neurasthenia and Pain in Modern China*. New Haven and London: Yale University Press.

Kleinman, A. 1988. *The Illness Narratives: Suffering, Healing and the Human Condition*. New York: Basic Books.

Kleinman, A. 1997. *Writing at the Margins: Discourse Between Anthropology and Medicine*. Berkeley: University of California Press.

Kleinman, A. and Kleinman, J. 1994. 'How Bodies Remember: Social Memory and Bodily Experience of Criticism, Resistance and Delegitimation Following China's Cultural Revolution', *New Literary History* 25: 707–23.

Kleinman, A. and Kleinman, J. 1996. 'The Appeal of Experience; the Dismay of Images: Cultural Appropriations of Suffering in our Times', *Daedalus* 125(1): 1–23.

Kolb, L. 1966. 'Soviet Psychiatric Organization and the Community Mental Health Care Concept', *American Journal of Psychiatry* 123(4): 433–39.

Kozlov, V.A. 1996. 'Denunciation and Its Functions in Soviet Governance: A Study of Denunciations and their Bureaucratic Handling from Soviet Police Archives, 1944–1953'. *Journal of Modern History* 68(4): 867–98.

Kraepelin, E. 1974. 'Comparative Psychiatry', and 'Patterns of Mental Disorder'. In Hirsch, S. and Shepherd, M. (eds). *Themes and Variations in European Psychiatry*. Bristol: John Wright.

Kultūras Fonda Izdevums. 1928. *Kultūras Fonds 1920–28*. Riga: A. Gulbis.

Kuper, A. 1988. *The Invention of Primitive Society: Transformations of an Illusion*. London: Routledge and Kegan Paul.

Kuper, A. 1991. 'Anthropologists and the History of Anthropology', *Critique of Anthropology* 11(2): 125–42.

Kynch, J. and Sen, A. 1983. 'Indian Women, Well-Being and Survival', *Cambridge Journal of Economics* 7: 363–80.

LaCapra, D. 1998. *History and Memory after Auschwitz*. Ithaca and London: Cornell University Press.

Lader, M. 1977. *Psychiatry on Trial*. Harmondsworth: Penguin

Laing, R.D. 1971. *The Self and Others*. Harmondsworth: Penguin.

Lallemand, J. 1847. *A Treatise on Spermatorrhoea*. Translated by McDougall, H.J. London: John Churchill.

Lang, B. 1992. 'The Representation of Limits'. In Friedlander, S. (ed). *Probing the Limits of Representation: Nazism and the 'Final Solution'*. Cambridge, Mass.: Harvard University Press.

Langer, L.L. 1991. *Holocaust Testimonies: The Ruins of Memory*. New Haven: Yale University Press.

Latvian National Foundation. 1982. *These Names Accuse: Nominal List of Latvians Deported to Russia 1940–1941*. Stockholm: Latvian National Foundation.

Latvijas Republikas Veselības Aizsardzības Ministrija. 1991. *Medicīniskās Aprūpes Kvalitātes Standarti* [Standards of the Quality of Medical Care], Riga. Latvijas Republikas Veselības Aizsardzības Ministrija.

Latvijas Republikas Labklājības Ministrija. 2000. *Sociālais Ziņojums* [Social Notification], Riga: Labklājības Ministrija.

Laub, D. 1992. 'Bearing Witness or the Vicissitudes of Listening'. In Felman, S. and Laub, D. *Testimony: Crises of Witnessing in Literature, Psychoanalysis and History*. London: Routledge.

Lavater, J.C. 1848 [1778]. *Essays on Physiognomy*. 5th edn. London: William Tegg and Co.

Lebensohn, Z.M. 1962. 'The Organization and Character of Soviet Psychiatry', *American Journal of Psychotherapy* 16: 295–301.

Le Roy Ladurie, E. 1979. *The Territory of the Historian*. Hassocks: Harvester.

Levitas, R. 1995. 'We: Problems in Identity, Solidarity and Difference', *History of the Human Sciences* 8(3): 89–105.

Lévy-Bruhl L. 1966. *How Natives Think*. New York: Washington Square Press.

Lewis G. 1976. *Knowledge of Illness in a Sepik Society. A Study of the Gnau, New Guinea*. London: Athlone.

Lewis, I. 1966. 'Spirit Possession and Deprivation Cults', *Man* 1(3): 307–29.

Lewis, I. 1971. *Ecstatic Religion*. Harmondsworth: Penguin.

Leydesdorff, S., Dawson, G., Burchardt, N. and Ashplant, T.G. 2002. 'Introduction: Trauma and Life Stories'. In Rogers, K.L., Leydesdorff, S. and Dawson, G. (eds). *Trauma and Life Stories: International Perspectives*. London and New York: Routledge.

Līce A. (ed.). 1990. *Via Dolorosa*. Riga: Liesma.

Lichtenberg, G. 1783. 'Fragment von Schwanzen', *Baldingers Neues Magazin für Aerzte 5*.

Lieven, A. 1993. *The Baltic Revolution: Estonia, Latvia, Lithuania and the Path to Independence*. New Haven and London: Yale University Press.

Littlewood, R. 1986. 'Russian Dolls and Chines Boxes: An Anthropological Approach to the Implicit Models of Comparative Psychiatry'. In Cox, J.L. (ed). *Transcultural Psychiatry*. London: Croom Helm.

Littlewood, R. 2000. 'Psychiatry's Culture'. In Skultans, V. and Cox, J. (eds.) *Anthropological Approaches to Psychological Medicine*. London: Jessica Kingsley.

Littlewood, R. and Lipsedge, M. 1982. *Aliens and Alienists*. Harmondsworth: Penguin.

Littlewood, R. and Lipsedge, M. 1997. *Aliens and Alienists*. 3rd edn. London: Routledge.

Loudon J. 1976. 'Introduction'. In Loudon J. (ed.) *Social Anthropology and Medicine*. ASA Monograph 13. London and New York: Academic Press.

Luhrmann, T. 2001. *Of Two Minds: The Growing Disorder in American Psychiatry*. London: Picador.

Lutz, T. 1995. 'Neurasthenia and Fatigue Syndromes'. In Berrios, G. and Porter, R. (eds.) *A History of Clinical Psychiatry: the Origin and History of Psychiatric Disorders*. London: Athlone.

Macdonald, M. 1981. *Mystical Bedlam*. Cambridge and New York: Cambridge University Press.

MacIntyre, A. 1992 [1981]. *After Virtue: a Study in Moral Theory*. London: Duckworth.

Maddock, A.B. 1854. *Practical Observations on Mental and Nervous Disorders*. London: Simpkin, Marshall and Co.

Malinowski, B. 1921. 'Review of McDougall's group mind', *Man* 21: 106–9.

Mandlebaum, D.G. 1988. *Women's Seclusion and Men's Honour. Sex Roles in North India, Bangladesh, and Pakistan*. Tucson: University of Arizona Press.

Mansbach S.A. 1997. *Modern Art in Eastern Europe: From the Baltic to the Balkans, ca.1890–1939*. Cambridge: Cambridge University Press.

Marcus, G.E. and Fischer, M. 1986. *Anthropology as Cultural Critique: An Experimental Moment in the Human Sciences*. Chicago: University of Chicago Press.

Maudsley, H. 1868. 'Illustrations of a Variety of Insanity', *Journal of Mental Science* 14: 149–62.

Maudsley, H. 1879. *The Pathology of Mind*. London: Macmillan and Co.

Mauss, M. 1979. *Sociology and Psychology*. Translated by Brewster, B. London: Routledge and Kegan Paul.

Medvedev, Z. and Medvedev, R. 1971. *A Question of Madness*. Translated by Kadt, E. de. London: Macmillan.

Meinig, D.W. 1979. 'The Beholding Eye: Ten Versions of the Same Scene'. In Meinig, D.W. (ed.) *The Interpretation of Ordinary Landscapes*. New York and Oxford: Oxford University Press.

Merkel, G. 1797. *Die Letten am Ende des Philosophischen Jahrhunderts*. Leipzig: H. Graff.

Merkelis, G. 1999. *Latvieši, Seviški Vidzemē, Filosofiskā Gada Simta Beigās*. Riga: Zvaigzne.

Merleau-Ponty, M. 1989. *Phenomenology of Perception*. London: Routledge.

Merridale, C. 1996. 'Death and Memory in Modern Russia', *History Workshop Journal* 42: 1–18.

Middleton, J. 1960. *Lugbara Religion*. London: Oxford University Press.

Miller, B.L. 1981. 'Autonomy and the Refusal of Life Saving Treatment', *Hastings Centre Report* 11(4): 22–28.

Miller, N.F. 1946. 'Hysterectomies: Therapeutic Necessity or Surgical Racket?' *American Journal of Obstetric Gynaecology* 51: 804–10.

Mills, C.W. 1970. *The Sociological Imagination*. Harmondsworth: Penguin.

Milton, J. 1854. 'On the Nature and Treatment of Spermatorrhoea', *Lancet* 1: 243–46, 269–70, 467–68, 595–96.

Mishler E.G. 1984. *The Discourse of Medicine*. Westport, CT: Ablex.

Misiunas, R.J. and Taagepera, R. 1993. *The Baltic States: Years of Dependence 1940–1990*. London: Hurst.

Mitchell W.J.T. 1994. *Picture Theory*. Chicago and London: University of Chicago Press.

Moore, H. 1988. *Feminism and Anthropology*. Cambridge: Polity Press.

Morison, A. 1824. *Outlines of Mental Diseases*. Edinburgh: MacLachlan and Stewart.

Morris, D.B. 2002. 'Narrative, Ethics and Pain: Thinking with Stories'. In Charon, R. and Montello, M. (eds.) *Stories Matter: The Role of Narrative in Medical Ethics*. London and New York: Routledge.

Mukarovsky, J. 1977. *The Word and Verbal Art: Selected Essays by Jan Mukarovsky*. Translated by Burbank, J. and Steiner, P. New Haven and London: Yale University Press.

Musil, R. 1997. *The Man Without Qualities*. Translated by Wilkinson, S. and Pike, B. London: Picador.

Myasischev, V.N. 1963. *Personality and Neuroses*. Translated by Wortis J. et al. Washington, DC: Joint Publications Research Service.

Nagel, T. 1991. *Mortal Questions*. Cambridge: Cambridge University Press.

Needham, R. 1962. *Structure and Sentiment: A Test Case in Anthropology*. Chicago: University of Chicago Press.

Newton-Smith, W. 1982. 'Relativism and the Possibility of Interpretation'. In Hollis, M. and Lukes, S. (eds.) *Rationality and Relativism*. Oxford: Basil Blackwell.

Nichter, M. 1981. 'Idioms of Distress: Alternatives in the Expression of Psychosocial Illness: A Case Study from South India', *Culture, Medicine and Psychiatry* 11: 289–335.

Nuckolls, C.W. 1992. 'Toward a Cultural History of the Personality Disorders', *Social Science and Medicine* 35(1): 37–47.

Nussbaum, M.C. 2001. *Upheavals of Thought: The Intelligence of Emotions.* Cambridge and New York: Cambridge University Press.

Obeyesekere, G. 1981. *Medusa's Hair: An Essay on Personal Symbols and Religious Experience.* Chicago: University of Chicago Press.

Ong, A. 1987. *Spirits of Resistance and Capitalist Discipline. Factory Women in Malaysia.* Albany: State University of New York Press.

Opler, M. 1969. 'Anthropological Contributions to Psychiatry and Social Psychiatry'. In Plog, S. and Edgerton, R. (eds.) *Changing Perspectives in Mental Illness.* New York: Holt Reinhart and Winston.

Orenstein, H. 1965. *Gaon: Conflict and Cohesion in an Indian Village.* Princeton, New Jersey: Princeton University Press.

Pabriks, A. and Purs, A. 2001. *Latvia: The Challenges of Change.* London and New York: Routledge.

Painter, C. 1996. *At Home with Constable's Cornfield.* London: National Gallery.

Parsons, T. 1951. *The Social System.* Glencoe, Ill.: The Free Press.

Passerini, L. 1987. *Fascism in Popular Memory: The Cultural Experience of the Turin Working Class.* Cambridge: Cambridge University Press.

Passerini, L. (ed.) 1992. 'Introduction' *Memory and Totalitarianism.* International Yearbook of Oral History and Life Stories. Oxford: Oxford University Press.

Penciks, A. 1967. *Nervu slimību un to profilakse* [Nervous Illnesses and their Prophylaxes]. Riga: Zinatne.

Pfleiderer, B. 1988. 'Ritual Healing in a North Indian Muslim Shrine', *Social Science and Medicine* 27: 415–24.

Plakans, A. 1995. *The Latvians: A Short History.* Stanford: Hoover Press.

Platt, K. 1996. 'Places of Experience and the Experience of Place'. In Rouner, L.S. (ed.) *The Longing for Home.* Indiana: University of Notre Dame Press.

Podrabinek, A. 1980. *Punitive Medicine.* Translated by Lehrman, A. Ann Arbor, MI: Karoma Publishers.

Popper, K.R. 1963. *Conjectures and Refutations.* London: Routledge.

Porter, R. 1991. 'History of the Body'. In Burke, P. (ed.) *New Perspectives on Historical Writing.* Oxford: Polity Press.

Poulet, G. 1963. *L'Espace Proustien.* Paris: Gallimard.

Putnam, R. D. 2000. *Bowling Alone.* New York: Touchstone.

Quine, W.V. 1960. *Word and Object.* Cambridge, Mass.: MIT Press.

Radcliffe-Brown, A.R. 1952. *Structure and Function in Primitive Society: Essays and Addresses.* London: Cohen and West.

Raeside, I. 1976. 'The Mahanubhavas'. *Bulletin of the School of Oriental and African Studies* 39(3): 585–600.

Rapport, N. 1997. *Transcendent Individual: Towards a Literary and Liberal Anthropology.* London and New York: Routledge.

Reich, W. 1984. 'Psychiatric Diagnosis as an Ethical Problem'. In Bloch, S. and Chodoff, P. (eds.) *Psychiatric Ethics.* Oxford, New York and Melbourne: Oxford University Press.

Ricoeur, P. 1976. *Discourse and the Surplus of Meaning.* Fort Worth: Texas Christian University Press.

Ricoeur, P. 2004. *Memory, History and Forgetting.* Translated by Blamey, K. and Pellauer, D. Chicago: Chicago University Press.

Riessman, C.K. 1993. *Narrative Analysis.* Newbury Park and London: Sage.

Rivers, W.H.R. 1917. 'Freud's Psychology of the Unconscious', *The Lancet* 95: 913–14.

Rivers, W.H.R. 1978 [1916]. 'Sociology and Psychology'. In Slobodin, R. *W.H.R. Rivers.* New York: Columbia University Press.

Robinson, D. 1971. *The Process of Becoming Ill.* London: Routledge and Kegan Paul.

Rogers, S.C. 1978. 'Women's Place: A Critical Review of Anthropological Theory'. *Comparative Studies in Society and History* 20: 123–62.

Rorty, R. 1989. *Contingency, Irony and Solidarity.* Cambridge: Cambridge University Press.

Rosaldo, M.Z. 1980. *Knowledge and Passion. Ilongot Notions of Self and Society.* Cambridge and New York: Cambridge University Press.

Rosaldo, R. 1993. *Culture and Truth: The Remaking of Social Analysis.* London: Routledge.

Rose, N. 1997. 'Assembling the Modern Self'. In Porter, R. (ed.) *Rewriting the Self.* London and New York: Routledge.

Rose, N. 1998. *Inventing Our Selves: Psychology, Power and Personhood.* Cambridge: Cambridge University Press.

Roskill, M. 1997. *The Languages of Landscape.* Pennsylvania: Pennsylvania State University Press.

Rossi, J. 1987. *The Gulag Handbook.* New York: Paragon House.

Rothman, D. 1971. *The Discovery of the Asylum: Social Order and Disorder in the New Republic.* Boston and Toronto: Little, Brown and Co.

Ryang, S. 2000. 'Ethnography or Self-cultural Anthropology? Reflections on Writing about Ourselves', *Dialectical Anthropology* 25: 297–320.

Ryle, G. 1949. *The Concept of Mind.* London: Hutchinson.

Sacks, O. 1998. *The Man Who Mistook His Wife for a Hat and Other Clinical Tales.* New York: Simon Schuster.

Schama, S. 1995. *Landscape and Memory.* London: HarperCollins.

Scheper-Hughes, N. 1992. *Death Without Weeping: The Violence of Everyday Life in Brazil.* Berkeley: University of California Press.

Scheper-Hughes, N. and Lock, M. 1987. 'The Mindful Body: A Prolegomenon to Future Work in Medical Anthropology', *Medical Anthropology Quarterly* 1: 6–41.

Scull, A. 1989. *Social Order/Mental Disorder: Anglo American Psychiatry.* London: Routledge and Kegan Paul.

Sedgwick, P. 1972. 'Mental Illness is Illness', *Salmagundi* (20): 196–222.

Seeman, T.E. 1996. 'Social Ties and Health: The Benefits of Social Integration', *Annual of Epidemiology* 6: 442–51.

Seligman, C.G. 1924a. 'Anthropology and Psychology: A Study of Some Points of Contact', *Journal of the Royal Anthropological Institute* 54: 13–47.

Seligman, C.G. 1924b. 'A Note on Dreams', *Journal of the Royal Anthropological Institute* 23: 186–8.

Shorter, E. 1992. *From Paralysis to Fatigue: A History of Psychosomatic Illness in the Modern Era.* New York: The Free Press.

Shotter, J. 2004. 'Expressing and Legitimating Actionable Knowledge from Within'. Unpublished paper.

Shweder, R.A., Nancy, C., Manamohan, M. and Lawrence, P. 1997. 'The "Big Three" of Morality (Autonomy, Community, Divinity) and Explanations of suffering'. In Brandt, A.M. and Roxin, P. (eds.) *Morality and Health.* New York and London: Routledge.

Siliņš, J. 1979. *Latvijas Māksla 1800–1914.* [Latvian Art 1800–1914]. Stockholm: Daugava.

Siliņš, J. 1990. *Latvijas Māksla 1915–1940.* [Latvian Art 1915–1940]. Stockholm: Daugava.

Silverstein, M. 1998. 'Monoglot "Standard" in America: Standardization and Metaphors of Linguistic Hegemony'. In Brenneis, D. and Macauley, R. (eds.) *The Matrix of Language*. Boulder: Westview Press.

Skae, D. 1863. 'A Rational and Practical Classification of Insanity', *The Journal of Mental Science* 9: 309–19.

Skujenieks, M. 1938. *Latvijas Statistikas Atlass*. Riga: Bureau Statistique de l'Etat.

Skultans, V. 1974. *Intimacy and Ritual: A Study of Spiritualism, Mediums and Groups*. London: Routledge and Kegan Paul.

Skultans, V. 1987. 'The Management of Mental Illness among Maharashtrian Families: A Case Study of a Mahanubhav Healing Temple', *Man. Journal of the Royal Anthropological Institute* 22: 661–79.

Skultans, V. 1995. 'Neurasthenia and Political Resistance in Latvia', *Anthropology Today* 11(6): 14–18.

Skultans, V. 1997. 'Theorizing Latvian Lives. The Quest for Identity', *Journal of the Royal Anthropological Institute* 3(4): 1–20.

Skultans, V. 1998a. *The Testimony of Lives: Narrative and Memory in Post-Soviet Latvia*. New York and London: Routledge.

Skultans, V. 1998b. 'Remembering Latvian Childhood and the Escape from History', *Auto/Biography* 6(1–2): 5–13.

Skultans, V. 2004. 'Narratives of Displacement and Identity'. In Hurwitz, B., Greenhalgh, T. and Skultans, V. (eds.) *Narrative Research in Health and Illness*. Oxford: Blackwell.

Skultans, V. 2007. 'The Appropriation of Suffering. Psychiatric Practice in ther Post-Soviet Clinic', *Theory, Culture and Society* 24(3): 27–48.

Smith, D.E. 1978. 'K is Mentally Ill: The Anatomy of a Factual Account', *Sociology* 12: 23–53.

Smith, D.E. 1993. *Texts, Facts and Femininity: Exploring the Relations of Ruling*. London and New York: Routledge.

Sokolowski, R. 1978. *Presence and Absence. A Philosophical Investigation of Language and Being*. Bloomington: Indiana University Press.

Sommer, D. 1996. 'No Secrets'. In Gugelberger, G. (ed.) *The Real Thing*. Durham and London: Duke University Press.

Sontheimer, G.D. 1989. *Pastoral Deities in Western India*. New York: Oxford University Press.

Spitzka, E.C. 1887. 'Cases of Masturbation', *Journal of Nervous and Mental Diseases* 33.

Stacey, J. 1991. 'Can There Be a Feminist Ethnography?' In Gluck, S. and Patai, D. (eds.) *Women's Words The Feminist Practice of Oral History*. London and New York: Routledge.

Stocking, G.W. 1986. 'Anthropology and the Science of the Irrational: Malinowski's Encounter with Freudian Psychoanalysis'. In Stocking, G.W. (ed.) *Malinowski, Rivers, Benedict and Others: Essay on Culture and Personality*. Madison: University of Wisconsin Press.

Sullivan, M. 1986. 'In What Sense is Contemporary Medicine Dualistic?' *Culture, Medicine and Psychiatry* 10: 331–50.

Švābe, A. 1930. *Agrarian History of Latvia*. Riga: Bernhard Lamey.

Švābe, A. 1950. *Latvian Encyclopaedia*. Stockholm: Tris Zvaigznes.

Szasz, T. 1971. *The Manufacture of Madness: A Comparative Study of the Inquisition and the Mental Health Movement*. London: Routledge and Kegan Paul.

Tambiah, S. 1970. *Buddhism and the Spirit Cults in North-East Thailand*. Cambridge: Cambridge University Press.

Taylor, C. 1985. *Human Agency and Language*. Cambridge: Cambridge University Press.

Thompson, J.B. 1984. *Studies in the Theory of Ideology*. Cambridge: Polity Press.

Thomson, A. 1998. 'Anzac Memories: Putting Popular Memory Theory into Practice'. In Perks, R. and Thomson, A. (eds.) *Oral History Reader*. London: Routledge.

Timpanaro, S. 1976. *The Freudian Slip: Psychoanalysis and Textual Criticism*. London: NLB.

Titavs, D. 1998. 'Viņi tika represēti likumīgi' [They Were Repressed Lawfully]. *Diena* April 14.

Tolstoy, L. 1980. *Anna Karenina*. Translated by Louise and Aylmer Maude. Oxford: Oxford University Press.

Tonkin, E. 1995. *Narrating Our Pasts: The Social Construction of Oral History*. Cambridge: Cambridge University Press.

Torpey, J. 1998. *Intellectuals, Socialism and Dissent: The East German Opposition and its Legacy*. Minneapolis and London: University of Minnesota Press.

Toulmin, S. 1988. 'The Recovery of Practical Philosophy', *American Scholar* 57: 349.

Tuan, Y. 1977. *Space and Place: The Perspective of Experience*. London: Edward Arnold.

Tucker, P.H. 1990. *Monet in the '90s: The Series Paintings*. New Haven and London: Yale University Press.

Turner, T. 1994. 'Bodies and Anti-Bodies: Flesh and Fetish in Contemporary Social Theory'. In Csordas, T.J. (ed.) *Embodiment and Experience: The Existential Ground of Culture and Self*. Cambridge: Cambridge University Press.

Turner, V. 1964. 'Symbols in Ndemba Ritual'. In Gluckman, M. (ed.) *Closed Systems and Open Minds: The Limits of Naivety in Social Anthropology*. Edinburgh: Oliver Boyd.

Turner, V. 1974. *Dramas, Fields and Metaphors: Symbolic Action in Human Society*. Ithaca, NY: Cornell University Press.

Turner, V. 1979. 'Preface', in Myerhoff, B. *Number Our Days*. New York: Simon Schuster.

Tylor, E.B. 1958. *The Origins of Culture*. New York: Harper Row.

Upleja, I. and Titavs, D. 1998. 'Vai Pienācis Laiks Vētīt Čekas maisus Latvijā?' [Has the Time Come to the Bags of the Cheka in Latvia?] *Diena* Oct. 26.

Ullrich, H. 1987. 'A Study of Change and Depression among Havik Brahmin Women in a South Indian Village', *Culture Medicine and Psychiatry* 11(3): 261–87.

Van Gennep, A. 1909. *Les Rites de Passage*. Paris: Emile Nourry.

Vatuk, S. 1980. 'The Aging Woman in India: Self Perceptions and Changing Roles'. In de Souza, A. (ed.) *Women in Contemporary India and South Asia*. New Delhi: Manohar.

Velmers, O. 1992. 'Medicine in Latvia'. Unpublished paper.

Velody, I. 1998. 'The Archive and the Human Sciences: Notes Towards a Theory of the Archive', *History of the Human Sciences* 11(4): 1–6.

Verdery, K. 1996. *What was Socialism and What Comes Next?* Princeton: Princeton University Press.

Virgil. 1980. *The Eclogues*. Translated by Lee, G. Harmondsworth: Penguin.

Waitzkin, H. 1991. *The Politics of Medical Encounters: How Patients and Doctors Deal with Social Problems*. New Haven and London: Yale University Press.

Weber, M. 1991. *From Max Weber: Essays in Sociology*. Gerth, H.H. and Mills, C.W. (eds.) London and New York: Routledge.

Wedel, J.R. (ed.) 1992. *The Unplanned Society: Poland During and After Communism*. New York: Columbia University Press.

Weiss, M.G., Desai, A., Jadhav, S., Behere, P.B., Gupta, L., Channabasavanna, S.M. and Doongaji, D.R. Year? 'Humoral Concepts of Medicine', *Social Science and Medicine* 27(5): 471–77.

Wessely, S. 1994a. 'The History of Chronic Fatigue Syndrome'. In Strauss, S.E. (ed.) *Chronic Fatigue Syndrome*. New York: Marcel Dekker.

Wessely, S. 1994b. 'Neurasthenia and Chronic Fatigue: Theory and Practice in Britain and America', *Transcultural Psychiatric Research Review* 31: 173–209.

Wiesel, E. 1996. 'Longing for Home'. In Rouner, L.S. (ed.) *The Longing for Home*. Indiana: University of Notre Dame Press.

Wieviorka, A. 1994. 'On Testimony'. In Hartman, G.H. (ed.) *Holocaust Remembrance: The Shapes of Memory*. Oxford: Basil Blackwell.

Wilkinson, R.G. 1996. *Unhealthy Societies: From Inequality to Well-Being*. New York and London: Routledge.

Williams, G.H. 1984. 'The Genesis of Chronic Illness: Narrative Re-construction'. *Sociology of Health and Illness* 6(2): 175–99.

Williams, G.H. 1993. 'Chronic Illness and the Pursuit of Virtue'. In Radley, A. (ed.) *Worlds of Illness: Biographical and Cultural Perspectives on Health and Disease*. London: Routledge.

Williams, G.H. and Wood, P.H.N. 1986. 'Common-sense Beliefs about Illness: A Mediating Role for the Doctor', *Lancet* 20(27): 1435–37.

Williams, R. 1993 [1973]. *The Country and the City*. London: Hogarth Press.

Wittgenstein, L. 2001. *Philosophical Investigations*. Oxford: Blackwell.

Woodward, S.B. 1835. *Worcester State Hospital Annual Report*. Mass.: Worcester State Hospital.

Yates, F. 1966. *The Art of Memory*. London: Routledge and Kegan Paul.

Young, A. 1995. *The Harmony of Illusions. Inventing Post Traumatic Stress Disorder*. Princeton: Princeton University Press.

Yudice, G. 1996. 'Testimonio and Postmodernism'. In Gugelberger, G. (ed.) *The Real Thing*. Durham and London: Duke University Press.

Zālīte, I. 2000. 'Ideoloģiskās Kontroles Mehānismi LPSR Augstskolās'. http://vip.latnet.lv/ lpra/ a-skol1.html. (accessed 6.5.2001).

Zborowski, M. 1952. 'Cultural Components in Responses to Pain', *Journal of Social Issues* 4: 16–30.

Ziferstein, I. 1972. 'Group Therapy in the Soviet Union', *American Journal of Psychiatry* 129(5): 595–99.

Ziferstein, I. 1976. 'Psychotherapy in the USSR'. In Carson S.A., O'Leary Carson, E. (eds.) *Psychiatry and Psychology in the USSR*. New York and London: Plenum Press.

Zīle, L. 1991. 'Latvijas Rusifikācija', In *Latvijas Vēsture* 1: 31–36.

Zola, I. 1966. 'Culture and Symptoms: An Analysis of Patients' Presenting Complaints', *American Sociological Review* 31: 615–29.

Zonabend, F. 1984. *The Enduring Memory: Time and History in a French Village*. Manchester: Manchester University Press.

INDEX

Foucault, Michel, 114; on language
hiding truth, 114
Frank, Arthur, 15; on 'thinking with
stories', 15
Freud, Sigmund, 97; on primitive
mentalities, 97; on primary and
secondary thought processes, 101,
113; on breakdown of division of
normal and abnormal, 114; on the
irrational, 115

G
Gadamer, Hans-Georg, 5; on learning a
first and second language, 5
Gaines, Atwood, 8; on illness and
visible saints, 8
Geertz, Clifford, 1; on 'being there',
108; on disciplinary boundaries, 6;
on enigmatical others, 110; on
'exemplary elsewheres', 110; on
experience-near and experience-far
categories, 4; on thick description,
10
Gellner, Ernest, 106
Gleason, Philip, 10; on identity 10–11
Goffman, Erving, 110; on his attitudes
to psychiatry, 110
Goldie, Peter, 2; on einfuelung and
empathy, 3
Group identity, 192

H
Hacking, Ian, 8, 9, 116; on ecological
niches and psychiatric diagnoses,
4; on new possibilities of
personhood, 9, 116; on the
sciences of memory, 116; on the
indeterminacy of the past, 116–17;
on semantic contagion, 120; on
the social construction of memory,
121; on transient mental illnesses,
162
Halbwachs Maurice, 117; on why we
remember, 117
Harvest metaphor, 192–94, 201–203
Humphrey, Caroline, 137; on evocative
transcripts, 137n3
Hypochondriasis, 31

Hysterectomies,45

I
International Classification of Diseases,
163

J
Jamesian model of emotion, 144
Jones Ernest, 97; on primitive
mentalities, 97
Jung, Carl, 97; on 'primitive man', 97

K
Kirmayer, Laurence, 6; on adamantine
and relational self, 6
Kleinman, Arthur, 104; on old and new
transcultural psychiatries, 104; on
somatization, 119
Kraepelin, Emil, 97; on primitive
society, 97; on empathy, 108
Kuper, Adam, 114

L
LaCapra, Dominic, 10; on memory 10
Latvian Cultural Foundation, 212–13
Latvian state archive, 227–35
Laub, Dori, 140
Lavater, Johann Caspar, 36
Levinas, Immanuel, 15; on face, 15
Levy-Bruhl, Lucien, 101, 104, 113
Lewis, Ioan, 1
Leydersdorff, Selma, 11; on trauma
and memory, 11
Littlewood, Roland, 106; on Russian
doll model of illness, 106; on form
and content of mental illness, 114
Luhrmann, Tanya, 6; 164; on mind
body dualism, 6

M
MacDonald, Michael, 99
Mahanubhavs, history, 60; affliction
and trance, 61–62, 87–91; carers
of mentally afflicted; gender and
mental affliction, 62–68, 84–87,
93–94; stigma and mental
affliction, 65–68

www.ingramcontent.com/pod-product-compliance
Lightning Source LLC
Chambersburg PA
CBHW072056020426
42334CB00017B/1525